WINTER BLUES

WINTER BLUES

Seasonal Affective Disorder
What It Is and How to Overcome It

NORMAN E. ROSENTHAL

THE GUILFORD PRESS
New York   London

Published by The Guilford Press
A Division of Guilford Publications, Inc.
72 Spring Street, New York, N. Y. 10012

The information in this volume is not intended as a substitute for consultation with healthcare professionals.

Each individual's health concerns should be evaluated by a qualified professional.

Printed in the United States of America

This book is printed on acid-free paper.

Last digit is print number: 9 8 7 6 5

Library of Congress Cataloging-in-Publication Data

Rosenthal, Norman E.
    Winter blues : seasonal affective disorder : what it is and how
to overcome it / by Norman E. Rosenthal. — Rev. & updated ed.
        p.   cm.
    Rev. & updated ed. of: Seasons of the Mind / Norman E. Rosenthal.
©1989
    Includes bibliographical references and index.
    ISBN 0-89862-149-6 (pbk.)
    1. Seasonal affective disorder.   2. Seasonal affective disorder—
-History.   I. Rosenthal, Norman E.   Seasons of the mind.
II. Title.
    [DNLM: 1. Affective Disorders—etiology—popular works.
2. Affective Disorders—therapy—popular works.   3. Phototherapy—
-popular works.   4. Seasons—popular.   WM 171 R815s 1993]
RC545.R67   1993b
616.85.'27—dc20
DNLM/DLC
for Library of Congress   93-30354
                                                                          CIP

For Leora and Joshua

Acknowledgments

I would like to acknowledge all those who helped make this book possible, but am prevented from doing both because so many people were involved and because some of them, the patients who generously permitted me to include personal details about their lives, are best thanked anonymously. Special thanks are due to my colleagues at the NIMH, Drs. Thomas Wehr and Dan Oren, for our many creative interactions that have helped to shape my thinking; to Drs. Rachael and Richard Heller, and Michael and Jiuan Su Terman, for reading large pieces of manuscript while on vacation and sharing their own clinical impressions and materials with me; to Neal Owens for providing photographs; to Bette Flax for her help in constructing the diets; to Abby Kohn and Patty Owen for their assistance in gathering materials; and to Jennifer Eastwood for her help in compiling the Resource Section. Many of my colleagues responded to my request for their opinions on the latest advances in the treatment of, and research on, Winter Blues, by providing me with their unpublished findings. Many are listed in the Resource Section of this book, but special acknowledgment is due to the following colleagues for their assistance that went way beyond the call of duty: David Avery, Paul Arbisi, John Booker, George Brainard, Charmane Eastman, Chris Gorman, Carl Hagfors, Siegfried Kasper, Raymond Lam, Alfred J. Lewy, Odd Lingjaerde, Ybe Meesters, Michael Norden, Barbara Parry, Chris Thompson, and Anna Wirz-Justice.

Contents

Part 4. Resources

PART 1

Seasonal Syndromes

CHAPTER 1

SAD and light therapy: Discovery or rediscovery?

> Four seasons fill the measure of the year;
> There are four seasons in the mind of man.
> —JOHN KEATS

Like the bears, squirrels, and birds, humans have evolved under the sun. We have incorporated into the machinery of our bodies the rhythms of night and day, of darkness and light, of cold and warmth, of scarcity and plenty. Over hundreds of thousands of years, the architecture of our bodies has been shaped by the seasons, and we have developed mechanisms to deal with the regular changes that they bring. We continue to respond to these rhythms in the way we feel and behave. For some of us, however, these changes can disrupt our lives.

The effects of the seasons on humans were all well known by the ancients, but were largely forgotten by modern medical practitioners until recently. Their importance was kept alive through the centuries by artists, poets, and songwriters. Shakespeare, for example, observed that "a sad tale's best for winter," while Keats wrote of a nightingale singing of summer "in full-throated ease," and the singer of a modern ballad calls his beloved the sunshine of his life.

In the past fifteen years, science has caught up with the arts, and the medical importance of the seasons has been recognized anew. Surveys have shown that most people experience some alteration in mood or behavior with the changing seasons, and that for as many as one in four persons, these changes are a problem. Natural and effective treatments have been developed to help people with marked seasonal problems, known as Seasonal Affective Disorder, or SAD. We are also aware of a milder version of this condition—the "winter blues"—and other forms of the condition, such as summer depression. Over the same period, our understanding of the emotional impact of the

3

seasons—of light and temperature—has advanced. We are now better able to understand our relationship to the physical world around us. How these developments came about, and what we have learned about the effects of the seasons on emotions and behavior, are the subjects of this book. I discuss the impact of seasons and light on our minds and brains, and how we can modify this impact when it causes problems.

There are indeed seasons of the mind, though they are not the same for everyone. Autumn may enchant some with its grand colors, but for others it carries the threat of winter. Winter, cheerless and forbidding for many, has associations with stagnation, decay, and loss. But some people experience a different type of winter—one that finds them snug and cozy by the fireside, with chestnuts popping. Spring brings buds and blossoms, rebirth, with sap stirring, feverish urges, and a longing to go on pilgrimages. But we are also told that "April is the cruelest month . . . mixing memory and desire." Summer yields a harvest of fruit and flowers, but in the words of the Bard, "sometimes too hot the eye of heaven shines." Had they heeded the words of the poets, twentieth-century physicians would have realized much sooner that the seasons can have a profound effect on the way we feel, and that we react to changing seasons in different ways.

States of mind evoked by the seasons and the weather form part of our language. A person is said to have a "sunny disposition," a "radiant smile," to be "warm" or "cold." Every news program carries a section on the weather. Our curiosity about the weather goes far beyond wanting to know whether to take along an umbrella or not. The weather and the changing seasons affect the way many of us feel, how we sleep, what we eat, whether we can concentrate on our work, and even whether we are able to love.

This idea seems so obvious now that it is hard to believe that there was a time when we paid no heed to the effects of the changing seasons on humans. Only twenty years ago, when I was in medical school, we were taught nothing about the effects of the seasons. According to the view handed down to us, human beings were seasonless creatures. Electricity provided us with light and heat. Food was available all year round. We were not like other animals, which have to cope with the challenge of the changing seasons.

Had we studied the ancients, we might have recognized that a seasonless view of human physiology and behavior is incorrect. Hippocrates, for example, observed in the fourth century B.C. that "whoever wishes to pursue the science of medicine in a direct manner must first investigate the seasons of the year and what occurs in them." Many physicians who followed him emphasized the effects of the different seasons on the mind and body. Apparently that wisdom was buried by the wonders of the Industrial Revolution. We forgot that we were once much closer to nature than we are today. We didn't realize that achieving some mastery over our physical environment did not eliminate our responses to the changing seasons, which are presumably programmed into our genetic code.

Artificial methods of escape from darkness, cold, moisture, and extreme heat have provided us with considerable protection from the effects of the seasons on our bodies, minds, and spirits. With this protection, the changing seasons are for many people merely the backdrops against which to go about their daily business. But others experience them with extreme intensity. Perhaps among these people are poets and artists who have seen the changing seasons as metaphors for our lives—whose emotional surges have produced some of the most beautiful products of the human mind.

However, there are also those for whom seasonal transitions trigger extreme changes in mood and energy, and produce sadness and despair. In this book I describe not only the types of marked responses that some people have to the changing seasons, but also how to recognize these problems and treat them. Of course, our responses to the changing seasons should not be examined only through the microscope of pathology. They are part of our response to our world as a whole, enhancing the range of our emotions. I also deal with this aspect of human emotional response, about which I have learned more from the intense experiences of my patients than from the most rigorous medical texts.

My Own SAD Story

I trained as a doctor in South Africa—a country that, for all the turbulence of its politics, can truthfully boast about its climate. In Johannesburg, where I grew up, there were really only two seasons: summer and winter. During summer you could swim outdoors and eat summer fruit: peaches, papayas, mangoes. During winter you could not do these things. It was warm outdoors during the day, though at night you needed a sweater. Spring and autumn were transition times. After several months of winter the blossoms would appear, and you knew it was spring. Similarly, when the long summer was over, the leaves would turn a simple brown and fall off the trees without much fuss or fanfare, and winter was there. But despite the mildness of the seasons, I was aware at some level of the effect they had on my mood. I had even considered writing a novel in which the mood of the central character changed regularly with the seasons. The novel was never written, but the seed of the idea stayed with me, germinating quietly. It required the intense seasonal changes of the higher latitudes to which I moved to activate that kernel of thought; it also required my encounters with some inspiring people, who are central to this story. I arrived in the United States in the summer of 1976 and began both my psychiatric residency at the New York State Psychiatric Institute and research into disorders of mood regulation. The summer days felt endlessly long, and my energy was boundless. I had never experienced such long summer days in Johannesburg, which is much nearer to the equator than New York City.

As the months passed, I was struck by the drama of the changing seasons. I had been unprepared for the brilliant colors of the autumn leaves in the north, the crisp days and cold nights, and—most of all—for the disappearance of the light. I had not anticipated how short the days would be. When the sun shone, its rays struck the earth at a strange, oblique angle, and I understood what the poet Shelley meant when he wrote:

> Bright Reason will mock thee
> Like the sun from a wintry sky.

Then daylight saving time was over and the clocks were put back an hour. I left work that first Monday after the time change, and found the world in darkness. A cold wind blowing off the Hudson River filled me with foreboding. Winter came. My energy level declined, and I wondered how I could have undertaken so many tasks the previous summer. Had I been crazy? Now there seemed to be no alternative but to hang in and try to keep everything afloat. I understood for the first time the stoic temperaments of the northern nations. Finally, spring arrived. My energy level surged again, and I wondered why I had worried so over my work load.

I registered all these impressions, but I did not put them together into a cohesive story—and I probably would never have done so, had it not been for the events that followed and the remarkable people I was to meet. At the end of my residency I went to the National Institute of Mental Health (NIMH) in Bethesda, Maryland, to undertake a research fellowship with Dr. Frederick Goodwin, whom I had heard speak on the topic of manic–depressive illness from both biological and psychological points of view. Dr. Goodwin made the subject come alive, describing how our shifting moods and fluctuating perceptions of the world correspond to certain changes in our brain chemistry. Since mind and brain seemed equally fascinating frames of reference, I wanted to use both models to try to understand mood disorders.

Shortly before my first visit to the NIMH, I met Dr. Alfred Lewy, one of several psychiatrists working with Goodwin at the time. Dr. Lewy had just developed a technique to measure the hormone melatonin, in collaboration with Dr. Sanford Markey. Melatonin is produced by the pineal gland, a pea-sized structure tucked underneath the brain. Each night, like clockwork, the pineal releases melatonin into the bloodstream in minute quantities, and continues to do so until dawn. The secretion of melatonin signals the duration of darkness, and thus serves as an important seasonal time cue in animals. Although it is unclear whether melatonin is instrumental in causing seasonal changes in humans, the research in this area proved to be a critical step in the rediscovery of SAD and light therapy.

Dr. Lewy and I spoke about our common interests and the various directions in which our research might take us. On occasion we chatted over a mass spectrometer, the instrument he had used to develop his technique for measuring melatonin. It looked like a very large washing machine. He injected samples of clear fluid into a small hole in the top, and reams of paper rolled off it, while inked pens traced out a graph upon the paper. He pointed to one blip on the graph and said, "That's melatonin." I was suitably impressed.

After I joined Goodwin's group, I was assigned to work most closely with Dr. Thomas Wehr, an outstanding clinical researcher, who had for some years been studying biological rhythms in an attempt to learn whether abnormalities in these rhythms might be at the basis of the mood disturbances in depression and mania. Shortly before my arrival at the NIMH, Drs. Lewy and Wehr had shown that bright light was capable of suppressing the secretion of human melatonin at night—a finding that was to have great influence over the events that followed. There was a buzz in Goodwin's group at that time—a sense of excitement—and I felt certain I had come to the right place.

A Light-Sensitive Scientist

Although many people were responsible for the rediscovery of SAD, our steps toward this end can all be traced back to the actions of one man: Herb Kern. In some ways, Herb might have appeared to be an unlikely person to initiate a new area of medical investigation, for he was not himself a medical professional, but a research engineer with a major corporation. I met Herb a year after I arrived at the NIMH. At sixty-three, he was a youthful-looking man with a wiry build, a crew cut, and a twinkle in his eyes. He was intensely curious, and he had noted in himself a regular pattern of mood and behavioral changes going back at least fifteen years. A scientist by nature and training, he had kept careful notes of these changes in numerous small notebooks. He observed that each year, from July onward, his energy level would decline and he would withdraw from the world. At these times he lacked energy, had difficulty making decisions, lost interest in sex, and felt slowed down and "ready for hibernation." He found it difficult to get to work in the morning, and once there he would sit at his desk, fearful that the telephone would ring, obliging him to have a conversation with someone. It is typical for a depressed person to withdraw—to have neither the desire nor the energy to interact with others. In fact, in many cases, he or she may feel that it is an impossible task. People who are depressed simply want to be left alone.

More bothersome to Herb than his social isolation was the decrease in his creative powers during his depressed periods. He would procrastinate at work because "everything seemed like a mountain" to him, and his productivity decreased markedly. It was only by grim perseverance that he was able to write up his studies from the previous spring and summer. His sleep was disrupted, and his characteristic enthusiasm for life evaporated.

The months would drag on like this for Herb until mid-January, when, over a two-week period, his energy would return. As he put it, "The wheels of my mind began to spin again." He had ample, even excessive energy at these times, and needed little sleep. Ideas came freely, and he was eager to communicate them to others. For five or six months he was very confident of his abilities and felt that he could "tackle anything." He was very efficient and creative, needed only four hours of sleep per night, was more interested in food and sex, and admitted to a "tendency to go overboard" in buying luxuries.

Herb had observed that his mood improved as the days lengthened and declined as they shortened, and he had actually developed a theory that this might be due to changes in environmental light. He attempted to interest several people in his hunch that his mood and energy levels were related to the time of year. One of these, Dr. Peter Mueller, a New Jersey psychiatrist in private practice who had a research background, listened to Herb and subsequently looked for other patients with a similar history. Herb was treated with several different antidepressant medications, all of which resulted in unacceptable side effects without correcting his symptoms. Herb eventually read about the work of Drs. Goodwin, Wehr, and Lewy and found his way to the NIMH, where he asked us to work with him on his seasonal difficulties.

Dr. Lewy suggested that we treat Herb by lengthening his winter day with six hours of bright light—three before dawn and three after dusk—in an attempt to simulate a summer day. He reasoned that since bright light is necessary for melatonin suppression in humans, it might similarly be necessary for altering mood and behavior. This reasoning was based on two pieces of information. First, the secretion of melatonin is an important chemical signal for regulating many different seasonal rhythms in animals. Second, the nerve pathways involved in the suppression of melatonin secretion by light pass through parts of the brain that we believe are important in regulating many of the physical functions that are disturbed in depression, such as eating, sleeping, weight control, and sex drive. If the suppression of melatonin required much brighter light than ordinary indoor fixtures provided, then perhaps bright light might also be necessary in order for the brain to perform other mood-related functions.

We asked Herb to sit in front of a metal light box, about two feet by four feet. The box emitted as much light as one would receive while standing at a window on a spring day in the northeastern United States. We chose full-spectrum fluorescent lights—a type that mimics the color range of natural sunlight coming from a summer sky—in order to replicate the conditions that appeared to bring Herb out of his winter depressions. We covered the lamps in the light box with a plastic diffusing screen, in order to create a smooth surface. Modern light boxes differ to some degree from the one we originally used in treating Herb. We now realize that it is unnecessary to use full-spectrum light, and that, in fact, the ultraviolet rays present in some full-spectrum lights may actually be harmful to the eyes and the skin. In addition, newer light box models are smaller and more portable. Some models are angled toward the patient's eye—an arrangement that has been found to have advantages over the original upright version. Specific details about light boxes are provided in Chapter 6, the "Light Therapy" section (pages 99–123) and in the "Resources" section (pages 261–262).

Within three days, Herb began to feel better. The change was dramatic and unmistakable. He was moving into his spring mode several weeks ahead of schedule. Did we dare to hope that we might have found a new type of treatment for depression? Intriguing as this possibility was, our excitement was immediately tempered by our scientific instincts. After all, Herb had had a heavy emotional investment in the light therapy. Might his response not have been due to something other than the light—the wish to feel better, for example, or the emotional impact of entering an experiment in which three research psychiatrists were studying the outcome of a treatment based on his ideas? This possibility—the so-called "placebo effect"—had to be seriously considered. The placebo effect has dogged behavioral researchers for years, and we could not rule it out in evaluating the antidepressant effects of light therapy on Herb.

A Human Bear

During the same winter that Herb was receiving light treatment at the NIMH, Dr. Mueller, in consultation with Dr. Lewy, tried artificial light treatment with another patient, whom I will call "Bridget." She also appeared to benefit from light, and had an unusually good winter that year. The following summer, as luck would have it, Bridget moved to the Washington metropolitan area, and Mueller suggested that she contact us. Bridget's history and ingenuity in fitting the details of her seasonal problems into a coherent story were as remarkable as Herb's. She described herself as a "human bear."

She was a professional in her mid-thirties, who had been aware of disliking winter since childhood. But it was not until her early twenties that a regular pattern of seasonal changes emerged. Bridget's problem would begin each year in August or September, as she anticipated the forthcoming winter with increasing anxiety. She was mystified about what subtle cues might be causing her premonitory dread, since this feeling began during the summer, when the days were still warm. She wondered whether it might be the fall catalogs, with their pictures of winter clothes, that triggered the memories of unpleasant winters of earlier years. Regardless, when the leaves began to change color, she would have a strong urge to take out her winter clothes and stock her cupboards with food, "like a squirrel getting ready for winter."

As winter approached, Bridget experienced many symptoms similar to those described by Herb, such as feelings of extreme fatigue a leaden sensation that made her want to lie down and sleep all day long. She would overeat at these times, and observed a marked craving for sweets and starches. As in Herb's case, Bridget continued to struggle in to work each day, though her productivity declined markedly. In addition to her seasonal mood problem, Bridget also felt depressed and irritable for a few days before each menstrual period, regardless of the season. When spring arrived, her depression lifted and was replaced by elation. In her earlier years she would forget her winter difficulties once they were over. "I was like the grasshopper, " she remarked (referring to the fable about the grasshopper and the ant), "singing and playing all summer long," indifferent to the next winter that was to come.

Bridget had also observed that other changes in the environment besides the seasons seemed to affect her mood. She had visited the

Virgin Islands during the two winters before her first light treatment. Both times she had been impressed by the marked improvement in her mood just days after her arrival on the islands, and the relapse a few days after her return to the north. She had lived for some years in locations at different latitudes: Georgia, New York, and Quebec. The farther north she lived, the earlier her depression began, the more depressed she felt, and the later her remission in the spring was. She began to suspect that something in the environment was influencing her mood, and that perhaps it was the light. Why else did she seem to crave it so? Why else did she hate her poorly lit office? She made up any excuse to seek out the brightly lit photocopying room. Light treatment made good sense to Bridget. She was eager to try it and was delighted to find that it worked for her.

In Search of SAD

Unusual individual cases have historically played an important role in medical research in general, and psychiatry in particular. We wondered whether Herb and Bridget might be examples of a special seasonal kind of depression, and whether they might help us understand how others respond to the changing seasons and environmental light.

Although single cases may be of great importance in generating new hypotheses, we generally need groups of patients to test them experimentally. Dr. Mueller said that he had encountered several other patients with seasonal depression. We wondered how common the problem was. Were there any other such patients in the Washington, D.C. area who might be interested in participating in a research program? I called a few local psychiatrists who specialized in treating depression, but they said they had not encountered the problem. I concluded that it must be quite rare and that the only chance we had of finding such a group was by publicizing our interest in the *Washington Post*.

Sandy Rovner, a journalist who specializes in health issues, sat across the room from me, tape recorder in hand, and listened to my story. She decided that it would be of interest to her readers and wrote an article for the *Post*, which launched an entire field of research. Rovner's article began with Bridget's own words: "I should have been a bear. Bears are allowed to hibernate; humans are not."

The response to the article took us all by surprise. Instead of hearing from a handful of afflicted people, we received thousands of responses from all over the country, and our phones rang for days . We sent out screening questionnaires, which were returned by the hundreds. I read them with a growing sense of excitement. In psychiatric research, "heterogeneity" is a major problem; in other words, the same condition may differ greatly in character from one patient to another. This has proven to be an enormous obstacle to psychiatric researchers, especially in the area of schizophrenia. As I read the questionnaires, it seemed as though Bridget had been cloned, as one person after another reported the symptoms of the condition that we went on to call SAD. I wondered whether this similarity in symptoms might correspond to a similar underlying disturbance in brain chemistry, which might imply a favorable response to light, as we had observed with Herb and Bridget.

We interviewed many people and admitted into our program all those with clear-cut histories of winter depression. During that summer, as expected, all the participants felt well and showed an unusually high level of energy. This generated considerable skepticism among some of my colleagues, who speculated that we might be dealing with a group of suggestible people who had read the article and persuaded themselves that they had the syndrome. That seemed unlikely to me, but I had no way of disproving it. I could not help feeling slightly uneasy when one of my colleagues pointed out that if none of the participants became depressed when winter arrived, we would all look a little foolish.

The First Controlled Study of Light Therapy for SAD

The days grew shorter, and in October and November, right on schedule, the participants began to slow down and experience their winter syndromes, just as they had described. Although I was clearly not affected to the same degree as my seasonal patients, I noticed that I too had to push myself harder to get anything done. It was more difficult to get up in the morning, and even the project did not seem so exciting as it had the previous summer.

We planned to treat the patients with light as soon as they became moderately depressed—just enough so that we would be able to measure an effect of the treatment, but not to such a degree that they felt incapacitated. We decided to use full-spectrum light, as we had with Herb Kern, for three hours before dawn and three hours after dusk. In any experiment designed to show the effectiveness of a treatment, it is important to have a "control" condition—one that incorporates all the ingredients of the "active treatment" condition, except the one believed to be crucial for achieving the desired effect. In this study we believed that the brightness of the light would be crucial, so we used dim light as a control. In order to make the control treatment more plausible, we chose a golden-yellow light—a color associated with the sun, and one to which the eye is highly sensitive.

We treated each patient with two weeks of bright light and two weeks of dim light, then compared the effects. This type of treatment design—called a "crossover" because the individual is "crossed over" from one treatment condition to the other—has since been used widely for light therapy studies. We presented the two conditions to the patients in random order. In other words, some began with the bright white light and others with the dim yellow light, so as not to bias the outcome. It is also important for psychiatrists evaluating the effects of a treatment not to be aware of which treatment a patient has received, so that their prejudices cannot be reflected in their ratings. For this reason, the treatment conditions were known only to me, not to my collaborators in this study, Drs. Wehr, David Sack, and J. Christian Gillin.

I will never forget the first patient who underwent the bright light treatment—a middle-aged woman, markedly disabled by SAD. During the winter she was barely able to do her household chores, get to work, or attend her evening classes. After one week of treatment, she came into our clinic beaming. She was feeling wonderful and keeping up with all her obligations. She also mentioned that her classmates were regarding her with a new competitive respect as she answered questions in her evening classes, as if to say, "Where have you been hiding all this time?"

The second patient who received the bright light condition was treated around Christmas. I called the ward from New York City, where I was spending the holiday with friends, and asked Dr. Sack how things were going with the study. He replied, "I don't know what treatment 'Joan' is receiving, but she's blooming like a rose."

And so it went. Nine patients responded to bright light, and the dim light proved ineffective. I began to use the lights myself and was sure that they made me feel better. Some of my colleagues requested them, too. After a few weeks I had to put a big sign in front of the dwindling stack of light boxes, asking anyone who wanted to borrow a fixture to discuss it with me first so that we would have enough for the study. A local psychiatrist, whom I had initially polled about the existence of SAD patients (and who had told me that he did not know of any), called to say that he had realized that he himself had the syndrome, and asked about how he might use the lights himself.

Many questions were raised by the results of our first study. Was it really possible that light was affecting mood? Could there be some explanation for the improvement, other than the light itself? Was it all a placebo effect? And if it was the light, how was it working? These were all important questions, and in due course, we and other researchers would address them, one by one. But as we reviewed the study in the spring of 1982, we realized that the patients had become depressed during fall and winter, as they had predicted they would. The light treatment had worked more dramatically than we had ever hoped it might. The azaleas and the dogwoods were in bloom. Spring had arrived and, at that moment, nothing else seemed to matter very much either to our patients or ourselves.

In the years that followed, we continued to treat new waves of SAD patients each winter, as did researchers at other centers. Light studies performed in other parts of the United States, Europe, and Japan corroborated our experience. SAD is common, and light treatment works. In view of this general consensus, the American Psychiatric Association recognized a version of SAD in its diagnostic manual, DSM-III-R, in the spring of 1987. In a brief six years since the first SAD patients were treated with light, a variant of depression that appeared at first to be a rare curiosity was recognized by the psychiatric community as an important clinical condition.

CHAPTER 2

SAD: The clinical profile

What exactly is Seasonal Affective Disorder (SAD)? What are its symptoms? Who tends to get it and when? How long does it last? How does it affect the way people function at home, at work, and in their relationships? How does SAD relate to the "winter blues" or "February blahs" that so many people complain about? These are some of the questions I address in this chapter.

We now know that the great majority of the population experiences some seasonal changes in feelings of well-being and behaviors, such as energy, sleep, eating patterns, and mood, to a greater or lesser degree. At one end of the spectrum are those who have few, if any, seasonal changes. Then there are those who experience mild changes that can easily be accommodated in the course of their everyday lives. A third group finds these changes a nuisance—not worth taking to the physician, but troublesome nonetheless. This group may be suffering from what is commonly known as the "winter blues" or "February blahs." At the far end of the spectrum are patients with SAD, whose changes in mood and behavior are so powerful that they produce significant problems in their lives.

Such changes were well expressed by "Jenny," who suffers from a typical case of SAD. She has observed that she feels like "two different people—a summer person and a winter person." Between spring and fall she is energetic, cheerful, and productive. She initiates conversations and social arrangements, and is regarded as a valuable friend, coworker, and employee. She is able to manage everything that is expected of her with time and energy to spare. During the winter, however, her energy level and ability to concentrate are reduced, and she finds it difficult to cope with her everyday tasks. She generally just wants to rest and be left alone, "like a hibernating bear." This state persists until the spring, when her energy, vitality, and zest for life return. It is easy to understand why she thinks of herself as two different people, and why her friends wonder who the "real Jenny" is.

This same theme is echoed by a variety of other seasonal people I have encountered. For example, a man from Missouri writes:

I feel as though I "live" only during the sunny months. The rest of the time I seem to shut down to an idle, waiting for spring, enduring life in general. This is no joking matter to those of us who are like this. We, in effect, live only half our lives, accomplishing only half of what we should. It is really rather sad, when you think of it.

One woman wrote about her elderly mother, who has suffered from SAD for her entire adult life:

In late spring or early summer she is full of energy, requiring only five or six hours of sleep. She talks incessantly and tries to do too many things. Then in late fall (occasionally she makes it to Christmas), her personality takes a complete turn. She sleeps twelve hours at night, cries all morning, and then takes a nap. She won't drive the car, seldom leaves the house, and won't answer the telephone.

Who are the victims of SAD? All sorts of people. The hundreds of SAD patients I have known have come from all different walks of life: different races, ethnic groups, and occupations. The disorder is four times more common among women than among men. Although people in their twenties through forties appear to be most susceptible, SAD occurs in all age groups. I have encountered children and adolescents with the problem, as well as the elderly.

My colleagues and I have estimated that approximately 6 percent of the population of the United States suffer from SAD, and that a further 14 percent have a milder form of the condition—the winter blues. Those rates are equivalent to a total number of ten million and twenty-five million people, respectively.

Just as the degree of seasonal difficulties may vary from one person to the next, so may the timing of the problem. For example, one person may begin to feel SAD symptoms in September, whereas another will feel well till after Christmas. A more severely affected person may only emerge from the winter slump in April, whereas a mildly affected one may feel better by mid-March. Many people can predict almost to the week when they will begin to experience their winter difficulties and when they will begin to feel better in spring, almost as one can predict when different flowers will begin to bloom.

The timing of the appearance of symptoms also depends on where a person lives. My colleague Dr. Carla Hellekson, when she worked in Alaska, noticed that the patients in her SAD clinic became depressed about a month earlier on average than my patients in Maryland, and began to feel better about a month later on average. "Terry," a thirty-eight-year-old realtor, is typical of many who have lived at different latitudes when she reports that during her years in Canada and New York, her problems began earlier than when she moved south to Washington, D.C.

"Merrill," an attractive vocational guidance counselor, sits in front of me, checking off on her fingers the symptoms she has during successive months. She has come to know her internal calendar well over the past eighteen years during which she has suffered from SAD. Since she is thirty-two years old now, these problems have been going on for more than half of her life.

I only feel good for two or three months: May, June, and July. By August my energy level has already begun to slip. I begin to sleep later in the morning, but I can still get to work on time. In September things are a little worse. My appetite increases, and I begin to crave candy and junk food. By October I begin to withdraw from friends, and I tend to cancel engagements. November marks the onset of real difficulties for me.

I become sad and worry about small things that wouldn't bother me at all in the summer. My thinking is not as good as usual, and I begin to make stupid mistakes. Other people notice that I am not looking well. Preparing for Christmas is always an enormous chore. I am bad about getting my cards off and my gifts wrapped. I tend to avoid the usual round of parties: I don't want people to think I am being rude, but I find it very difficult to pretend to be cheerful and make conversation when all I feel like doing is going home and sleeping.

January and February are my worst months. On many days it's all I can do to get in to work, and often I don't. I call in sick. Once I'm there, it's very hard to get my work done. I procrastinate as much as possible and hope that I'll be able to handle things later.

In March and April my energy begins to come back, and that's a relief, but my thinking is still not back to normal and I continue to feel depressed at times. They are tricky months because you never know what the weather will be like. You can feel good for a few days, and then, wham, you're down again. And then it's late spring and summer, and once again I feel myself again: friendly and happy. I can do my work and can be available to the people I care for. But it's so hard to have to cram everything you want to do into three months.

In Washington, D.C., November seems to be the month when people begin to feel really bad. Again, this differs from one person to the next. Merrill's sense of dread at having the joy of summer slip away, only to be replaced by the grim drudgery of winter, is very familiar to those who have experienced it or seen it in others. Henry Adams, the famous chronicler of American life, wrote from Washington to Charles Milnes Gaskell, in November 1869, a description of his feelings about that month. It sounds remarkably similar to the sentiments I have heard many times from patients with SAD:

> Dear Boy:
> I sit down to begin you a letter, not because I have received one since my last, but because it is one of the dankest, foggiest, and dismalest of November nights, and, as usual when the sun does not shine, I am as out of sorts as a man may haply be, and yet live through it. . . . This season of the year grinds the very soul out of me. My nerves lose their tone, my teeth ache, and my courage falls to the bottomless bottom of infinitude. Death stalks about me, and the whole of Gray's grisly train, and I am afraid of them, not because life is an object, but because my nerves are upset. I would give up all my pleasures willingly if I could only be a mouse, and sleep three months at a time. Well! one can't have life as one would, but if I ever take too much laudanum, the coroner's jury may bring in a verdict of willful murder against the month of November.

The three months during which most patients with SAD would like to be mice or bears and sleep are December, January, and February. These months could well be called the SAD months. Then comes the thaw of March, April, and May. People emerge from their low winter state in different ways. Some glide gracefully through April and May into feeling cheerful and well in June and July. Some have a bumpy course over the spring, especially in places where the weather is dark, stormy, and unpredictable. Others emerge into an exuberant state where they may be excessively energetic, needing little sleep, and feeling "wired" or "high." At times this state of excessive energy, known clinically as "hypomania," can constitute a problem in its own right. A final group of people with SAD never quite emerge completely from their winter depressions and remain somewhat down all year round, though less so in the summer.

Profiles of SAD

Below are four profiles of SAD patients whose symptoms include the full range of seasonal changes. The first two, Neal and "Angela," suffered from milder and more common forms of SAD. The second two patients, "Peggy" and "Alan," suffered more severely and have participated in the Seasonal Studies Program at the National Institute of Mental Health (NIMH) for several years. Although such severe SAD symptoms are less common, they are capable of interfering markedly with the lives of those who suffer from them, and it is particularly important that they be recognized and treated.

Neal and Angela: Light for a Living and Light to Write By

Neal Owens is currently the president of the SunBox Company, which sells lights for the treatment of SAD. He is in his mid-thirties and has had difficulties during the winter for the past several years. His problems occurred mostly in the sphere of his work as a sales representative, as he found his productivity declining markedly in the winter months. He would sleep late, cancel appointments, and spend much of the day at home, depressed. It is not surprising that for a salesman, who needs to be upbeat, energetic, and eager to interact with others and promote his product, the symptoms of SAD would be rather disabling.

He consulted a psychiatrist at the urging of his girlfriend, and was given a series of antidepressants, none of which proved helpful. After seeing a television documentary about SAD, he mentioned light therapy to his doctor, who was not supportive of the idea. He then obtained information about it from the NIMH, constructed his own light box, and began therapy on his own. He switched therapists and improved noticeably, using a combination of light and psychotherapy. Neal's positive experience with light therapy inspired him to change careers and start a business to help others, by selling light boxes and providing information on SAD. He recently married and feels very hopeful about the future, now that his winter depressions are under control.

Angela is a sixty-year-old writer, with a long history of winter difficulties too mild either to meet criteria for a diagnosis of SAD or to lead her to seek medical help. Since her childhood she has disliked winter and dark climates and places, which she has avoided whenever possible. She thought of herself as entering a "little hibernation" in the winter, when she would feel less creative than usual and "slightly melancholy," if not actually depressed. She had never consciously associated her low energy states with the quality of winter light, but when she first heard about SAD, she immediately identified herself as having a minor version of the condition.

Angela first found out about light therapy when she was writing a magazine article on the subject, for which she interviewed me. But she did nothing about her own winter problems until four years later, when she had strenuous writing deadlines to meet. She installed a set of lights on her desk, and they have been there ever since. She uses the lights both summer and winter, whenever she happens to be working—at least when she is living in Washington, D.C. She observes:

> Since I started using the lights in winter, my brain seems to be clearer, I seem to be happier, and the writing goes better. Not only am I much more productive, but I also seem to be much more creative. The words come more easily and I seem to get more images. I also don't mind being at my desk and writing as much as I did before. When I used to think of having to write in the winter, it was a great effort. I felt almost as though I would have to pull the resistant words out of my head by force and sheer will. Now I have a much lighter feeling about it. It's more fun.

In the past few years Angela has been so successful in her writing that she has purchased a second home in a popular Florida resort, where she spends much of her time—and she's happier and more creative than ever.

Peggy: Forty-One Grim Winters

Peggy is an attractive, youthful-looking woman in her late fifties, with blue eyes, fair skin, and silver-gray hair. She worked as a medical statistician for many years before retiring from that job. She was married twice and now lives alone. She grew up in the Midwest and has had difficulty with the winter since she was eleven years old. She would start out particularly well at school in the fall semester, but when winter came, there were always problems. Her teachers, who regarded her as one of their best students, would register surprise and dismay at the sudden change in her work. Her parents would also become "disgusted" with her performance, which would decline for no apparent reason.

This seasonal problem in school performance increased over time. In her senior year of high school she was an honors student, and was given the responsibility for keeping a log of student aid contributions. The task involved simply putting a check mark next to the name of every student who had donated a nickel. Although she applied herself to the job enthusiastically in the fall, by the time November came she found it overwhelming. Having such difficulties with so simple a task was confusing for Peggy, but typical of her state of mind every winter. She scored above the 99th percentile in intelligence tests, but when she had difficulties with simple things, she believed that she was a fraud and that the test results must have been wrong; her teachers, she assumed, must have given her good grades just because she was a nice person.

Peggy is sure that her mother had SAD as well. During the winter her mother would nap most of the day, whereas in summer she was energetic and vivacious. Both Peggy and her sister were conceived in August. Winter seemed like a low time for the whole family, and Peggy's own difficulties went unnoticed by the other family members. These troubles reached a crisis during her junior year of high school:

> It was mid-January. There had been a string of gray days but nothing bad had happened. I hadn't failed any exam or lost a boyfriend, but I felt so weighed down and in such a state of despair that I saw no future for myself. Everything I looked at was wrong. I went down into the basement, found a water pipe, got a piece of clothesline and tried to make a noose out of it, but I was unable to do so. I just didn't have the energy to figure out how to do it properly or the strength to do it.
>
> I went back upstairs to the bedroom I shared with my sister, and lay down on my bed crying, disgusted that I couldn't even commit suicide properly. I kept the whole thing to myself. The next day was sunny and I said to myself, "Had you committed suicide yesterday, you wouldn't be alive to see this beautiful day," and I felt better. I always thought that it was a miracle that the sun was shining the next day. I wonder what would have happened had it been cloudy. That experience taught me not to try and predict the future—that one day can be bad and the next day good.

Although Peggy had thoughts of killing herself on several subsequent occasions, that was the only time she ever came close to trying.

During adulthood Peggy's seasonal cycles continued. She would begin to prepare for winter in September, buying a six-month supply of toilet paper and all other nonperishable goods, "like a squirrel about to hibernate." In November, she notes,

> The physical difficulties start first: eating more, sleeping more, and the slowing down of brain functioning. Initially, I'm not sad. I can still sit down and laugh with friends and enjoy my favorite TV shows. As it becomes obvious that I'm less able to function at work or with friends, mental depression starts taking over. I have trouble writing Christmas cards, which adds to my depression, since I am unable to communicate with people I really care about. Even

though I really don't want to lose touch with them, I simply want to be left alone from December until April.

Needless to say, this wish to withdraw caused Peggy difficulties both at work and in her personal relationships:

I worked in an office where there was a lot of gift giving. I would feel very upset with people who got their gifts out before December 20. I would wonder, "Why can't I get my gifts out on time?" By then I was closing the door to my office. I didn't want anyone to come in, and I would select only those phone calls I wanted to take. It was okay if people just wanted to chat, but I would hate it when they wanted me to dig up data, or worse still, to do a computer run. In the summer, doing that stuff was like a game. It was fun to sit in front of the computer. But in the winter any task was daunting.

The winter changes also caused problems in Peggy's relationships with men, in part because of her irritability and fault finding—common early signs of her winter depressions. She would drive to work in the winter "cussing out the other drivers." It was hard for her to believe that this was the same morning commute that she found enjoyable during the spring. The same relationships to which she was open in the summertime seemed unappealing in the winter:

I had several relationships with men I met in the fall, during the beautiful, sunny October days, and managed, because of the early passion of each relationship, to make it through the first winter. Summer was great. Then the next winter came along and the relationship would collapse. During the winter, when someone canceled an evening social engagement, I generally felt relieved that I was spared the guilt of having canceled the engagement myself.

The memory and thought-processing problems that troubled Peggy during her school and college days continued to cause difficulties later on. She would fail to set her burglar alarm, forget where she had put the keys, and lose track of other things that she would take for granted in the summer. Every chore seemed to take much longer in the winter, and complex tasks, which were easy for her in the spring and summer, were impossible during the winter months. She would become anxious at her failures and irritated by her ineptitude, and would accuse herself once again of being a fraud.

She would eat more in the winter, particularly carbohydrates. When she lived in the Northeast, she would have to drive home from work for an hour each evening through the gray New England land-scape; when she finally reached home, as she confessed to the minister at her church one Lent, she would not be able to resist gorging on cookies. Was she not guilty of gluttony?

Her energy level stayed low all winter long. Over the years, she developed strategies for coping. For example, she would buy lots of winter clothes and let the laundry pile up for months until the spring, when she could finally face doing it all.

Peggy's sex drive was low during the winter. She recalls with amusement how there were two workmen in the house one winter day. In the late afternoon, she was unable to stay awake, so she retired to bed and asked them to tell her husband that he could find her there when he got home from work. When he returned he was incensed, "as though I were this terrible seductress who had gone to bed, tempting the workmen in the house. He felt as though I had destroyed his honor. I laugh when I think of it now. All I wanted to do was sleep, and the last thing I was interested in was seducing those men."

Peggy was in classical psychoanalysis for three years, "five days a week, every month of the year except for August," but the seasonal pattern of her problems never emerged as an issue for discussion in the analysis. She had no other formal treatment for her seasonal difficulties.

During the summer she would often feel even more energetic and enthusiastic than the average person. Her high energy level would keep her working in the garden till nine at night, and she would stay awake until two in the morning. She required only six hours of sleep. She recalls with amusement the summer day when she went rowing on a lake with a very large man. She felt so energetic that she did all the rowing, and the sight of a small woman rowing a two-hundred-pound man across a lake caused a group of passing fishermen to whistle catcalls at him.

It was her winter depressions, not her summer highs, that brought Peggy to the NIMH Seasonal Studies Program. She was beginning to enter her November decline when she received a tax audit notice. The thought of having to collect and submit all the necessary records threw her into an intense depression and induced her to seek psychiatric help. She was fifty-two at the time and had suffered regular winter depressions for forty-one years, though she had never recognized them as such. On being asked how that could have happened, she replied, "I thought it was normal to feel like that in the winter."

Peggy has been treated successfully with light therapy for the past several years and has participated in a number of studies of light treatment. Shortly after treatment was first started in January, she managed to refinance her house within a week—something she would never have been able to do before during the winter months. Since finding out about her seasonal problem, Peggy has learned to take winter vacations in the sun. She also moved into a house with large windows and decorated it in light colors. She entered weekly psycho-therapy to deal with a variety of psychological issues. Having retired from her former job, she undertook a new career, working with elderly people, and became a founding member of the National Organization for Seasonal Affective Disorder (NOSAD), a support group for patients with SAD (see the "Resources" section, page 276). As a result of her treatment, Peggy now feels fulfilled and much happier with her life than ever before.

When she thinks of what her understanding of SAD and her light treatment have given her, Peggy concludes:

> Now I don't have to blame myself for what happened in past winters. It's liberating to know that SAD is a physical disorder— not my fault. I can give myself some leeway for what happens now. I don't have to be so critical of myself. I have a tool to make myself feel better.

Alan: Too Low or Too High

Alan is a divorced electronics technician in his late thirties. Well-built, dark, and handsome, he has a wry smile, a twinkle in his eyes, and a cynical attitude toward life. This view of the world may have been partially shaped by his SAD and its consequences. Since about age seven, he has had winter difficulties—times when he didn't want to be around people, accompanied by changes in sleep and appetite. He was considered a "moody" child. His greatest early difficulties were in relation to school, where his dyslexia was aggravated during the winter. He remembers reversing numbers and letters, writing on the wrong side of the page, and having great difficulty spelling. Yet somehow he managed better in the summer and fall. In winter his increasing difficulties made him panicky about going to school, which he perceived as "an institution where I would have to go in order to be humiliated."

By age twelve he was refusing to go to school on a regular basis. He was taken to a psychiatrist and given electroshock therapy, apparently to cure him of his "fears, phobias, and dread of going to school." Not only was it unhelpful, but Alan has grim memories of the experience. By thirteen, the problem was so severe that reform school was considered; later, when his parents agreed to go regularly to see a psychiatrist with him, the county provided him with a tutor a few days a week. With this help Alan was able to pass seventh and eighth grades. Eventually, the tutor was dropped, and Alan played hooky regularly until he was fifteen. By then he was aware that his problems were related not only to school, but in some way also to the changing seasons, as he continued to feel bad in the winter.

At fifteen, Alan began to work; after a series of jobs, he became an electronics technician. He dated girls extensively in his late teens, and at age nineteen, entered into a stormy marriage that was to last eight years. The turbulence in his work and domestic life was dictated to a large extent by his dramatic responses to the seasons:

By October I would definitely start to feel a little gray. My performance at work would start falling off, as would my strength, and my sleep would begin to increase. At work, my output would suffer, and I'd begin to start charging less for the same job. I lost confidence in the quality of my work. I'd start worrying about everything and ask myself, "Why the hell am I doing this? What's the use?" It was somewhere between apathy and panic because I knew something was going wrong, but had no idea at the time what the heck it was.

His difficulties at work caused Alan to lose jobs on a regular basis, usually around Christmas. Four to five months of unemployment would follow, when he would live on the money he had earned and saved.

During that time I would feel very depressed. My wife would do all the grocery shopping. In the early years she was worried and panicky, and would try to come home and be a cheerleader. I was usually so disagreeable to be around that she didn't say anything about my behavior. If anybody said, "What's the matter? Why aren't you up getting a job?" I would get very upset, scream, and yell. Usually, after one of those encounters, people would stay clear of me.

If money ran out, Alan would "get some kind of a job, moving pianos, driving semis, fixing cars, collecting loans, or bouncing at night-clubs"—anything except work at electronics repairs. He was unable to figure out the logic of the circuitry, diagnose a problem, and find a solution to it—all things that came easily to him during the summer months.

During the winter, Alan found little pleasure in anything. Occasionally he would forget himself and his misery for a few minutes, but would soon be engulfed again by helplessness and despair. He considered suicide many times. Standing by the roadside, he would think of walking in front of a truck; or he would stand on a balcony or bridge and consider "flopping over onto the asphalt below." While taking a bath or shaving himself, he would contemplate his razor and think of cutting his wrists. On one occasion in the winter, Alan actually tried to kill himself. His winter problems had been getting worse during his late twenties and early thirties, and during that particular winter he felt the worst ever—"incapacitated, hospital material." One day he sat for a long time with the barrel of a gun in his mouth, the hammer cocked and his finger on the trigger. He still doesn't know exactly what stopped him from pulling the trigger.

By mid-March Alan would be aware of a difference in the way he was feeling, and by mid-April he would begin to emerge from his depression. Between spring and summer he would move "along a pretty even curve" from depression to exuberance or even mania.

Usually by the time something was green, I was beginning to feel better. It's frightening at first. You begin to wonder, "Is it a teaser? Am I going to feel better for a few days and then bad again?" By May I was feeling pretty damn good. By June and July I was feeling like it was very urgent to do things. With a lot of enthusiasm and exhilaration, I'd think, "I beat the beast again." I felt fantastic compared with how hellacious I had felt in the winter.

By July 4 I would really begin to accelerate, to feel extremely strong and healthy, definitely virile. I was much more likely to be at all the parties. I'd work as much overtime as I could get. I was on top of the world. By August things were going even faster, and I was needing less sleep. A lot of people thought I was doing speed during the summer, especially at that time when a lot of people were doing speed. People were amused, shocked, or irritated. For example, at the beach or a party, if I wanted to go into the water nude, I would just do it. But I wasn't using drugs; my mood was simply high—it was summer, after all.

My sex drive would increase and become just about my reason for being. Trying to find one individual who had the same drive was kind of tough to do. I usually ended up seeing a lot of people during the summer months.

By August my temper was much worse. If nothing drastic happened, I would generally get through the summer with just a couple of fights. If I really got speeded up, which happened one particular year, I got into trouble with the police. By September I'd mellow out a little. I'd usually be licking my wounds from what happened in July and August.

Although Alan had made a connection between his changing behavior and the seasons, he had never specifically connected his behavioral changes to the light. But he had always been fascinated by light: "colored light, sunlight, white light, reflections, and, in the sixties, strobe lights." He even built some colored strobe lights for himself. However, he was skeptical when his psychiatrist recommended the NIMH Seasonal Studies Program to him. It sounded "absolutely bizarre—right up there with shock treatments and sleeping under the full moon. It was kind of a lunatic idea." But antidepressants, lithium, and psychotherapy had been of no help to him, so he thought he had little to lose.

His first light treatment was given as part of a study on an inpatient unit. He recalls,

About the third day I said to one of the nurses, "I feel kind of funny, light-headed. Something's happening." I got the dose of light that night and I knew what the feeling was—exhilaration. It was like compressing two or three months into four days. By the fourth day, I asked a nurse to marry me or something, and by five days I was higher than a kite.

Although formerly skeptical, Alan is now convinced that light has a real biological effect on him and is not just a placebo. He was asked to stop using the lights on a number of occasions as part of the research program, and he became depressed each time. When he restarted light treatments, he observed that the effects were not immediate; it took a day or two before he began to feel good again. If he used them for too long, he would get a tingling feeling in his hands and feet, and become "wired" and overactive.

Alan has used lights for the past several years. He had special sets at work, where he had no windows, and at home. After starting light treatment he functioned well at his job and worked consistently. Financially, it made a big difference for him to be working twelve months a year instead of nine. He was able to establish friendships and hold on to them "without having to start over again in the spring because I've insulted people or disappointed them or just felt too bad to have anything to do with them." He was also able to spend time on hobbies he enjoys, such as carpentry. Curiously, he was no longer troubled by manic symptoms in the summer, probably because his light environment became more constant across the seasons. Because Alan's mood was more even all year round, he found life easier and less unpredictable. He became more optimistic and was able to enter into more stable, long-term relationships.

The Range of Seasonal Problems

We now recognize that most people experience some changes in mood and behavior in conjunction with the seasons. These vary widely across the population. At one end of the spectrum are those who experience hardly any changes at all. At the other end are those, like Peggy and Alan, whose lives before they began treatment were severely disrupted by the influence of the seasons on their mood and behavior. Neal's life was not as severely disrupted by the seasons. He was lethargic, sad, withdrawn, and unproductive during the winter, although he was never completely dysfunctional either at work or socially, nor did he ever feel suicidal. Nevertheless, along with Alan and Peggy, Neal would qualify for a formal diagnosis of SAD because of the severity of his symptoms.

Angela's winter problems were on the milder side of the spectrum of seasonal change. They never led her to seek medical attention, nor was she conspicuously depressed. Nevertheless, the lethargy and dullness she experienced during the winter interfered with her ability to function as a creative writer. Since this was her chosen career, such interference had a serious and discouraging impact on her life. Although she was not severely affected enough to qualify for a diagnosis of SAD, she could be described as suffering from the "winter blues" or, as it is more technically termed, "subsyndromal SAD." Like Angela, many people with this milder form of the condition can benefit from enhanced environmental light, even though they do not meet the more stringent criteria for SAD.

All of the people described in this section benefited from therapy with bright light. Peggy and Alan received this in a formal treatment setting, whereas Neal and Angela undertook treatment on their own. Both Neal and Angela believe that they made mistakes as a result of not having had their treatment properly supervised. In Neal's case, he used the lights for too many hours each day. As a result, he felt "wired"— excessively activated and uncharacteristically irritable. Through trial and error, he finally found out how much light he needed. In Angela's case, she did not realize that she should sit within three feet of the fixture, and thus did not experience the full benefit of the light for some time.

The four people described in this section are very different individuals, united by one particular trait—marked physical and emotional responses to the changing seasons. Although their symptoms will sound familiar to all SAD sufferers, individual experiences are colored to a large degree by a person's particular personality and life situation. The following chapter will show you how to evaluate your own degree of seasonality, and whether you might stand to benefit from light therapy.

CHAPTER 3

How seasonal are you?

"It is certainly very cold," said Peggotty.
"Everybody must feel it so."
"I feel it more than other people," said Mrs.
Gummidge.
—CHARLES DICKENS, *David Copperfield*

In the charming exchange from *David Copperfield* quoted above, both characters are correct, at least to some degree. Although all people have some reaction, both physical and emotional, to extreme seasonal or climatic changes, some people really do experience them more severely than others. Such sensitivity is often experienced as a change in mood and behavior. As I have noted, seasonality exists as a spectrum within the population. Patients with SAD find themselves on the extreme end of this spectrum, whereas others have extremely low degrees of seasonality. The purpose of this chapter is to help you evaluate how seasonal you are, what your pattern of seasonality is, and how it compares to those with diagnosed cases of SAD or the winter blues.

My colleagues and I at the National Institute of Mental Health (NIMH) set out some years ago to develop a scale to measure an individual's seasonality. Questions from this scale, called the Seasonal Pattern Assessment Questionnaire (SPAQ), are shown below in Figure 1. The SPAQ has been found to be a valid way of measuring seasonality in many different populations. Although a person's seasonality is to some degree inherent, it also depends on where he or she lives. For example, someone who shows marked seasonality in Alaska may show none in Hawaii. In order for you to obtain a stable and accurate assessment, it is necessary for you to think back over a period of time—say, three years—when you have lived continuously in one climatic region. Since seasonality can change over time, and the most recent years are generally clearest in one's memory, think of the most recent three years during which you have lived consistently in one area when answering the questions below.

Instructions for Completing the Seasonal Pattern Assessment Questionnaire (SPAQ)

The purpose of the SPAQ (see Figure 1, below) is to find out how your mood and behavior change over time. Please fill in all relevant circles. Note: Answer according to *your* experience—not that of others you may have observed.

How to Score the SPAQ

1. *Establishing your pattern of seasonality*: You can determine your pattern of seasonality by examining your answers to question 1, which asks during which months of the year you feel best and worst, eat most and least, gain and lose the most weight, sleep most and least, and socialize most and least. In practice, we generally evaluate the pattern of seasonality only according to when you feel best and worst. Answers to the other parts of this question provide us with additional information regarding some other typical symptoms of SAD.

> If you feel worst in December, January, or February, you have a winter seasonal pattern.
> If you feel worst in July or August, you have a summer seasonal pattern. If you feel worst at both of these times, you have a summer–winter pattern.
> If there is no time of year when you generally feel best or worst, you have a nonseasonal pattern.
> There are other, less common seasonal patterns. For example, some people feel worst in the spring; others feel worst in spring and fall.

2. *Establishing your degree of seasonality*: You can determine your degree of seasonality by examining your answers to question 2, which asks to what degree you experience seasonal changes in six different functions: (A) sleep length, (B) social activity, (C) mood (overall feeling of well-being), (D) weight, (E) appetite, and (F) energy level.

Each of these functions should be scored according to the five possible levels of severity. Score each item as follows:

The purpose of this form is to find out how your mood and behavior change over time. Please fill in all the relevant circles. Note: We are interested in <u>your</u> experience; <u>not</u> others you may have observed.

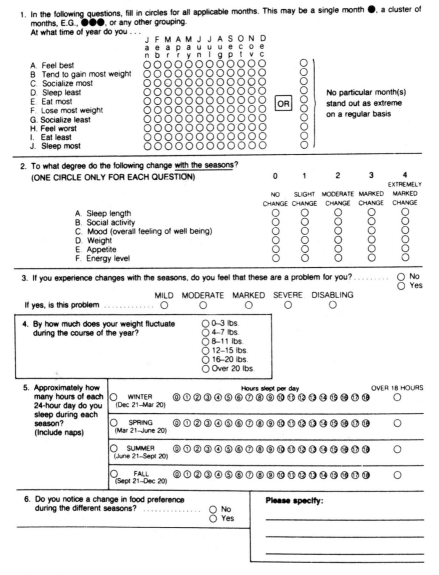

Figure 1. Questionnaire for evaluating your degree of seasonality (modified from the Seasonal Pattern Assessment Questionnaire [SPAQ] of N. E. Rosenthal, G. Bradt, and T. Wehr).

No change	0 points
Slight change	1 point
Moderate change	2 points
Marked change	3 points
Extremely marked change	4 points

In order to calculate your level of seasonality, add up your scores for all six items, thereby deriving your overall seasonality score.

3. *Determining whether seasonal changes are a problem for you, and, if so, to what degree*: This information is derived from question 3. If seasonal changes are a problem for you, you may regard them as mild, moderate, marked, severe, or disabling.

4. *Evaluating other information derived from the SPAQ—not for scoring purposes*: Answers to questions 4, 5, and 6 provide information about the actual number of pounds you gain and lose during the year, the number of hours you sleep during different seasons, and whether you have any change in food preference through the year. Although these questions are not taken into account for scoring purposes, they are of interest to clinicians and researchers who treat SAD, and may be of interest to you as well. For example, we have found that patients with SAD report sleeping an average of 2.5 hours more in winter than in summer. Corresponding figures for people with the "winter blues" and the general population in the northeastern United States are 1.7 hours and 0.7 hours, respectively.

How to Interpret Your Scores on the SPAQ

1. *Establishing your pattern of seasonality*: Almost half of all people in the northern United States report that they feel worst during the winter, and can be said to have a winter pattern of seasonality. This pattern is more marked among people who live in the higher latitudes. For example, a higher percentage of people dislike winter in New Hampshire (42° north) than in Sarasota, Florida (27° north). On the other hand, as one examines locations closer to the equator, more people say that they dislike the summer. By the time one reaches Sarasota, Florida, more people report disliking the summer than the winter, presumably because of the heat and humidity. This information is derived from surveys in which the SPAQ was used as part of a collaboration among the NIMH, the New York State Psychiatric Institute, and the Psychiatric Institutes of America.

Most winter types report eating most, sleeping most, and gaining the most weight in the winter months and, conversely, eating and sleeping least and losing weight during the summer months. They also find it easiest to socialize during the summer. Although they often join in the round of parties that takes place at Christmas, they find it hard to muster up the spontaneous pleasure of summer get-togethers, where they feel a true desire to mix with people. Rather, winter celebrations often take on the quality of a chore, a command performance, asked of people who would much rather be left alone with a dish of sweets. Indeed, people with SAD often report a strong preference for sweets and starches during the winter months—an exaggeration of an eating trend observed in the general population. People also commonly report preferring "heavy" foods (stews and casseroles) during the winter months, whereas salads, fresh fruit and vegetables, and protein-rich foods are preferred in the summer months. Summer types, by definition, mark the summer months as the time when they feel worst. Some of them like the winter months best, but others—the summer–winter types—also mark January and February as months when they feel bad. This last group may only enjoy the spring and fall. People who dislike summer may tend to socialize least at that time. Unlike winter types, they often do not overeat, oversleep, and gain weight during the time of year when they feel the worst. Instead, they tend to eat less, lose weight, and sleep less. As more people learn to control their winter symptoms by modifying their environmental light, and as the world's climate heats up as a result of the greenhouse effect, I would predict that the percentage of those who dislike summer will increase and the percentage of those who dislike winter will decrease.

Some people report very few seasonal changes at all. These people will generally mark most of the items in question 2 as not changing with the seasons. They often have a hard time understanding why their more seasonal friends and relatives are making such a fuss about the cold or heat, the humidity or cloudiness. They may be tempted to see these exaggerated responses as character defects. These nonseasonal people should understand that they are blessed with a constitution well-insulated against seasonal changes, and that this is a biological gift, not a moral virtue.

The pattern of seasonal behavior changes seen in SAD patients—sleeping and eating more and gaining weight in the winter—is also seen in the general population. What distinguishes people with SAD and the winter blues from the general population is the overall seasonality score, which is greater in the first two groups than in the general population.

2. *Establishing your overall seasonality score:* Since there are six items on which this score is based, and you can obtain a score of 0 to 4 on each item, the overall seasonality score has a possible range of 0

to 24. The behaviors that make up this score—sleep length, social activity, mood, weight, appetite, and energy level—vary seasonally, particularly in SAD patients, but also in those less severely affected and in the general population. The extent to which they vary is reflected in the overall seasonality score.

An average overall score ranges from 4 to 7 points. If your score is 8 to 11, you may fall into the category of "subsyndromal SAD," also known as the "winter blues" or "February blahs"; if your score is 11 or more, you may well qualify for a formal diagnosis of SAD. More specific guidelines to help you evaluate whether you may be suffering from these conditions are outlined later (see Table 1). People with higher seasonality scores are more likely to regard the changing seasons as a problem (see question 3); tend to show greater changes in weight and in the number of hours they sleep per day during different seasons (see questions 4 and 5); and are more likely to report a seasonal change in food preference (see question 6).

The seasonality score may change over time, and also according to where you live. For example, someone who has difficulty with the winter is likely to have a higher seasonality score when living farther from the equator. The reverse is true for someone with a summer problem.

According to a population study conducted by Dr. Siegfried Kasper and colleagues in the Seasonal Studies Program at the NIMH, women in their late thirties are likely to have the highest seasonality scores, and these scores tend to decrease as they get older. There is less evidence that the seasonality score changes with age in men.

We still do not understand why certain people are more seasonal than others, although a tendency to develop SAD does seem to run in families. It is possible that the genetic vulnerability to seasonality may be expressed as an abnormality in visual information processing or in certain light-sensitive areas of the brain.

3. *Determining whether seasonal changes are a problem for you, and, if so, to what degree:* The answer to this question should be related to your overall seasonality score. The higher your score, the more likely it is that the changing seasons are a problem for you. Almost all people accepted into the NIMH programs as either SAD or subsyndromal SAD patients rated their seasonal changes as being at least a mild problem. Approximately 25 percent of individuals in the general population surveyed in the northern United States report that the changing seasons are a problem for them. Most of these complain of winter rather than summer difficulties, and could benefit by increasing their environmental light exposure during the winter months.

The section that follows should help you evaluate whether you suffer from one of two conditions that have been found to respond to bright environmental light: SAD and the winter blues. It is important to remember, however, that the SPAQ has been developed as an instrument for population surveys, as well as to screen patients in a clinical setting—but not as a diagnostic test. For that reason, you should not depend upon the test results alone as a guide to diagnosis. If, after completing this questionnaire, you think you may have a significant problem with the changing seasons, I would encourage you to follow up by scheduling a detailed clinical evaluation. Guidelines are provided on the following pages to help you decide when it may be appropriate to consult a doctor.

Estimating Whether You Are Suffering From SAD or the Winter Blues on the Basis of the SPAQ

Your answers to questions 1–3 on the SPAQ can give you a rough idea as to whether you have suffered from SAD or the winter blues. Remember that these conditions are not clearly demarcated from each other. A person may have the winter blues when living in one type of climate (say, southern California), but this may develop into a full-blown SAD after the person moves (say, to Michigan). The same person may be free of all symptoms after relocating permanently to an equatorial climate, such as the Galapagos Islands. Guidelines for making diagnoses of SAD and the winter blues are provided below in Table 1.

In providing a diagnostic guidelines based on a questionnaire, we decided on cutoff scores that include most people who have the condition in question, and exclude most people who do not have the condition. The guidelines outlined below in Table 1 tend to be a little on the strict side, especially for diagnosing the winter blues. In other words, studies have shown that some people may not meet SPAQ criteria for these conditions, but may be found to have SAD or the winters blues on the basis of clinical evaluation. Those people with SAD will generally, at the very least, meet SPAQ criteria for the winter blues, however, may not qualify for any diagnosis, according to the SPAQ criteria. People tend to rate themselves differently—more or less strictly—which may account for some of the discrepancies between self-rating and clinical evaluation. If your diagnosis, based on your SPAQ responses, differs from your perception of yourself as someone with SAD or the winter blues, remember that the SPAQ is only a guide, not a hard-and-fast diagnostic test. Table 2 below shows how

Table 1. Diagnosing SAD and the Winter Blues on the Basis of the SPAQ

	SAD	Winter blues

Question 1
Seasonal pattern:
    During which months
    do you feel worst?
	Winter type
	(Feel worst in months
	between December and
	February)
		Winter type
		(Feel worst in months
		between December and
		February)

Question 2
Overall seasonality score:
    To what degree do
    the following change
    with the seasons:
    sleep length; social ac-
    tivity; mood; weight;
    appetite; and energy
    level? (Obtain score
    as indicated above)
	11 or more	8–10

Question 3
Are seasonal changes in
    mood and behavior a
    problem for you? If
    yes, is the problem
    mild, moderate,
    marked, severe, or dis-
    abling?
	Yes, at least moderate	At least mild, if score on
		question 2 is 8 or 9; you
		may answer "no" if score
		on question 2 is 10.

clinicians go about making the diagnoses of SAD and the winter blues, and may provide you with further insight into whether you may be suffering from one of these conditions.

The Implications of Your SPAQ Results

The main practical value of knowing how seasonal you are and what your pattern is relates to how likely you are to benefit from increasing the level of light in your living environment. Many research studies have shown that most people with marked winter difficulties—those suffering from SAD—will benefit from enhancing their environmental lighting. Recent studies have shown that the same is true for those suffering from milder winter changes—the "winter blues" (see Chapter 4). On the other hand, in a series of studies at the NIMH, we have shown that people with little or no seasonal change are unlikely to experience an elevation in mood from light therapy when it is administered in the same way in which it has been given to SAD

Table 2. Clinical Guide to Distinguishing SAD from the Winter Blues

	SAD	Winter blues
Winter changes last at least four weeks	Yes	Yes
Regular winter problems (at least two consecutive years)	Yes	Yes
Interferes with functioning (work or interpersonal)	To a significant degree (productivity decreases markedly; marked loss of interest or pleasure; withdrawal from friends and family; conspicuous changes in energy, sleeping, or weight)	To a mild degree (less creative; slightly less productive; less enthusiastic about life; less enthusiastic about socializing; slight decrease in energy or bothersome weight gain)
Have seen doctor or therapist about winter problem (or others have suggested it)	Yes	No
Have felt really down or depressed in winter for at least two weeks	Yes	No

patients. In fact, some people have even found that light therapy makes them feel uncomfortable!

When to Seek Medical Advice

It is likely that in the future, more and more people will become aware of comparatively minor, subtle seasonal difficulties and will attempt to modify their environmental lighting to cope with them. You should definitely seek medical help under any of the following circumstances:

1. *Your functioning is impaired to a significant degree.* For example, you should seek help if you develop problems at work, including:

- Difficulty getting to work on time on a regular basis
- Marked reduction in your ability to think and concentrate
- Difficulty completing tasks that you could previously manage

Problems can also occur in your personal life. For example, you may feel that you want to be left alone and withdraw significantly, which can cause difficulties with friends or family. Your spouse or partner may feel that you are distant and unavailable.

You should also suspect that your ability to function is slipping if you begin to fall behind with bills and other necessary chores.

2. *You experience significant feelings of depression.* These may include:

- Regularly feeling sad or having crying spells
- Feeling that life is not worthwhile, or wishing you would not wake up in the morning
- Thinking negative thoughts about yourself (e.g., that you are a bad person, incompetent, unreliable, an impostor), which you would regard as inaccurate descriptions of yourself at other times of the year
- Feeling guilty much of the time
- Feeling pessimistic about the future

3. *Your physical functions are markedly disturbed during the winter.* For example:

- You require several more hours of sleep per day, or have great difficulty waking up in the morning
- You just want to lie around for much of the day
- You feel you have no control over your eating and weight

All of these symptoms are indications that you should have the situation checked out by a qualified professional. If light therapy is required, a qualified professional should supervise the treatment. People with mild winter changes may choose instead to increase the lighting in their homes or workplaces. This topic is discussed in greater detail in Chapter 6.

Besides the seasonal changes noted above, some people react strongly to a variety of climatic conditions. Most people enjoy sunny days and dislike gray, cloudy days; most prefer dry to humid weather. The difference between seasonal types is primarily in the degree to which they dislike certain types of weather or climate. Winter types strongly prefer long, sunny days and abhor short, dark ones. Summer types, on the other hand, strongly dislike the heat and greatly prefer cool weather.

Obviously, various external factors can produce changes in mood or physical symptoms on a seasonal basis that do not imply SAD. For example, people with allergies have trouble during certain seasons. Pollen appears in high concentrations at different times of the year, and your specific allergy may determine when you are most miserable. I mention this mainly to point out that if a problem occurs seasonally, this simply provides a clue that some seasonally changing variable may be causing distress or difficulty. This might include a psychological or work-related factor. For example, an accountant may be most stressed at tax season, and an air-conditioning salesman during the summer. In all of these cases, the changing seasons are like some giant sorting machine, sorting out different types of people according to their specific biological or occupational vulnerabilities.

Seasonality as a Dimension of Human Experience

Through most of this chapter and this section, I have considered seasonality insofar as it indicates illness and needs to be reversed. I believe it is important that we do not regard seasonality only as a disease—as one might regard diabetes or asthma. Especially in its less marked degrees, seasonality provides us with a shifting way of experiencing our world—a richness and color that most people would not wish to do without. There is evidence that some artistic and creative people experience marked shifts in moods and energy with the changing seasons, and many of them regard these as necessary or integral to their work. But even in those of us not given to creative work, the internal shifts associated with the changing seasons may be a source of joy and inspiration. If this is the case, there is clearly no reason to alter them. But if the effects of certain seasons create more pain and havoc than fulfillment, the good news is that there is now a way to alleviate them.

CHAPTER 4

SAD: An owner's and parent's manual

What are the risk factors that predispose people to getting SAD? What do we know about the biological and physiological basis of the various symptoms? What is it like to have the winter blues, as opposed to full-fledged SAD? How does SAD manifest itself in children and adolescents? How common is the problem? These are some of the most frequently asked questions about SAD. Many of them have been addressed to some degree already, but for those who want a fuller understanding of the subject, here are some of the answers, based on my clinical experience and the latest research.

What Predisposes People to Getting SAD?

The symptoms of SAD result from factors in the environment that act upon a vulnerable individual, resulting in the problems already described. What is it about certain people that makes them vulnerable to these environmental effects? Which environmental effects are important?

If we can find out those influences that are important in producing the symptoms of SAD, then perhaps we can modify them. This line of thinking was the key to recognizing the critical role of light deprivation in the development of winter depressive symptoms, and to the use of light in reversing these symptoms. Both clinician and patient should be continually watchful for fluctuations in harmful environmental influences, such as light deprivation, even after these have been initially identified. It is surprising how often such a simple explanation for clinical deterioration can escape even an experienced clinician or a sophisticated patient. For example, let us suppose that a man with identified SAD begins to feel badly during the bright summer weather. Because it is summer, neither the patient nor his therapist realizes at first that this is happening because he is spending most of the day developing film in a darkroom. Among the other environmental influences that should be considered in understanding the development of symptoms in SAD patients are psychological and interpersonal stresses.

The three keys to the development of depression in SAD are these:

- Inherent vulnerability
- Light deprivation
- Stress

Inherent Vulnerability

Although SAD affects all types of people, women are most vulnerable, and the twenties through the forties seem to be the prime ages for this problem. SAD runs in families, and most patients have at least one close relative with a history of depression (often SAD) at some time in the past. An example of familial transmission has been described by a woman in Tennessee with a long history of SAD. She notes: "We have identified [my SAD] as coming to me through my paternal grandmother, being carried by her seven sons, and showing up as active illness in the females of my generation."

Are certain ethnic groups more likely to suffer from SAD? This frequently asked question is often inspired by the idea that SAD may have evolved as an adaptive mechanism—a condition that conferred a survival advantage on the sufferer. Perhaps among those in the far north, where winter conditions are harsh and food is especially scarce during the cold months, it was advantageous to be inactive, overeat, store body fat, and withdraw during winter. Maybe the symptoms of SAD had an energy-conserving function, like the hibernation of bears. If this were the case, perhaps we would find more SAD in those of Scandinavian origin—fair-skinned, blond-haired, and blue-eyed people—rather than in those with dark hair, dark eyes, and darker complexions who hail from Africa and the shores of the Mediterranean. So far there is no evidence that this is the case, and I have seen SAD patients from a broad variety of ethnic backgrounds.

This theory about the energy-conserving functions of SAD might also be used to explain the preponderance of women patients. In primitive societies it might have been adaptive for the women, who stayed at home, pregnant or breast-feeding or raising children, to evolve such energy-conserving behaviors, while the men—the hunters—needed to have a ready supply of energy all year round in order to carry out their functions. Again, there is no direct evidence for such speculations, and an opposite argument can actually be made. According to this line of reasoning, SAD may represent the failure of intrinsic mechanisms for coping with the changing seasons. Such mechanisms may have developed most powerfully in people who have evolved at very high latitudes. This latter argument is supported by one survey by Dr. Andrés Magnússon in Iceland, who found that although SAD certainly occurs in his country (see below), it may actually be less common among Icelanders than it is in the United States. In other words, an argument could be made that suffering from SAD actually interferes with being able to survive at very high latitudes, thus putting those with the condition at an evolutionary disadvantage.

We really don't know why women are more vulnerable to SAD, but we suspect that it is related to the cyclical secretion of the female sex hormones, estrogen and progesterone. Support for this theory comes from population surveys in both adults and children. Dr. Siegfried Kasper, in his survey of adults in Maryland, found that women showed a greater tendency to seasonal changes between their twenties and their forties—in other words, during their reproductive years. After the menopause (when there is a profound decrease in the cyclical secretion of female sex hormones), the tendency to experience seasonal changes was no greater in women than in their male counterparts. It would be interesting to know whether estrogen and progesterone replacement, which has become so common nowadays, affects the tendency of postmenopausal women to experience seasonal changes. This question has not yet been studied.

Support for the relationship between seasonal changes in women and the secretion of female sex hormones was also provided in a survey of Maryland schoolchildren by Dr. Susan Swedo and colleagues. Young girls report a marked increase in seasonal changes after puberty. In boys, on the other hand, there was not such a clear-cut relationship between seasonal changes and the onset of puberty. Female sex hormones may predispose affected individuals to seasonal changes by acting directly on certain brain centers. There is good evidence that receptors for sex hormones are present in the brain, and hormones may act on these centers to differentiate the responses of men and women to the type of light deprivation that occurs during the winter.

Although women are more susceptible to seasonal changes than men, most women do not experience the marked seasonal changes typical of patients with SAD. We believe that there are certain genetic factors that make some people - both women and men—vulnerable to this condition. Since SAD was first described, clinicians have observed that the condition tends to run in families. Further support for a genetic basis for SAD comes from a recent study by Dr. Pamela Madden and colleagues, who surveyed several thousands of individuals from the Australian twin registry. The responses of these twins (both identical and fraternal) were analyzed by sophisticated mathematical techniques, which revealed a clear-cut genetic influence on seasonality. Even though we strongly suspect a genetic basis for SAD, we do not as yet know which genes are responsible. With the rapid growth in our understanding of the human genome, however, it is probably only a matter of time before the genes for SAD are identified.

Environmental Considerations

The most important environmental factor to consider when a patient with SAD becomes depressed is light deprivation, in all its forms. Many people experience feelings of low energy and sadness, similar to those that SAD patients report in the winter months, as a result of light deprivation—no matter at what time of year this may occur. A change in latitude is a common cause of light deprivation, triggering winter depressions that may not previously have been a problem. For example, a young physician who moved from Texas to New York City and became depressed the following winter might have been suffering from light deprivation and SAD, rather than from problems of adjustment to big-city life. The following letter provides a good description of how one middle-aged woman looks back on her experiences at different latitudes:

> The last two winters have been miseries of depression for me. About February I begin to regain hope as spring approaches (in Florida), and I am truly euphoric by May. Yet even now, as I revel in July's bright days and in my own comfortable stability, I am inwardly dreading next winter.
>
> I grew up in Canada, and of course it is worse there—it depresses me even to visit there now. But even in Florida there is a different quality to the daylight in winter: it seems as though it takes something really wonderful to make me happy during the winter, whereas in summer it takes something pretty bad to make me sad.

Another cause of light deprivation, which often goes unrecognized, is a move from a brighter to a darker home. For example, a thirty-year-old secretary who moved from her twentieth-floor apartment, where the sun streamed in every morning, into a basement apartment suffered the effects of diminished environmental light and became depressed. Recognizing this relationship between mood and the environment, a student from Minnesota writes:

> I have often wondered over the past several years why it is that when I go home I lose all energy and have a strong desire to sleep. This occurs all year round for me, although it is more pronounced during the winter months. My house is exposed to very little direct sunlight and is quite gloomy. I have also noticed that when I go and stay at a certain friend's house that is exposed to a lot of sunlight, my mood lightens drastically.

People with SAD are particularly susceptible to moving into dark places in the summer, when the prospective home may seem quite adequately illuminated, and the memories of SAD may be far away.

Moves from a well-lit to a darker workplace can create similar problems. One schoolteacher from Minneapolis writes: "In many of our area schools, windows are being closed over to conserve energy, bringing the effect of winter darkness all year round. No wonder I found my classroom depressing after the windows were sheeted up; it was darker." Even in sunnier places, however, working people are often exposed to very little bright light. For example, Dr. Daniel Kripke and colleagues in sunny San Diego measured light exposure in working adults and found that on average they were exposed to only half an hour of bright light per day. In recent years there has been a tremendous increase in the number of windowless buildings, apparently designed in response to concerns about energy conservation. Even in offices with windows, the glass is often coated with a light-absorbing substance—again in an attempt to conserve energy. Unfortunately, electrical energy is conserved at the expense of human energy, at least in those who suffer from SAD or even from less severe degrees of low energy in the winter.

An amusing incident occurred recently when a contractor was hired to cover the windows of a large government building with light-blocking film to conserve energy. Workers began to apply the film to the top story of the building and worked down from there. When they reached the floor that housed mental health workers, the occupants objected. Their awareness of the behavioral and emotional impact of light deprivation enabled them to predict the adverse effects that the film would have on their mood and energy levels. If more people were aware of this relationship, a great deal of unnecessary suffering in the workplace could be avoided.

Apart from changes in season, latitude, and indoor lighting environment, certain weather patterns, regardless of when they occur, may deprive us of light. It is fascinating to sit each week in the seasonal disorders clinic and listen to patients as they come in, one after the other, each a living weather vane. If there has been a sunny streak, all will be fine. If there has been a long spell of cloudy days, all will be amiss. Small inconveniences will feel like major disruptions, and there will be an abundance of symptoms, both physical and psychological. These symptoms may occur even in the summer if there has been a string of rainy days. Conversely, a clear snap in the winter may result in unseasonable remissions.

A woman who writes to me from the Northeast clearly associates light deprivation rather than season with her symptoms:

> On gray or stormy days (no matter the season!) I become very depressed. The longer the duration of this weather, the lower I feel. As soon as the sun appears, my mood drastically improves. I do not like a dark environment and will seek out bright areas. Dark rooms are oppressive to me.

I have received several letters from San Francisco, where fog abounds and obliterates the sunlight in many areas of the city. One street may be foggy, while over the next hill it may be sunny. Apparently the price of real estate depends in part on these patterns of sunlight and fog; given the powerful effect that light can have on mood, this is not surprising. For individuals who live and work in fog-ridden pockets, it might as well be winter all year round. One self-diagnosed "sun worshiper" wrote to me:

> I live in the coastal region of San Francisco, where it is often foggy, overcast, and windy. I often feel depressed about the lack of sun in our area. While this depression is not strong enough to be incapacitating, it does make me irritable and somewhat of a "complainer." My husband simply cannot understand my feelings. When we spend a day or two in an area such as Sacramento, where the temperatures remain in the hundreds during most of the summer, I feel alive. But my husband can hardly wait to get back to San Francisco, to what he and many others refer to as the "naturally air-conditioned city." It is encouraging to find support for my theory that fog, wind, and cold can get some people down while others can thrive on it.

Light deprivation is a problem in many parts of the world. As one might expect, SAD has been described in Scandinavian countries, where recognition of the problem was accepted as part of the culture even before the condition was described in modern times. In Iceland, for example, the condition of *skammdegistunglyndi*, or "short-days depression," was described in medieval epics. In Tromsø, a Norwegian city 125 miles north of the Arctic Circle, all manner of ills are blamed on the *mørketiden*, or "murky times"—the forty-nine days of total darkness around the winter solstice (see Chapter 14). Light deprivation is not confined to these countries of legendary darkness, however. Though it may be less common elsewhere, SAD has been described in sunnier countries, such as Italy and Japan and, in the Southern Hemisphere, Brazil, Australia, and South Africa. Even in tropical countries where winters are sunny, there is frequently a cloudy, wet, monsoon season, during which the country's inhabitants are often light-deprived and may experience the symptoms of SAD. Even in Hawaii, which many of us think of as eternally sunny, colleagues have reported cases of SAD—especially in residents of those parts of the islands less well known to tourists, which are often covered with clouds.

An unusual cause for the emergence of SAD symptoms came to my attention recently when I was consulted by an engineer in his early sixties, who had developed SAD some three years earlier. It is rather extraordinary for a man of that age to develop such symptoms out of the blue, and I quizzed him about all the usual triggering factors. Had he moved north recently, changed homes, or changed his working environment? "No," he answered. It was only toward the end of the consultation that it emerged that he had injured one eye about four years previously, and a cataract had grown across the lens. This greatly decreased the amount of light entering the eye and had apparently pushed him over his threshold of vulnerability for SAD.

No studies have yet been performed on the rate of SAD among the visually impaired. Such research would certainly be worthwhile, for the more we understand about the many different effects of light deprivation on brain function, the more likely it seems that in understanding and treating the blind, we will need to take into account not only their loss of vision but also the loss of these other light-related functions.

Stress

Light deprivation is not the only environmental factor that can trigger feelings of depression in the winter. Stressful events may also contribute to them. For example, a young sales manager had a sales conference scheduled in January, just at a time when the extra hours of work and preparation required for this major event were most difficult for him. During previous winters he had felt quite well, experiencing only mild drops in energy and productivity. But this time the high level of stress and the demands of work, coming in the middle of the winter, combined to precipitate him into the depths of a depression.

A young mother with SAD was required to start a stressful new job during December. Although she was normally a quick study, she was unable to learn the new skills that the job required, in addition to running her household and coordinating her day care arrangements. She became progressively more depressed. When she was able to analyze the difficulties, she concluded that she would have been able to handle all those stresses during the summer, or the household and family ones during the winter, but the combination of stresses occurring in winter rendered her unable to function adequately either at work or at home.

The Symptoms of SAD

SAD as an Energy Crisis

"Jenny," a middle-aged housewife, makes the point succinctly:

> I don't really feel depressed. I just feel like all my systems have been turned off for the winter. I feel leaden and heavy and just want to lie around all the time. It's only when I am expected to do something out of the ordinary, and I realize I cannot do it, that I feel my mood being pulled down.

Jenny's description provides us with an important clue to the understanding of SAD, and of depression in general. Many of the symptoms of depression involve physical functions: sleeping, eating, activity levels, sex drive. Disturbances in these functions produce physical symptoms, and their presence is an important clue that someone is suffering from a clinical depression, not just ordinary sadness. Often, in fact, the sadness and gloom that we associate with depression are not the most prominent parts of the general picture. So important are the physical symptoms that modern diagnostic systems do not permit the diagnosis of depression if there has not been a history of at least some physical symptoms.

Almost all people with SAD have problems with their energy level, and they often express it in similar ways. Here are a few of their voices:

"The fatigue is agony. I feel I have to drag myself from one place to the next."

"Everything seems like more of a chore in the wintertime."

"I have to use all my willpower just to get up in the morning, go to work, be pleasant to people, pay my bills, and put my dishes in the dishwasher."

Changes in Eating, Sleeping, and Sex Drive

Most people with SAD eat more in the winter. They also report a change in their food preference from the salads, fruits, and other light fare of summer to high-carbohydrate meals: breads, pasta, potatoes, and sugary foods. Many have told me that eating carbohydrates actually makes them feel better, more energetic. "Laura," a musician in her forties, describes her seasonal change in eating patterns:

By September and October, I feel like I am constantly feeding and gnawing. My winter diet consists mainly of pastas, macaroni and cheese, rice casseroles, and chicken and mushroom soup—heavy, heavy food. Things that take a long time to cook so you smell them. Stews and pot roast with potatoes and gravy . . . lots of gravy on everything. And dessert—heavy dessert.

Two research groups have actually tried to record the eating habits of people with SAD at different times of year. Dr. Judith Wurtman at MIT and Dr. Anna Wirz-Justice in Basel, Switzerland have confirmed that the increase in carbohydrate consumption reported by so many patients does, in fact, occur. This pattern seems to be an exaggeration of the eating patterns in the population as a whole. One study performed in the cafeteria of the National Institutes of Health found that people eat more carbohydrates in winter and more salads in summer. Recently, the same patterns were reported in a population study in Montgomery County, Maryland.

Surprisingly, people with SAD report that eating carbohydrates seems to give them *more* energy, because research with people who don't have SAD shows just the opposite. Drs. Bonnie Spring and Harris Lieberman both showed that carbohydrates actually make non-depressed people feel more drowsy. In an NIMH study, my colleagues and I gave high-carbohydrate meals (six big cookies) and high-protein meals (a plate of turkey salad) to people with SAD and nonseasonal people. We found that the patients had been correct in their reports, for the high-carbohydrate meal did indeed make the SAD group feel more energetic, whereas the nonseasonal group felt more fatigued. This would suggest that there is a basic difference in the brain chemistry of seasonal and nonseasonal individuals, resulting in this difference in response to carbohydrates.

We don't yet know what this biochemical difference is, but studies of serotonin, a nerve chemical messenger that is of widespread importance in brain functioning, may provide some answers. Drs. John Fernstrom and Richard Wurtman showed that in animals, carbohydrates increase the production of serotonin in the brain. Further studies show that this mechanism may also be important in humans. One reason why patients with SAD may crave carbohydrates and consume them in excessive quantities may be an instinct to correct an abnormality in their brain serotonin concentrations.

Drs. Rachael and Richard Heller, researchers at Mount Sinai Hospital in New York, have taken the concept of carbohydrate craving one step further by calling it "carbohydrate addiction." They note that like other types of addicts, people who are carbohydrate addicts generally don't feel satisfied with only small amounts of their preferred substance—carbohydrate-rich foods. Portions that would satisfy most people's desires for sweets and starches actually make the carbohydrate addict want to eat more of the same type of food, until so many calories have been consumed that the addict's diet is ruined for the day. They suggest that carbohydrate addicts may secrete too much of the hormone insulin from the pancreas, which would cause blood sugar levels to drop precipitously, resulting in a craving for more carbohydrates. It is not known whether patients with SAD do in fact secrete too much insulin in response to eating carbohydrate-rich foods. But whatever the cause, the Hellers' description of carbohydrate addiction certainly seems to fit many SAD patients I have known and has some interesting dietary implications, which are discussed in greater detail in Chapter 7, on pages 141–143.

Considering the changes in diet and the low levels of activity that occur in the winter in SAD patients, it is not surprising that they tend to gain weight, often quite dramatically. One physician with SAD tells me that his winter trousers are two sizes larger than his summer ones, and this is not unusual. I have seen people gain up to forty pounds in the winter and lose all of the weight the following summer. Unfortunately, some people do not lose it all, and become steadily heavier from year to year. This "yo-yo" pattern of weight loss and weight gain is associated with serious medical conditions, such as diabetes, heart disease, and certain cancers.

People with SAD complain as much about changes in their sleep patterns as they do about their eating. Common problems are difficulties with getting up in the morning, making it to work on time, and getting the children off to school. Those with SAD generally sleep more but don't feel refreshed on waking. Sleep is often interrupted and of low quality. Laura, the musician mentioned above, recalls seasonal changes in sleep patterns from her school days:

> I can remember being unable to get up in the morning during the winter as I was growing up, during high school and junior high. My mother would scream at me to get up and get ready for school. I would drag myself up. In contrast, during the spring, I would go out in the yard every morning before school started and look for a flower to wear in my hair or in my buttonhole. Obviously, I had to get up early enough to go and get the flower, and to have the desire to do that. In winter, I'd have a terrible time staying awake. . . . I used to work in the cafeteria, and I would get these baking powder biscuits at dinner. You could take home whatever was left over after dinner. So I would take a pile of these biscuits and a Coke. If you put a bite of biscuit and a sip of Coke in your mouth it reacts and fizzes—that was how I stayed awake to study in the evening after I would get back. I gained a lot of weight, but in the summer the weight would come off—without dieting.

"Flora," an editor in her forties, describes somewhat different sleep patterns:

> I'm tired all the time during my depressions, but I do have a little trouble going to sleep, so I'll read in bed for a long time. I never knew how often I woke up in the middle of the night until I started keeping track of it, but when I'm untreated, that's what I do. Then I would find it impossible to get up in the morning and would sleep through the alarm clock. Once, in college, I slept through a fire drill, which made my dorm mates very angry. The bell was right outside my room, and they all went out in the cold and stood there. But since I didn't go out, they had to repeat the fire drill. . . . This was in the winter.

Studies performed at the NIMH actually show differences between the way people with SAD and nonseasonal people sleep at different times of the year. In the winter, people with SAD sleep longer, as measured by electrical recordings of their brain wave activity. They also have a decrease in a type of deep sleep called "slow-wave sleep." The decrease in this component, as well as the tendency to more sleep disruptions during the winter, may account for SAD patients' daytime drowsiness, despite their increased duration of nighttime sleep.

In most people with SAD, sex drive decreases markedly during the winter. Many people report not wanting to be touched or to exert themselves in any way; they just want to curl up and be left alone. I have heard many reports of women who wear long flannel nighties to bed during the winter. Although these garments are worn mainly for warmth and comfort, they send out a strong signal to the women's partners that the SAD victims have little interest in sex. Male patients with SAD may be similarly affected by a lack of sexual interest. Of course, marked changes in sex drive affect not only a person who experiences them, but his or her partner as well. The partner can easily feel rejected because of the lack of sexual interest shown by the person with SAD. When spring and summer arrive and the SAD patient's sexual interest picks up again, the couple will have to adjust to the new equilibrium, which is often difficult. The patient with SAD, forgetting that he or she has been uninterested in sex for several months, may be surprised at the aloofness of his or her partner. The partner, having felt rejected or, at the very least, frustrated during the winter months, may eye the renewed sexual interest with suspicion or anger. An understanding that marked shifts in sexual interest are a common feature of SAD—together with communication between the partners about this problem—can greatly ease the tensions that tend to result.

"Sylvia" and "Jack" are a middle-aged wife and husband who have had to learn to deal with Sylvia's seasonal changes over their twenty years of marriage. Their sex life suffers in the winter, when Sylvia just wants to be left alone. She retires to bed before Jack does, and by the time he gets there, she's asleep. He has learned to let her sleep at those times because, as she puts it, "I wouldn't be much fun if he woke me up." For the rest of the year the couple enjoys an active and satisfying sex life.

The effect of SAD on relationships is not confined to the sexual arena. Again, people with SAD often just want to curl up in a secluded place and be left alone. A person who may be a social butterfly in the summer often wants no company in the winter. Conversations are avoided and invitations are turned down. Anything that requires expending the energy involved in social contact is experienced as an overwhelming demand, to be avoided if at all possible. Many people with SAD (like Bridget, described in Chapter 1) compare themselves to hibernating bears. Although this is not a scientifically sound comparison, it accurately conveys the feeling of wanting to be left alone.

As one might expect, there are considerable social costs to such behavior. Friends may become annoyed. A marriage may come under strain, as the spouse experiences withdrawal and distancing on the part of the seasonal person. Lovers may be lost, although at the time this may be experienced as a relief, since it results in a welcome decrease in personal and sexual demands. I know many seasonal people (like Peggy, described in Chapter 2) who have consistently started relationships in spring and summer, but failed to keep them through the winter.

Cognitive Problems

As the seasonal people you have already met in this book have testified, problems in thinking are among the most troublesome symptoms of SAD. Generally, concentration and information processing are things we do automatically. It is only when we are unable to do these things that we really notice them. I am sure you can remember a time when you were not thinking properly—for example, when you were very tired. This is how people with SAD often feel during the winter months. They tend to have problems with thinking clearly and quickly. It's very difficult, if not impossible, for them to summon up the information and knowledge needed for their work—or even for casual conversations. They are not able to keep up with what is going on around them or what needs to be done.

A scene from Charlie Chaplin's film *Modern Times* comes to mind. A factory worker is working away quite well on an assembly line, when suddenly the conveyor belt begins to move faster. The worker rallies in an attempt to keep up with the increased challenge, but eventually the rate at which he is called upon to perform is accelerated so rapidly that it is impossible for him to continue. This provides a wonderful vehicle for Chaplin's madcap antics. In reality, however, the feeling of having information coming at you faster than you can handle is an overwhelming, and even frightening, experience.

In SAD, the ability to concentrate and process information varies greatly over the course of the year. In summer it's a snap; everything goes "click, click, click" and gets done. In winter it's a drag, with minor tasks taking on major proportions. I have heard many patients say, "I begin to make stupid mistakes in the fall."

These mistakes can become apparent even in the performance of relatively simple tasks. Routine chores, such as doing the shopping or cooking a meal, involve several steps that need to be performed in a certain sequence. People with SAD often feel unable to focus on the task—to remember all its different parts and to carry them out in the correct sequence. Patients often say, "I just can't get my act together. Simple things seem so difficult." In all the patients profiled in Chapter 2, a combination of low energy, low motivation, and especially difficulty in thinking impaired their ability to function at work, which was a major complaint. In children, this combination of symptoms results in school difficulties, which may be the first problem to come to a parent's attention. The effects of SAD in children and adolescents are discussed in greater detail below.

Many business executives and professionals with SAD complain that during the winter they are unable to take the necessary steps to handle the tasks that await them. Instead they hide behind their office doors, shuffling papers around on their desks, creating the appearance of getting work done. Secretaries and assistants, who aren't fortunate enough to have personal offices in which to hide, often call in sick and say they have the flu—a more acceptable excuse than depression.

Tasks involving logic are often especially difficult, but some people even complain of difficulties in estimating distances. One woman reported that while driving during the winter, she had a hard time estimating the distance between her car and the one in front of her. A young tree surgeon with SAD found it hard to estimate the length of a branch he was sawing off, and injured himself as a result.

Dr. John Docherty, who has had extensive experience with SAD in Boston and New Hampshire, has estimated the frequency of the different work-related problems encountered by his patients with SAD. They are as follows, in order of frequency: decreased concentration, productivity, interest, and creativity; inability to complete tasks; increased interpersonal difficulties in the workplace; increased absences from work; and simply stopping work. This is quite a staggering list of problems.

One exciting research development in the area of information processing was reported by Dr. Connie Duncan and her colleagues at the NIMH, who have measured the brain wave pattern responses to visual stimuli. A certain part of the brain wave response corresponds to a person's ability to attend to a stimulus. These researchers showed that this part of the brain wave increases in strength in patients with SAD after they have been successfully treated with light therapy. This change occurs at the same time as people begin to feel better and their ability to think improves. Dr. Charles Mate-Kole in Nova Scotia has found that SAD patients are less able to deal with spacial information, for example, recognizing faces, than their nonseasonal counterparts. It is very reassuring for patients to realize that their ability to think can be objectively measured and shown to change after light therapy. It helps them to recognize that they are suffering from a problem in brain functioning and that their cognitive difficulties are not their fault.

Mood Problems

As I have mentioned earlier, many people with winter problems may feel physical changes long before any feelings of sadness occur. Some people may experience only physical changes with the changing seasons and never feel depressed. These people are comparatively lucky because the emotional aspects of depression are among the most painful experiences known to humankind.

"John" is an engineer who has just turned fifty. A well-groomed man, with gray hair and blue eyes, he sits in my office trying to control himself, as he has always been told he should. But the depression breaks through his mask and the tears begin to roll down his cheeks. He feels sad, he says, but doesn't know why. Life has no meaning for him any more. His wife, children, and job have all ceased to give him any pleasure. He feels that he is just a burden to his family and that they would be better off without him. He feels guilty—he has let them down, been a bad father and husband. He thinks back on his childhood and feels that even then he failed to come through for his parents when they needed him. He goes to work each day wracked with anxiety. Small problems become overwhelming. How will he get it all done? Perhaps the best thing would be to end it all, but that is against his religion. He contemplates a spot on the freeway where the road veers sharply to the right, and there is a steep decline to the left. Sometimes he thinks about driving his car over the edge if the pain gets too bad.

John expresses feelings that are typical of depressed people, and, indeed, he is severely depressed. His thoughts—that he is a failure as a father, husband, and worker—are not shared by his children, his wife, and his supervisor, all of whom feel that he is caring, devoted, and hard-working. John's thoughts can legitimately be regarded as distortions of reality, though they certainly feel real to him. A serious symptom of severe depression is losing touch with reality.

A college student in her late twenties described the loss of perspective that occurs in depression:

A patient with diabetes knows that his pancreas is disordered, and that's not so hard to understand. But when you're depressed, your mind and heart and soul are disordered—everything that makes you a human being—and that's not so simple to understand, especially when you are in the middle of it.

The anxiety that John reports often occurs in depression, and treatment often helps it, as well as the sadness. People with SAD also complain of being snappy, irritable, and unpleasant toward others.

Depressed people, including those with SAD, often distort reality by blaming themselves unfairly. Another type of cognitive distortion that may occur involves blaming others—or one's life circumstances—for problems that are really the result of SAD. A woman may say, for example, "My marriage is going wrong because my husband is inconsiderate and too demanding," while the major reason may be that she is depressed and unable to meet his needs. Another may say, "This job is not right for me. It's causing me distress and feelings of failure." Although a difficult job can aggravate the symptoms of SAD, the main cause of the problem at work may be the SAD itself. I often counsel patients not to make important decisions while they are depressed if they can possibly avoid doing so. Decisions made hastily by a depressed person are often the result of mistakenly attributing problems to life circumstances, and they are often regretted later. The best way for a depressed person to handle problematic life circumstances either at work or at home is to have the depression treated first, and then to decide on the best course of action.

Physical Illnesses and SAD

People with SAD may suffer all sorts of physical problems during the winter months—from backaches, muscle aches, and headaches, to different types of infections. Many people with SAD feel as though they suffer from the flu all winter long. We don't really know whether having SAD or being depressed actually makes people more likely to get the flu or whether it just feels worse for them to be sick when they are already suffering from SAD. Fibromyositis, a condition of muscular aches and pains (especially in the neck and shoulder areas), typically gets more severe in the winter, is associated with sleep difficulties, and responds to treatment with antidepressants. Researchers have speculated that it may be somehow related to SAD, and it would be interesting to find out whether it responds to light therapy. The idea that the mind or brain exerts an influence on the human body in general and the immune system in particular is gaining increasing acceptance in scientific circles and is an exciting new area of developing research. The possible relationship between SAD and physical afflictions has yet to be fully explored.

Premenstrual Difficulties

At least half of all menstruating women with SAD report that they have suffered from emotional and physical problems related to their periods, usually in the week before a period begins. Some of the patients may be suffering from "premenstrual syndrome" (PMS). Some women experience PMS all year round, but most severely in the winter.

Others have PMS only in the winter. Many women say that during their premenstrual period they feel a bit like they do when they have SAD.

"Sharon" is a housewife in her early thirties and the mother of two teenagers. She is aware of eating too much, craving sweets and starchy foods, gaining weight, and sleeping more during the four or five days before her menstrual period. She tends to retain fluid, and her rings feel tight on her fingers around that time. She also has abdominal cramps. But most distressing to her and her family is her irritability at those times. She will tend to pick fights with her husband, with whom she normally gets along rather well. This was especially bad before they recognized the cyclicity of their arguments and their biological origin. Now they have learned to be careful during the week before her period, and have resolved to postpone all contentious topics until after it has passed. Even her children have learned to tread carefully during those premenstrual days. Irritability is more typical of PMS than of SAD, where people more commonly feel lethargic and sluggish. One woman pointed this out to me in colorful terms when she noted: "My premenstrual problem is like a black cloud hanging over me; the winter problem is more like being in a blue funk—it's a condition inside of me that I walk around with."

Not every episode of premenstrual phase is necessarily the same for a particular woman. During some cycles, a period may arrive unexpectedly without any symptoms of PMS. Yet at other times, unpredictably, these difficulties may be rather severe. In a similar fashion, the severity of episodes of SAD may also vary from cycle to cycle, from one year to the next.

Hunger for Light

Even before any formal studies of light therapy had been performed, some patients had made a connection between light and mood. For example, one woman would routinely sit in front of her plant lights, because she found she felt better there. Another would wander through brightly lit supermarkets at night, while a third would seek out the photocopying room at work because it was well lit. It is common for people with SAD to want to turn on all the lights in the house during the dark winter days. One middle-aged woman was nicknamed "Lights" by her husband because of this habit. For some people with SAD, the wish to turn on all the lights in the house has led to arguments about the high cost of electricity from spouses who have not understood the biological nature of the SAD sufferers' need.

In their search for light, some people have instinctively chosen winter vacations in the south, year after year. Others have relocated permanently. In many instances, the people involved may not have realized how medically important it was for them to move; they may just have done so instinctively. Not all patients with SAD have made the association between their symptoms and the amount of available environmental light. Some have reacted by lying down in darkened rooms, thereby inadvertently aggravating their symptoms. It is important to recognize that SAD is a condition where the patient's behavior can have a profound effect on how he or she feels. Light-seeking behavior can do much to alleviate symptoms. Conversely, avoiding the light can make matters much worse.

Self-Treatment with Drugs: Alcohol, Caffeine, Nicotine, and Others

> Stay me with flagons, comfort me with apples
> For I am sick of love.
> —*Song of Songs*

Since Biblical times, people have realized the mood-altering effects of food and wine. In an attempt to feel better, depressed people often resort to commonly available drugs, some of which may compound the problem. I have already discussed the use of sugar and starches as mood regulators by people with SAD, but obviously the effects of food go beyond its carbohydrate content. Many people specifically crave chocolate, perhaps seeking the combination of sugar and caffeine that it contains. Others crave stews, pastas, and "heavy" or "crunchy" foods. One woman with SAD actually craved broccoli in the wintertime. We cannot explain these idiosyncratic choices, but it is possible that these cravings may represent the physiological need for a particular nutrient. Gratifying this need may result in an improved sense of well-being.

Caffeine is a mood-altering drug that often appeals to people who feel sluggish, lethargic, and unable to get anything accomplished. Flora, mentioned above, recalls her caffeine addiction during her depressed times:

I used to drink eight, ten, or twelve mugs—tremendous amounts of coffee steadily all day: espresso, made by the drip method. At times the amount of coffee it took to keep me going was enough to upset my stomach.

Caffeine is such a widely available and accepted stimulant that patients with SAD naturally gravitate toward the coffeepot or the teakettle. When these are not available, caffeinated sodas are a common substitute. People often drink many more cups of tea or coffee in the winter than in the summer. Although the immediate stimulant effects of caffeine can be quite useful in certain circumstances, it also has distinct problems and limitations. These are becoming more widely appreciated, as evidenced by the growing number of calls for decaffeinated coffee. Besides indigestion and abdominal cramps, caffeine can cause jitteriness, palpitations, and insomnia. In addition, people frequently become tolerant of its effects, so they may have to drink increasing amounts to get the same energy boost. Nevertheless, the problems associated with caffeine should not be overstated; some people drink it with impunity, and for them a few cups of tea or coffee a day may be helpful. I should remind those who want to stop drinking tea or coffee that abrupt discontinuation of caffeine can cause withdrawal symptoms, which include sluggishness and headaches.

Alcohol is another substance to which depressed people at times resort—"drowning their sorrows in drink," as the saying goes. One patient who comes to mind is John, the fifty-year-old engineer mentioned above. During the fall and winter, he feels increasingly depressed as he becomes less able to function effectively at work. His regular routine of exercising usually falters at this time, and he tends to drink to obliterate his painful feelings of failure. Not surprisingly, the heavy drinking becomes a problem in its own right, and causes him further difficulties at work and at home. Drinking too much alcohol can, of course, cause many problems, a detailed description of which goes beyond the scope of this book. Suffice it to say that excessive alcohol use can be physically harmful, disrupt relationships, kill others (as in driving while intoxicated), and ruin the life of the addicted individual.

I have also seen people turn to marijuana in the wintertime. One young man—a tennis instructor greatly concerned with his physical health—turns to marijuana each winter, despite his awareness of its potential physical dangers. He is an enthusiastic and upbeat person in the summer, sought out by friends and employees for his support, understanding, and counsel, but he feels desolate and bleak in the wintertime. Life loses all of its charms, and nothing seems to give him any pleasure. At these times he smokes marijuana to escape into a haze in which his daily cares seem far removed. He does not feel happy with this solution to his problems and is eager for alternative approaches.

Even smoking tobacco may seem more appealing in the winter. One physician in his mid-forties, who hardly needs any lectures on the harmfulness of tobacco, takes up smoking during the winter, even though he has given it up the previous spring.

So it is that many people seek refuge from the pain of SAD in commonly available substances. Some, like pasta and cookies, may be innocuous unless eaten to great excess. Others, like alcohol, can be extremely destructive, creating problems that far exceed those for which they are consumed. Why some people resort to alcohol, while others resort to cookies or chocolates, is not understood at all. It may be a feature of an individual's peculiar individual biochemical makeup, or a result of what the person was conditioned to associate with comfort from childhood. For example, one friend of mine recalls being comforted with sips of brandy when she woke up at night as a child feeling sick. In other families, ice cream or candy may be the standard remedy. In general, these "drug" solutions are regarded as unsatisfactory by those who adopt them. For better solutions, I refer you to Part 2 on treatments for SAD.

Other Conditions That May Resemble SAD

In medicine, it is always important to question a diagnosis. Could a person have a condition other than the one the doctor suspects? In evaluating whether someone is suffering from SAD, we need to consider other conditions that produce similar symptoms, such as lethargy, overeating, carbohydrate craving, weight gain, and depression. Many physical illnesses can cause lethargy and depression, which is why it is important for people who think they are suffering from SAD to be thoroughly examined by a physician. However, it is unusual for other conditions to appear in the winter and leave in the summer, year after year. Even so, if you think you have SAD, it is better to be on the safe side and have a physical examination and the necessary blood tests, since you could have another illness as well as SAD.

Specific illnesses that need to be considered are as follows:

1. *Underactive thyroid function (hypothyroidism)*: In this condition, people feel sluggish and cannot tolerate the cold weather. The thyroid gland, situated centrally in the front of the neck, is responsible for producing hormones that regulate the rate of metabolism. Underactivity of the thyroid can usually be treated simply by taking thyroid hormone in the form of pills.

2. *Low blood sugar (hypoglycemia)*: People with this condition feel weak and light-headed at times, usually one to two hours after a meal. At times they may feel very hungry and crave sweets. This condition

can usually be treated by dietary regulation. People with hypoglycemia should avoid foods containing high concentrations of sugar in forms that are rapidly absorbed into the system. Examples of these "simple" carbohydrates are candies and other very sweet things. Instead, people with this condition should eat combinations of proteins and complex carbohydrates, such as fruit, rice, and pasta.

3. *Chronic viral illnesses:* SAD symptoms can resemble those of the Epstein–Barr (E-B) virus (which is responsible for infectious mononucleosis) or even the flu. Some people are susceptible to viral conditions, which may be most prevalent during the winter. It is not uncommon for people to feel lethargic and debilitated for some time after a bad attack of flu. Similarly, the E-B virus, which has attracted a fair amount of media attention recently, may cause long-term lethargy and fatigue.

Unfortunately, chronic viral illnesses are very difficult to diagnose precisely, and there are no specific treatments for them. Blood tests showing antibodies against the E-B virus simply indicate that a person has been infected in the past—not that the virus is necessarily responsible for the present symptoms. Luckily, however, most cases of chronic E-B virus infection get better with time.

Although viral conditions may masquerade as SAD, the occurrence winter after winter of typical SAD symptoms, which improve in spring and summer, points strongly toward SAD. In any event, since the presence of viral infections is difficult to document and there are no specific treatments for them, and since there are specific treatments for SAD, it usually makes sense to treat the problem as SAD.

4. *Chronic fatigue syndrome (CFS):* This disabling condition is thought to occur following viral infections, at least in some cases, but its causes are poorly understood. Whatever its cause, the patient is often left in a state of disabling fatigue. Dr. Mark Demitrack, formerly at the NIMH and now at the University of Michigan, surveyed a group of CFS patients for a history of seasonal variations in their symptoms and found that they reported significant seasonal changes, though these were no greater than those occurring in the general population. This suggests that CFS patients suffer from a condition quite separate from SAD, and that on top of the fatigue that is the hallmark of this condition, they are also susceptible to the ordinary seasonal changes in energy that affect a high percentage of the general population. It is unknown at this time whether light therapy is of any benefit whatsoever in these individuals.

SAD in Children and Adolescents

Some time ago, a middle-aged woman walked into the NIMH clinical center and asked me if I knew of any articles on SAD in children. I said

I did indeed have an article, and wondered why she was interested in the subject. "My son asked me to stop by and find out more about the condition," she said. "He thinks he has it." It emerged that her twelve-year-old son had seen a television program on the subject and had identified with the patients.

I was reminded of "Jason," another smart twelve-year-old, who had seen both of his parents suffering from SAD and being treated with light therapy. One winter he approached his father, saying that he thought he was also suffering from SAD, as he had noticed that he was eating more candies. His father dismissed this observation with a psychological explanation—the boy was clearly identifying with his parents, and what child doesn't eat too much candy? But Jason, normally a fine student, began to have increasing difficulties with his schoolwork. One day his father, finding him dozing over his homework, asked him again what the problem was. "Dad, I think it's the winter," Jason replied. And he was right. Light therapy has since reversed the problem to a large degree.

Although some children and adolescents with SAD are able to recognize that they have a seasonal problem, many others do not understand what is wrong. Often they are not even aware that the change is internal, but blame it instead on the world around them, which they experience as having turned cruel and uncaring. In their view, teachers have become excessively strict and parents unfairly demanding. Many adults similarly misperceive the source of their SAD symptoms and seek external explanations to account for the dramatic difference in the way they feel when they are depressed.

I first started looking for children and adolescents with SAD because about one-third of our adult patients reported symptoms going back to these early years. In addition, many of the adult patients reported similar symptoms in their children, which is not surprising, considering the high familial incidence of the disorder. SAD in children has many similarities to the adult form—for example, there is often difficulty in waking up on time in the morning and accomplishing tasks, particularly schoolwork. One difference is that children appear to show more irritability during their winter depressions than do adults.

Drs. Susan Swedo, A. J. Allen, and I have studied children and adolescents with seasonal difficulties at the NIMH. We have surveyed students in junior high and high schools in Montgomery County, Maryland, and have found that seasonal problems are by no means uncommon in these age groups. Although SAD appears to affect only about 1 percent of children in the lower grades, there is a dramatic increase in prevalence in the last three years of high school. This marked increase corresponds to the onset of puberty and is more pronounced in girls than in boys, suggesting that cyclical secretion of female sex hormones may be one factor in the development of the symptoms of SAD, as proposed earlier in this chapter.

By the senior year of high school, approximately 5 percent of students report seasonal problems severe enough to qualify them as suffering from SAD, which makes the problem almost as common as it is for adults surveyed in the same geographical area. When all students from ages nine to seventeen are considered together, the overall percentage of SAD sufferers is about 3 percent. If those numbers can be applied to students across the country, it would mean that at least a million children and adolescents suffer from SAD.

In a separate study, Drs. Mary Carskadon and Christine Acebo at Brown University surveyed the parents of children in grades four through six for a history of seasonal changes. They found that almost half of all parents observed some seasonal changes in their children's behavior, and that, depending on how it was calculated, the proportion of children with seasonal problems ranged from 4 to 13 percent. These researchers also found that, as with adults, children's seasonal problems are more marked in locations that are farther north. "Given the potential therapeutic benefit of light therapy in children with such seasonal patterns," they noted, "a careful assessment of seasonality is merited when evaluating children who present with mood and behavior problems in the winter."

If you would like to find out whether a child or adolescent you know meets the criteria for SAD, as developed by researchers at the NIMH, you can do so by consulting the Seasonal Pattern Assessment Questionnaire for Children and Adolescents (SPAQ-CA) presented below in Figure 2. It is important to recognize that these criteria have been used only for research purposes and do not coincide fully with clinical criteria. A proper diagnosis of SAD can only be made by a qualified clinician. Nevertheless, the answers on this questionnaire do provide useful information and guidance as to whether it is worth having a child or adolescent evaluated more fully for SAD. A simpler and more straightforward guide for parents who suspect that their child may be suffering from SAD is provided on page 65.

How to Interpret Scores on the Seasonal Pattern Assessment Questionnaire for Children and Adolescents (SPAQ-CA)

1. *Establishing the pattern of seasonality:* If a child or adolescent is suffering from winter SAD, he or she should report feeling worst during

1. Please circle the × under the month(s) when the following happen:

	Jan	Feb	Mar	Apr	May	Jun	Jul	Aug	Sep	Oct	Nov	Dec	All the same
I have the least energy	×	×	×	×	×	×	×	×	×	×	×	×	×
I am the most irritable	×	×	×	×	×	×	×	×	×	×	×	×	×
I feel my worst	×	×	×	×	×	×	×	×	×	×	×	×	×

2. For you, do any of the following vary with the seasons? (circle the ×)

	No (0)	A little (1)	Sort of (2)	Pretty much (3)	A lot (4)
Length of sleep	×	×	×	×	×
Getting in trouble	×	×	×	×	×
Social activity	×	×	×	×	×
Substance abuse (drinking, smoking, drugs)	×	×	×	×	×
Mood	×	×	×	×	×
School performance					
a. Difficulty	×	×	×	×	
b. Grades	×	×	×	×	×
Weight	×	×	×	×	×
Irritability	×	×	×	×	×
Energy level	×	×	×	×	×
Appetite	×	×	×	×	×

3. If you experience change with the seasons, do you feel this is a problem for you?

Yes: _____   No: _____

If yes, is this problem (circle one):

Not bad   Pretty bad   Very bad   So bad I have trouble functioning

Figure 2. Seasonal Pattern Assessment Questionaire for Children and Adolescents (SPAQ-CA; adapted by S. Swedo and J. Pleeter from the SPAQ of N. E. Rosenthal, G. Bradt and T. Wehr).

January or February on at least one of the items noted in question 1—namely, "I have the least energy," "I am the most irritable," or "I feel my worst."

  2. *Establishing the degree of seasonality*: The global seasonality score can be obtained from question 2 simply by adding up all the individual item scores. Since there are 11 items and each item score ranges from 0 to 4, the global seasonality score will range from 0 to 44 for each individual. In our school survey, we used 21 as a cutoff score for diagnosing SAD. It is important to remember that this score is somewhat arbitrary, and children or adolescents with lower scores may

also suffer seasonal problems. One of the problems with self-administered questionnaires such as this one is that they require accurate memory and the recognition of a seasonal pattern; such a pattern may be quite difficult to reconstruct, especially for younger children. In fact, many of the children and adolescents diagnosed as suffering from SAD at the NIMH had cutoff scores below 21.

3. *Determining whether SAD is a problem:* In order to make a diagnosis of SAD, we require that a child or adolescent rate the problem with the seasonal changes as being at least "pretty bad." Here again, as researchers we have to be strict so as not to overdiagnose the condition. From the point of view of a concerned parent, however, it might be worth taking note if a child or adolescent reports that seasonal changes are a problem at all. The young person may be underestimating the degree to which these changes are a problem, and even if the changes are minor they may respond favorably to a simple intervention, such as making sure to go outdoors for at least half an hour each day.

In summary, a child or adolescent may well be suffering from SAD if you find all of the following responses on the SPAQ-CA:

- In January or February he or she feels least energetic, worst, or most irritable.
- The global seasonality score is 21 or more.
- Seasonal changes are experienced as a "pretty bad" problem.

Most patients with childhood SAD first come in for treatment when they are about fifteen or sixteen, having experienced an average of six winters of symptoms. There are several reasons why it takes so long for children and adolescents to get diagnosed. First, some of the symptoms of SAD fit the stereotype of what people might expect to find in adolescence, such as lethargy, irritability, and lack of motivation. Research indicates that this stereotype is a myth and that adolescence is frequently a happy and stable time. Second, many physicians are still unaware of SAD, especially in its childhood and adolescent forms. Third, it takes several years for a seasonal pattern to emerge, so that the reason for the first few difficult winters is quite likely to be missed. Fourth, children or adolescents may be less adept than adults at recognizing the seasonal pattern. Finally, it is easy to attribute school difficulties to other causes, such as psychological problems. It is particularly important, however, to distinguish SAD from these other types of problems, since it is eminently responsive to light therapy in young people just as it is in adults. At present, children too often suffer needlessly for several winters before getting appropriate help.

Telltale Signs of SAD in Children and Adolescents: A Guide for Parents

The single biggest clue that your child may be suffering from SAD is that he or she develops problems at the same time each year: during the fall and winter. This particular point may be more important than the actual symptoms themselves, which may be atypical; the problems may manifest themselves, for example, as anxiety or school avoidance. Children or adolescents with SAD often do well at school in the first few months after returning from their summer vacations and generally do not experience seasonal problems until December or January. When the problem does hit, however, its effects are often very marked, and parents are frequently surprised to find how much of a struggle schoolwork can become for a young person who was a fine student in the early part of the semester. Adolescence is often a time when sleeping and eating habits change, so reports of changes in these behaviors are less helpful in making the diagnosis of SAD than are problems with concentration, schoolwork, energy, and mood.

Common symptoms of SAD in children and adolescents are the following:

- Feeling tired and washed out
- Feeling cranky and irritable
- Temper tantrums
- Difficulty in concentrating and doing schoolwork (this may manifest as either slipping grades or the need to work harder to maintain grades at pre-existing levels)
- Reluctance to undertake chores and other responsibilities not previously regarded as a problem
- Vague physical complaints, such as headaches or abdominal pains
- Marked increase in cravings for "junk food"

Several young people with SAD come to mind. "Michael," a twelve-year-old swimming champion, had swim times that invariably deteriorated during the winter and improved during the summer. "Susan," an eight-year-old with long, flowing blond hair and a wistful gaze, had suffered from pronounced seasonal rhythms since infancy. Her parents noticed marked differences between her sleep length during the short summer nights, when she would wake up with the first rays of the sun, and the long winter nights, when she would sleep for hours and hours. Her problems began in nursery school, when teachers noticed that she would withdraw from friends and be uninterested in the usual routine of daily activities during January and February. "Jeannie," a thirteen-year-old, not only had the usual difficulties with schoolwork and social activities in the winter, but became overactive in the summer. At that time her activity level would increase, she would need little sleep, and she would tend to be impulsive and show poor judgment. On one occasion her father found her cavorting about on the roof, enjoying the night air, apparently unaware of the danger of falling.

College Freshmen: A Population at Risk

"Jackie's" story is a familiar one; I can think of several others like hers. She was an upbeat young woman and a good student in high school, with many friends and varied hobbies and activities. Although she suffered from asthma, this condition was well controlled by medications, which she took regularly. In retrospect, winters were somewhat difficult for her, but not severely enough to interfere with her participation in sports, her social life, or her grades. Things changed when she went to college in New England. The beginning of the first semester went well. She enrolled in several difficult classes, participated fully in college life, and continued to thrive until December. After returning to college after the Thanksgiving break, she began to have trouble waking up in time for her morning classes and fell behind in her studies. She felt exhausted in the early evening and was unable to turn in her papers on time or to prepare for examinations.

For Jackie, failure was a new experience, and it caused her to question all the assumptions she had previously made about herself— namely, that she was a competent, successful, and popular person. She wondered whether she could have fooled herself and everybody else all through high school. Now that she was in the real world, could life be showing her up for what she was—a second-rate mediocrity and an impostor? She lay around in bed a good part of the day and neglected many aspects of her life, including regular visits to the health center to have her asthma monitored. When her medications ran out, she didn't refill them, became physically ill, and had to drop out of school.

A careful history revealed that Jackie's SAD had been the leading edge of the problem. After receiving appropriate treatment for it (light therapy, psychotherapy, and antidepressant medications), she returned to school in the spring, when she did very well. During the summer, she caught up on the work she had missed the previous winter and entered the fall semester armed with extensive knowledge about SAD, a referral to a knowledgable psychiatrist close to her college, and a game plan for managing the fall and winter quarters. This game plan included the following elements: (1) a schedule of relatively easy courses, none of which required early morning classes; (2) a light box, which she planned to use regularly; (3) a dawn simulator to help her wake up in the morning; (4) plans to exercise outdoors regularly during the daylight hours; and (5) regular scheduled sessions with her psychiatrist.

Jackie did well until mid-January, when her SAD became problematic despite all the preventive measures outlined above. At that time her psychiatrist put her on a course of fluoxetine (Prozac), which she continued to take until the end of March. Although it would be an exaggeration to say that she actually enjoyed the winter, Jackie felt well throughout the semester; she continued to take her asthma medications and had no relapse of this condition, and she closed out the year with a feeling of accomplishment and a fine grade point average.

Jackie's story illustrates several points that are important to bear in mind in planning for college freshmen who have a history of problematic seasonal changes. First, the move to college often involves a change of latitude or climate, which may enhance the tendency to SAD. Second, when at home, a young person is often woken up and bundled off to school by parents. This makes it less likely that classes will be missed, and ensures exposure to natural early morning light. This support does not carry through to college, where the student, left to his or her own devices, may lie for hours in a dark dorm room and miss both classes and sunlight. Finally, the newly experienced demands of college often pose a much more stressful challenge to the freshman than the familiar routine of high school. Although these stresses may be relatively easy to handle in fall and spring, they may prove too burdensome in winter, when the vulnerable student becomes less resourceful and resilient; accordingly, they may bring on or aggravate the symptoms of SAD. Once these symptoms emerge, they compound the problem further, which frequently leads to failure and (as in Jackie's case) to dropping out of school. Although her tendency to develop asthma was specific to Jackie, many individuals have special needs that require extra attention, and these are often sacrificed when energy and concentration decline in the winter months.

It is particularly important to target vulnerable individuals in high school, since good planning can prevent predictable misfortune. I can imagine a time not too far from now when school counselors routinely screen high school seniors for a history of problematic seasonal changes and counsel those at risk. Those who know they are at risk may even consider geography as one of several factors to take into account in their choice of colleges.

Attention Deficit Disorder and SAD

A school problem called "attention deficit disorder" may look like SAD in some instances, but it should not appear regularly in fall and winter unless the child has a seasonal problem as well. Indeed, I have encountered patients with both problems. One young girl I treated suffered from attention deficit disorder all year round, for which she was treated with a stimulant drug, methylphenidate (Ritalin). During the winter she experienced typical symptoms of SAD, apparently inherited from her mother, who suffered from similar problems. Thirty minutes of treatment with bright light in the morning reversed all her symptoms and helped her wake up and get to school on time, which had previously been a serious problem for her.

Nonseasonal depression may also occur in children and may resemble SAD, but, by definition, it should not occur only in the fall and winter months.

Treatment of Children with SAD

A crucial element in the treatment of SAD in children and adolescents is the attitude of the significant adults in their lives. If it is difficult for adults to accept that they have psychiatric problems, it is even harder for children and adolescents, who are very eager not to seem different from their peers. If they are to accept their seasonal problems, it is therefore critical to present them in a nonstigmatizing way as simply a variant of the seasonal changes that affect many people and, indeed, all of the natural world.

Treating SAD optimally requires organization, which is difficult to muster when one is tired and unfocused. The child or adolescent with SAD will therefore need the help of adults in getting organized. This can easily result in a power struggle between parent and child if the matter is not empathically and tactfully handled. Things are often easier if one of the parents is also seasonal, since there are many opportunities for parent and child to empathize with each other and share strategies for coping. But even if a parent is not seasonal, it is valuable to point to the diversity in nature and the many ways that different people and animals adapt to our changing world. Depending on the nature of the child or adolescent, it may be sufficient to make this point in passing. If your child has an inquiring mind, however, it may be fun and useful to engage him or her in activities involving the changing seasons and the responses they elicit in nature. You could construct a sundial in the garden, for example, and chart the annual course of the sun across the sky. Projects involving plants, insects, or animals are ideal for studying the natural effects of the seasons. It is even possible to study the effects of seasons on human mood and behavior. In fact, the results of the NIMH survey of Maryland students mentioned above resulted from a school science project, developed by a talented high school senior.

Once the presence of SAD is accepted, destigmatized, and regarded as a manageable fact of life, and once the child or adolescent is recruited as a collaborator in the treatment process rather than the object of it, all specific suggestions become much easier to implement. Such specific suggestions are not in principle different from those outlined in the adult treatment section (Part 2 of this book). They include the following:

- Helping the child or adolescent wake up in the morning
- Ensuring that he or she is exposed to sufficient light, either natural or artificial
- Helping him or her manage stress
- Reminding him or her that many of the difficulties encountered are a result of the seasonal problem rather than signs of failure
- Encouraging him or her through the difficult months
- Asking the doctor about antidepressant medications, if the above interventions are insufficient

In a follow-up study of six children who had been diagnosed as having SAD seven years before, Dr. Jay Giedd and colleagues at the NIMH found that two children had been successfully treated with the antidepressant fluoxetine (Prozac) (see Chapter 9, pages 162–178, for further details about this and other antidepressant medications). A knowledgeable and sympathetic psychiatrist or other therapist can be invaluable in helping you and your child negotiate the difficult winter months, and should be involved on a continuing basis if light therapy is used. In addition, a psychiatrist should certainly be consulted before any medications are initiated.

Waking up in the morning is generally the first battle of the day for a child or adolescent with SAD (as it is for many adults). This will be much easier if the child wakes up in the light. A bright bedside lamp, attached to a timer, will be helpful in this regard. Although the more expensive and sophisticated dawn simulator (see Chapter 6, pages 124–127), which provides a more graduated artificial dawn, may be superior, it has not yet been directly compared to the simpler arrangement with the bedside lamp on a timer. A radio alarm clock may also be very useful. By helping to wake the child up, it will result in earlier exposure to the light of morning, either real or artificial. If possible, it is best if the child or adolescent can assume responsibility for waking up, as struggles centering around this issue start the day off on a bad note.

A child or adolescent with SAD may either have his or her own light box or share a light box with other members of the family. I recall a mother and daughter, both of whom suffered from SAD, who would enjoy sitting and talking together by their light box each morning. As with adults, light treatment can be administered to good effect either in the morning or the evening, and in conjunction with homework or other sedentary activities. Since childhood and adolescent SAD is a more recently recognized and studied entity than adult SAD, there is less research on the use of light in these age groups. My experience suggests that children may need shorter treatment sessions than adults—perhaps as little as fifteen to twenty minutes per day. It is particularly important than the light source emit as little ultraviolet light as possible, since the lens of a child's eye does less to filter out these potentially harmful wavelengths than the lens of an adult. As far as we know, conventional light fixtures, used under the supervision of a professional, are quite safe. More information about the potential long-term effects of bright light is provided in the discussion of light therapy for adults (see Chapter 6, pages 110–111). *Besides formal light therapy, children should be encouraged to spend at least half an hour a day out of doors, so that they can derive the benefit of natural light as well.* It may also be useful to enhance bedroom lighting in an informal way, as described in Chapter 7, pages 134–135.

Activities that the child or adolescent with SAD handles easily in summer and fall often become burdensome in the dark months. Gentle assistance with organizing schedules and with anticipating and managing stress is often necessary at those times. A young person with SAD should perhaps leave demanding and time-consuming extracurricular activities, such as participating in a school play or working on the school newspaper, to the spring and fall months. Sports activities, on the other hand, can relieve the symptoms of SAD, because they combine aerobic exercise (which may be useful in itself) with exposure to outdoor light. Tasks associated with deadlines should be anticipated well ahead of their due date and tackled as early as possible to prevent last-minute crises. Just sitting down with your child and reviewing his or her schedule can be experienced as supportive and can serve as an early warning system for potential trouble down the road.

A review of the adult treatment section will provide further insights and tips for helping your child. Remember, you will be working against resistance. A child or adolescent does not want to think that he or she is suffering from an illness, so tact and creativity are necessary in broaching the topic. On the other hand, he or she knows very well that there is a problem. Recognizing it, giving it a name, and outlining practical solutions will generally be appreciated. By setting an example in this way, you are instilling in your child the capacity to take charge of the problem and overcome it—a skill that will be critical in the years to come.

The Flip Side of Depression: Spring Fever

Mania and Hypomania

Although many people with SAD feel normally cheerful during the summer months, it is quite common for individuals to report feeling exceptionally energetic and creative at this time. Herb Kern, the first patient with SAD to be treated at the NIMH, was exceptionally productive in his scientific work during the summer—so much so that his boss was happy to let him plod through his less productive winter months. Artists and writers may also get most of their creative work done during the summer, and may leave the more humdrum aspects of their work for wintertime.

Such enhanced productivity is not universal for those who develop extra energy in the summer. In some people this acceleration goes too far and may result in major problems—bank accounts overdrawn as a result of excessive spending, difficulties in getting along with friends and colleagues, and even trouble with the law. This state is referred to clinically as "mania."

An exaggerated sex drive caused by a midsummer high resulted in problems for "Marie," a housewife in her twenties, who was at home with her two young children. Although she was a faithful wife under ordinary circumstances, one summer she could not resist the attentions of a carpenter who was installing bookshelves for her husband. This dalliance caused her a considerable amount of guilt until she understood that her abnormal mood state had disrupted her usual level of responsibility and judgment, while at the same time increasing her sex drive.

Some manic patients may spend large sums of money that they can ill afford on items that, at other times, would seem extravagant.

They may show poor judgment in their driving and speed along the highway, assured that their lightning reflexes make them invulnerable to accidents. Or they may suddenly and impetuously decide to undertake some long journey for reasons that to the outsider would seem frivolous.

The degree of acceleration does not have to reach manic proportions in order to be considered a problem by an individual or, more commonly, by the person's partner, friends, and colleagues. These people may complain that they are unable to get a word in edgewise, or are interrupted repeatedly during a conversation. This condition—less severe than mania—is known as "hypomania," and it often impairs efficiency. Although hypomanic people have a great deal of energy, they have so many ideas for projects that they find it difficult to focus on any single one. As a result, their energies are scattered; their attention darts from task to task; and, fueled by grandiosity, they are often left with several unfinished projects at the end of the summer.

Summer Highs: Scenes from a Marriage

Although Jack and Sylvia have some problems with each other when Sylvia is in her "low" winter state, her summer highs present the couple with more serious difficulties. The following excerpts from an interview with the two of them, conducted during the summer, illustrate some of these.

JACK: During her lows Sylvia really gets down. She will say, "I don't know how anyone can love me," or "I'm so slow, I hate myself." And then in the summer, when she gets in the high, she'll say, "Aren't you fortunate to have somebody with my personality?" It's just a complete reversal. I'm amazed—sometimes the highs are more trying than the lows. A day can make a huge difference. In just one day she can come alive.

Most of our arguments come in the early spring, when she comes alive and wants to do all kinds of things. I remember going to Wolf Trap [an open-air amphitheater near Washington, D.C.] with some friends; she was so excited that everyone said, "Look at Sylvia, she's so high." She became the focal point of her friends because of her excessive energy. It is difficult for me because Sylvia gets after me to join in on her whirlwind of activities. Just the other day I said to her, "Look, I can't be as high as you unless I take cocaine, and I don't plan to take cocaine." At Wolf Trap she just bounced around—it was unreal. I thought she could fly, and I think Sylvia and all her friends thought she could, too!

Jack documents many incidents that have occurred during the summer as evidence of Sylvia's hypomanic state. She spends money on projects that he regards as unnecessary, but that she feels are interesting or creative. For example, she bought an expensive video camera so that her sons could learn to make films. On another occasion, she bought a pet iguana, capable of growing to a length of eight feet. While Jack regarded the animal as a bizarre nuisance, Sylvia identified with its love for the sun. She remembers, "When he would get out of the house and I couldn't find him, I would wait for the sun to start going down and know that he would be in that one spot in the yard where the sun was still shining."

Although they have generally been able to resolve their financial difficulties amicably, Jack actually suggested taking Sylvia's credit cards away from her during the summer on one occasion. She became extremely angry and threatened to leave him, and he backed down.

They discuss their seasonal problems further:

SYLVIA: There's a kind of power struggle that goes on between us, because for six months you can just lead me anywhere, and then in the summer I want to lead. And Jack is not the kind of person who likes a boss.

JACK: In the winter Sylvia would be really down, and I'd feel really sorry for her and try to keep her spirits up. Then in the spring she'd almost turn on me. I almost got the feeling she didn't like the person she was in the winter, and the fact that I cared for that person in the winter was held against me in the spring. And I couldn't believe that. I think to myself, "I've done all kinds of things for you in the winter, driven you around, made excuses for you to your friends, but because you hate that Sylvia, you hate me, too."

SYLVIA: Jack's reactions to me have always worried me. I like myself in the spring and summer, but I don't think Jack really enjoys me then.

When asked how she feels about Jack's having helped her and taken care of her during the winter, Sylvia replies: "I don't like to think about it."

"Do you forget it, put it out of your mind?" I ask.

"I certainly do. I want to think about happy things," she replies.

Jack comments: "The heck with that! Next winter I'm going to let her take care of herself."

Both Jack and Sylvia agree that she becomes short-tempered in the summer and is most likely to have run-ins with other people then.

On one occasion, when Jack's mother came to visit during the month of May, she and Sylvia had an argument from which Jack says it took his mother two years to recover. As a result, Jack makes sure to keep the two women apart during the summer. Sylvia also has to stay away from meetings at her church then, as she is likely to monopolize them and antagonize some of the other church members with blunt and tactless remarks. She relates this with a certain amount of enjoyment and little evidence of regret.

Although Sylvia's high periods are a source of frustration for Jack, there are aspects of them—the humor, creativity, and liveliness—that he enjoys as much as she does. In the past year or two, however, Sylvia has become worn out during her high periods from lack of sleep and excessive activity. She has been reluctant to take any medications for this, and I have treated her by having her wear dark glasses during the summer days. This treatment has been quite successful, and at times she has even slept with eyeshades on to prevent herself from waking up with the first rays of dawn.

Jack and Sylvia have benefited greatly from marital therapy as well, which has helped them to identify the symptoms of SAD, understand that biological processes are at work, and help them cope with these changes. Jack sums it up: "I think we're like ships passing in the night. We're very seldom at the same level. She's either below me or above, and only momentarily do we see eye to eye."

Dysphoric Hypomania

Although hypomanic individuals often feel euphoric, as in Sylvia's case, hypomania may also be an extremely unpleasant or "dysphoric" state. Like euphoric hypomanics, people with dysphoric hypomania also feel acivated, experience racing thoughts, and speak in a pressured way. But unlike their euphoric counterparts, they feel uncomfortable both physically and emotionally, and long for something to bring them down from their hypomanic state. To this end, they may resort to alcohol or cigarettes in an unavailing attempt to calm themselves down. They are irritable and snappy with those they come into contact with. As a consequence, friends and family often avoid them at such times, which may cause them to feel rejected and isolated. A few patients I have encountered with dysphoric hypomania in spring and summer have also complained of physical aches and pains.

These symptoms may be a result of the impact of the rapidly increasing spring light levels on the oversensitive eyes and brains of individuals who have become accustomed to the low levels of environmental light typically found in winter. One young woman consulted me on a spring evening for her problems with dysphoric hypomania. Over the course of the consultation, she became increasingly agitated. I noticed that the lights in my office were very bright, and suggested that we experiment by dimming them. Over the next half hour her agitation subsided dramatically—so much so that I suggested she try treating herself with light restriction. She called me a week later in a state of elation, and reported that she had become able to manage her hypomania without using the tranquilizers that she had previously needed, simply by going into a darkened room for a short period of time whenever she felt overexcited. This rapidly acting, nondrug treatment that she was able to regulate herself not only relieved her symptoms, but also gave her a sense of personal mastery over them. Other ways of restricting one's light exposure include wearing eyeshades while asleep to avoid exposure to early morning light; wearing wrap-around dark glasses when outdoors; and avoiding brightly lit indoor environments in the evening. If these measures don't work, effective medications are available to lessen the uncomfortable and problematic aspects of this condition.

Although spring and summer hypomanias may cause problems, I should emphasize that for many people with SAD, hypomanias are joyful and creative times that do no harm and don't require treatment.

The Winter Blues or February Blahs

Soon after we first encountered patients with SAD, it became clear that there were many people with a milder form of the condition. These people would not generally seek out medical help for their winter difficulties, but when asked specifically about them, would recall that they had some problem each winter—for example, lack of enthusiasm or decreased productivity. In order to study this question, Dr. Siegfried Kasper and I undertook a study of what we called "subsyndromal SAD," or the "winter blues," at the NIMH. We established criteria for this condition, which are outlined in Chapter 3 (see Table 1), and set out to find people who met the description.

"Jeff," a typical victim of the winter blues, read an article of ours in the *NIMH Record*, which gave a checklist of symptoms that people with this variant of SAD experience: low energy, difficulty with concentrating and getting one's work done, and tiredness—in short, a syndrome that was milder than the depression previously described as responding to light. Jeff was in his mid-forties and was a well-informed mental health professional, but he had never quite recognized the basis of his seasonal problem.

As he looked back on his difficulties, it was clear to him that his ability to concentrate would decline each winter. A self-declared workaholic, he was always less productive during the winter months than during the rest of the year. During the winter, he felt tired and attributed it to a lack of sleep, even though he was actually sleeping more than he did during the summer. He had never been formally treated for this winter problem. He treated his low energy level with cups of coffee and found that if he put several very bright lamps on his desk, it helped him concentrate. He also found that if he had to meet a deadline, he could sometimes do so by sleeping from 7:00 P.M. to midnight, and working straight through the night and the following day. Sleep restriction is a known treatment for depression and is discussed later in this book.

Curiosity led Jeff to take part in the NIMH research program—curiosity and a hope that maybe there was an explanation and a simple treatment for his recurrent winter difficulties. He entered the program with great skepticism. His expectations of the effects of the light treatment were very low. But the treatment worked dramatically for him, and he has used bright light at his desk ever since.

Dr. Kasper has shown that bright light is effective for most people with the winter blues, which seems to affect at least twice as many people as SAD does, though not as dramatically. Nevertheless, this milder winter syndrome does interfere with the quality of life in those who suffer from it and decreases their productivity. Since it is easily reversible in most cases, it is important that we identify these people and offer them information and treatment.

Scientists believe that SAD and the winter blues are two broad categories of problematic seasonal change to which many people are susceptible. Although some clearly fall into one category or another on the basis of the severity of their winter problems, many fall into a gray zone between the two. The important point is that bright light can help those in either category. The distinction between the two is that those who meet the criteria for SAD should seek out professional help and receive light treatment as part of a comprehensive evaluation and treatment plan. Those who are affected by only mild winter changes may be able to obtain satisfactory relief of symptoms simply by increasing the amount of light in their living and working environments. Since SAD and the winter blues have been described, an increasing number of individuals are recognizing that they experience subtle decreases in energy in the winter and are considering light therapy, even though they have never experienced themselves as having problems with the winter. Guidelines are provided in Chapter 3 to help the interested reader decide when a physician should be consulted.

Commonly Asked Questions About SAD

1. How common is SAD? How many people suffer from it? Does it get worse the farther north you go?

This question has been studied by several researchers, many of whom have used versions of the SPAQ, just like the one you may have used to rate your own seasonality (see Chapter 3, Figure 1). Studies done in several different parts of the United States suggest that the farther north you go, the more common are both SAD and subsyndromal SAD (the winter blues). Table 3 below shows the percentages of the population thought to be affected by SAD and subsyndromal SAD at different latitudes.

As one might gather from Table 3, the projected rates for SAD and subsyndromal SAD (winter blues) in the United States are high. Dr. Leora Rosen and colleagues have estimated that the prevalence of SAD for the entire U.S. population is 6 percent, or eleven million people; for subsyndromal SAD, the corresponding figures are 14 percent, or twenty-five million people. If one examines the entire population likely to benefit from enhanced environmental lighting—namely, a group consisting of SAD plus subsyndromal SAD sufferers—the estimated figures are 20 percent of the population of the United States, or thirty-six million people.

These estimates may be a little high for the most northern latitudes, since a recent study in Fairbanks, Alaska (64° north) by Drs. John Booker and Carla Hellekson found a 9 percent prevalence of SAD and a 19 percent prevalence of the winter blues. Although these are lower than the figures one would have predicted from the study by Dr. Rosen and colleagues, the Alaska study confirms that SAD and the winter blues are extremely common in the North.

For comparison with Table 3, latitudes for some European countries are as follows:

60–55° Denmark, southern Norway, Sweden

50–55° The British Isles, northern Germany

45–50° Northern France, northern Italy, Switzerland, Austria, Romania, northern Yugoslavia, Hungary, Czechoslovakia, southern Germany

40–45° Southern France, Yugoslavia, northern Spain, northern Portugal, Albania, Bulgaria

35–40° Southern Portugal, southern Spain, Greece

Table 3. Estimated Prevalence of SAD and Subsyndromal SAD at Different Latitudes in the United States and Canada

Latitude	States/cities	SAD(%)	Subsyndromal SAD(%)
45–50°	Washington, Montana, North Dakota, Minnesota, northern Michigan, Maine; southern Quebec, southern Ontario, Manitoba, Saskatchewan, Alberta, and British Columbia	10.2	20.2
40–45°	Oregon, Idaho, Wyoming, South Dakota, Nebraska, Iowa, northern Indiana, Massachusetts, Ohio, Wisconsin, Pennsylvania, New York, Vermont, New Hampshire, Rhode Island, Connecticut, New Jersey	8.0	17.1
35–40°	Northern California, Nevada, Utah, Colorado, Kansas, Oklahoma, Missouri, southern Illinois, Tennessee, Kentucky, West Virginia, Maryland, Delaware, Virginia, Washington, D. C., North Carolina	5.8	13.9
30–35°	Southern California, Arizona, New Mexico, Texas, Arkansas, Louisiana, Mississippi, Alabama, Georgia, South Carolina	3.6	10.6
25–30°	Mexico, south Texas, Florida	1.4	7.5

Note. This table is based on a collaborative study by the NIMH, Psychiatric Institutes of America, New York State Psychiatric Institute, and Walter Reed Army Institute of Research. The rates at different latitudes were calculated by Dr. Leora N. Rosen, based on only four sites: Nashua, New Hampshire; New York City; Montgomery County, Maryland; and Sarasota, Florida. Generalizing these rates to other parts of the United States and Canada may not be valid.

2. I have heard that the commonest seasons for suicide are the spring and summer. How does this tie in with SAD's occurring in the fall and winter?

This question is answered in greater detail in Chapter 5. In most studies there is a peak incidence of suicide in the spring and summer. The reason for this paradox seems to be that those who suffer from SAD and those who are at risk for committing suicide in the summer appear to be two distinct groups, with completely different patterns of response to the seasons.

3. Is SAD the same as the "holiday blues" or "Christmas depression" that we hear so much about?

For therapists in clinical practice, it is not unusual to see some feelings of sadness around the time of the holidays. Although this is a time when people are supposed to be happy, and many are, there are some for whom the expected happiness does not arrive. Lonely people, people without family or friends, feel lonelier than ever when they see celebrations going on all around them. It is a time for nostalgia—perhaps for remembering holidays when things were better. It is also a time for missing people, such as relatives or friends, who have passed away during previous years.

The holidays present a special problem for individuals who grew up in dysfunctional families—families where the atmosphere was full of conflict, anger, violence, or abuse. When these people were growing up, the holidays might have been particularly confusing and difficult times. Other families were conspicuously enjoying themselves, but their families clearly were not. Their parents might have expected them to go along with the external trappings of festivity, but a genuine holiday spirit of good cheer was plainly lacking. When these people become adults, they often re-experience similar conflicts with their new families at the holiday time. They feel pressured to create a holiday atmosphere, but are suffused with feelings of sadness, anger, and confusion when they are reminded (at times unconsciously) of the unhappy holidays of their childhood.

I have seen such individuals, when they enter psychotherapy, begin to understand the origins of their unhappiness, anger, and confusion. Once this first step is accomplished, they may permit themselves to avoid any pretense at celebration when they don't truly feel like celebrating; they often regard this as extremely liberating. As they progress in their recovery from the emotional injuries of their childhood, they may begin to feel that they really want to celebrate—not necessarily in ways that they have been told they ought to, but in their own individual fashion. These new celebrations feel quite different from those of their childhood since they are spontaneous feelings of joy, rather than stereotyped responses extracted from them as a matter of duty. This particular form of the holiday blues is thus eminently treatable with psychotherapy.

The common element of sadness between SAD and the holiday blues is where the resemblance between these two conditions usually stops. When we refer to "depression" as a clinical term, as opposed to the sadness that arises out of psychological conflicts or as part of our ordinary lives, we think of a sustained state lasting several weeks that is accompanied by physical changes—for example, in eating, sleeping, energy level, and daily functioning. There is no evidence that most people reacting to Christmas or the holidays exhibit this picture, whereas it is typical for SAD patients to show all of these features.

Although a number of studies have looked for the holiday blues by examining, for example, the incidence of visits to the emergency room for psychiatric help, or admissions to psychiatric units during the holiday season, none has been able to find evidence of "Christmas depression" as a psychiatric entity. In fact, one study showed that presentations to psychiatric emergency rooms decreased in the few days before major holidays and increased in the few days after them. It is as though people did not want to spoil their holiday by going to the emergency room, so they waited until the holiday was over before doing so. Although the holiday blues may not be accompanied by physical changes and do not show up in studies of emergency room visits, they can be a source of real psychological pain as well as a clue to unresolved problems from the past. Such a clue is well worth following up by consulting a therapist, because these problems can be helped greatly, enabling people to enjoy the holiday season and other times of celebration more fully.

4. What about the possibility that people may regularly feel bad at a certain time of year because something bad once happened at that time of year in the past?

In clinical practice, we certainly see patients who experience symptoms that appear on or near the anniversary of some traumatic event. Sigmund Freud recognized these, and in his description of Fraulein Elisabeth von R. in 1895, he wrote: "This lady celebrated annual festivals of remembrance at the period of her various catastrophes, and on these occasions her vivid visual reproduction and expressions of feeling kept to the date precisely." The poet Longfellow also recognized the "secret anniversaries of the heart, when the full river of feeling overflows." These anniversary reactions tend to be experienced rather specifically around the date of the anniversary and do not typically last for weeks or months, as is the case with SAD.

In many cases of SAD I have seen attempts on the part of the patient or therapist to explain symptoms in terms of some anniversary. For example, patients may say, "I always thought it was because school began at that time of the year," or may recollect a loss that occurred in October or February. For example, one patient with SAD observed that his mother had died in September. His therapist tried to understand his winter problems in terms of the anniversary of this sad event, but the patient experienced this interpretation as unsatisfactory. In my experience, such explanations don't usually stand up to careful scrutiny. If the symptoms of SAD last for five months (almost half the year), it stands to reason that there would have been a high percentage of unpleasant occurrences during those months. In addition, why should an anniversary reaction for something that occurred in January or February begin in September or October? Finally, one would not expect anniversary reactions to respond to treatment with bright light.

5. Are there people who develop symptoms in the evening, when the sun goes down?

Indeed there are. One psychoanalyst recognized this symptom and called it "Hesperian depression" after the Greek name for the evening star, Hesperus. Some patients with SAD complain of this problem. For example, one observed that she could not keep working after the sun went down. Another felt unable to make love to her husband except during the day, when the sun was shining.

It's a curious symptom because it suggests an immediate response to the light. This coincides with the experience of some patients using light therapy, in whom I have seen an increase in energy occur even within the first half hour of light treatment.

CHAPTER 5

"Summer SAD" and other seasonal afflictions

> Of natures, some are well or ill adapted for summer, and some for winter.
>
> —HIPPOCRATES

The Summertime Blues

Although the commonest form of recurrent seasonal depressions in northern countries is the winter pattern of SAD, it is by no means the only one. In response to the first newspaper articles on SAD, approximately one in twenty people with seasonal depressions mentioned a pattern of mood change just the opposite of the pattern that had been described in the articles: They regularly became depressed each summer and felt better when fall arrived. Studies indicate that most people in the northern United States dislike winter more than summer. When you look as far south as Florida, however, the pattern is reversed and more people dislike the summer. In our NIMH survey of seasonal changes in Maryland, we found about five cases of winter SAD for every case of summer SAD. In sunnier countries, such as Italy and Australia, there may be nearly equal numbers of these two different forms of SAD. If the greenhouse effect is occurring, as disturbing evidence suggests may be the case, and the world is becoming progressively hotter and hotter, summer depressions may become increasingly common in future.

Characteristics of Summer SAD

Dr. Thomas Wehr has studied several patients with summer SAD. One of Dr. Wehr's original summer-SAD patients, "Marge," was a retired government administrator in her mid-sixties when she came to the NIMH for help. She had suffered from regular bouts of depression for the previous forty-five years, but had not recognized that her moodiness, lethargy, and irritability were out of the ordinary until the last fifteen years. For her, summers were always the worst times, except once when she went on vacation with her family for a few weeks to the Finger Lakes in upper New York State. She recalls swimming two or three times a day, "in that deep, dark, cold water. After a few days of that, my mood lifted, and that summer at least the depression never came back."

Although she knew her depressions were related to summer, she was never really sure why this was so. Perhaps, she thought, it was related to being on vacation. During the summer she was "too down and lethargic" to think about it, "and when fall came, I felt so much better I didn't bother because I had so many other things to do. When it goes away, you don't expect it to come back. But it always comes back in the spring." When she first saw Dr. Wehr in the summer, she said that her depression had apparently remitted spontaneously a day or two before the consultation. This coincided with an unusual cold front of air that had moved into the Washington, D.C. area, changing its usual sweltering and humid summer days into cool and pleasant ones.

Dr. Wehr postulated that it might be the heat of the summer that was triggering this patient's depressions, and that the cool air and her swims in the cold, spring-fed lakes of the north might have exerted a therapeutic influence on her mood. He observed that temperature changes had been suggested as a cause of depression since the time of Aristotle. On the basis of this hypothesis, Dr. Wehr suggested that Marge stay in her air-conditioned apartment for a week and avoid the summer heat completely. She followed his suggestion and showed a markedly positive response to this treatment.

As often happens in clinical work, it took a very interesting prototypical patient to make researchers wonder exactly what caused these recurrent summer depressions. Marge played this role for summer SAD. Following Marge's successful treatment, Sandy Rovner ran an article in the *Washington Post* in which she described the summer version of SAD, and mentioned that a new research program at the NIMH was looking into the condition. Numerous responses followed, and Dr. Wehr evaluated the histories of these patients.

In general, there are many similarities between people with summer and winter depressions. Most of the patients are women, and feelings of low energy are once again a prominent part of the picture. Many are not aware of experiencing any actual mood changes, but, according to Dr. Wehr, they regard themselves as "being in a holding pattern." They just want to be left alone. As one of Dr. Wehr's patients put it, "I'm just not running on all cylinders." Just as in the case of winter depressives, a notable proportion of family members of summer depressives have also suffered from mood disorders.

In contrast to winter-SAD patients, who tend to eat more and crave sweets and starches during depressions, summer sufferers tend to eat less and lose weight. These differences have also been observed by two Australian researchers, Drs. Philip Boyce and Gordon Parker, who sent out questionnaires to those responding to an article in a women's magazine, and received responses from both winter- and summer-SAD patients. Whereas the winter-SAD patients feel physically slowed down during depressions, summer-SAD patients are often agitated. In addition, those with summer SAD express more suicidal ideas than their winter counterparts, and may be at greater risk for harming themselves or taking their own lives. This is in keeping with studies showing that the peak time for suicide in the general population is the spring and early summer (see below).

Summer depressives frequently ascribe their symptoms to the severe heat of summer, whereas winter depressives more often attribute their symptoms to a lack of light—influenced perhaps by the publicity surrounding research in this area. Some winter depressives feel that the extreme cold of winter may also play a role in their symptoms, but this possibility has not yet been explored. Conversely, it is possible that some summer depressions may be triggered by the intense light, rather than the heat, of summer. One of my patients with summer SAD, a woman in her late thirties, experienced one of her typical "summer" depressions after a heavy snowstorm. Since temperatures were below freezing outside, we speculated that the bright light reflected off the snow might have been responsible for the unseasonable onset of that particular depression.

Curiously, some patients report having both regular summer and winter depressions. For these people, spring and fall are the only times when they feel good. Flora, for example, the editor in her mid-forties mentioned previously, recalls having had winter depressions since age sixteen, which last "from Thanksgiving until the daffodils begin to bloom in April." It's only in the last fifteen years that she has become aware of having summer depressions. Before then she lived in upstate New York, where temperatures do not often go above 85 to 90° F—the point at which she has observed that she begins to feel "slowed down and stupid and forgetful and depressed." Her summer depressions usually last from the middle of June until the middle of September. She has become aware of this because, as a keen gardener, she has noticed that "I garden pretty seriously through June. Then I look up in September, and the garden is full of weeds." In her professional life, she is least proud of the editing she does in the summer.

Flora has noticed many similarities between her summer and winter depressions. She feels lethargic, needs more sleep, craves candy bars, and gains weight in both seasons. She has used light treatment for several winters, but has not as yet been treated for her summer depressions. One difference between the two types of depression that Flora has noted is the rapidity and ease with which they can be reversed. "During my summer depression, I feel better instantly if I go north. In the winter, on the other hand, if I am separated from my lights, it takes me several days to feel better again after I return to them."

The winter depressions tend to be longer and deeper for Flora. In the summer, she notes, "I never get so far from reality that I lose track of how it actually is. I can't always deal with it at that moment, but I don't think that I get really buffaloed, while in the winter I think I actually lose touch with reality; I begin to get kind of paranoid."

One big problem for people with both summer and winter depressions is that they have to cram as much as possible into the spring and fall. Flora notes that because of her depressions, "I go through cycles of letting things slide, and then, when I feel better, I scurry around, pay my income taxes and bills, clean my basement and weed my garden, make new friends, and start a whole bunch of projects."

"Gary" is another person who has suffered from both winter and summer depressions since he was ten years old. A tree surgeon in his early thirties, he loves outdoor activities, particularly rock climbing. In spring and fall he is lean and fit and strong, "like a horse let out of a starting gate." But when winter comes along, he gains up to thirty pounds and feels slowed down and sluggish. "I can't fight it. It's as if a switch has been thrown. Each time you think you've conquered the beast, the depression starts again." Summer sets him back in just the same way, derailing his plans, frustrating the hopes that come with the spring:

> You think, "Look how far I've come since winter." Friends come up and tell me how good my body is looking. And I can feel it. I'm stronger and fitter. Projecting the curve up, I think of how well I can do if it just keeps going that way. Unfortunately, that's usually exactly the time when I begin to get depressed again.

Gary has responded very well to light therapy during the winter. In summer his depressions have been successfully prevented by his taking the antidepressant fluoxetine (Prozac) (see Chapter 9). Because of his outdoor work, it is impossible for him to avoid the intense heat of a Washington summer.

In my experience, most SAD patients retain the same pattern of seasonal depressions throughout the course of their lives. But I have encountered one patient who started off experiencing depressions only in the winter, and later developed only summer depressions. Some people who have one form of the depression have relatives with the other form, or with depressions that are not seasonal at all. These observations raise questions as to how the different types of depression may be related to each other.

Patients with regular spring depressions seem to be quite rare. One such person whom I have treated did not respond to light therapy, but did well when given appropriate medications.

Treatment of Summer Depressions

At this time, no specific physical treatments for summer depression have been properly developed. Researchers have considered trying to keep patients cool or to restrict their levels of environmental light. Although some patients (like Marge, mentioned above) have found that traveling to cooler climates, swimming in cool water, and staying in air-conditioned rooms have alleviated their symptoms, others have found such measures to be either impractical or ineffective. Regular aerobic exercise can be helpful for summer SAD, as for other types of recurrent depressions. The value of nonpharmacological approaches, administered either individually or in combination, has clearly not yet been fully explored and deserves more thorough-going investigation. In the meanwhile, the mainstay of treatment remains antidepressant medications. My colleagues and I have had some success in treating summer SAD patients with antidepressants, notably selective serotonin reuptake inhibitors, such as Prozac, Zoloft, and Paxil (see Chapter 10 for more details). In some cases, we have observed further improvement by combining an antidepressant with nonpharmacological treatments and with other types of antidepressants.

Understanding Recurrent Depressions

How can we understand the recurrences and cycles of mood, energy, and behavior that occur in some individuals? What is the nature of this vulnerability? How is it that different people become depressed at different times of year and in response to different types of stresses and stimuli?

Claude Bernard, a great pioneer in the field of physiology, stressed the concept of constancy of the interior environment. According to this idea, all animals, humans included, are designed in such a way as to keep their internal environments constant. This includes body temperature, the concentrations of bodily chemicals, the rate of metabolism, and all manner of other essential functions. We now know that the internal environment does not really remain constant, but that it varies in a regular and predictable way over the course of the day, the menstrual cycle, and the year. Such predictable internal changes take place despite challenges from our external environment—for example, alterations in temperature and light.

Areas of the brain, most notably the hypothalamus, help us to adjust to these external fluctuations, almost as a thermostat in a house helps to keep the indoor temperature constant. In people who are susceptible to seasonal depressions, the capacity to react appropriately to these changes in the environment appears to be impaired. We have not as yet discovered the exact location of this abnormality, but in the case of winter SAD the problem may reside somewhere between the eye and the hypothalamus. In summer-SAD patients the problem presumably resides elsewhere—perhaps in the neuroanatomical pathways involved in the body's response to heat. Clearly, this is the sketchiest of explanations, and further research will be needed to define the abnormal circuitry more precisely.

Some medications seem to correct the regulatory abnormalities in SAD and restore normal functioning, as long as they continue to be used. An exciting new development in the treatment of seasonal depressions, however, involves altering the physical environment in such a way as to induce the brain and body (perhaps via the hypothalamus) to behave normally. Thus, exposure to bright light may correct abnormal responses to light deprivation, and cooling the environment may correct abnormal responses to high temperatures. There are several attractive features of these nonpharmacological approaches. First, the side effects that often go along with medications can be avoided. Second, new and better treatments—including medications—can be developed through an understanding of the environmental changes that cause or reverse the symptoms of these conditions. And finally, these treatments are wonderful tools for helping us understand the abnormalities that underlie seasonal depressions.

Effects of the Seasons on Behavior in the Population

> For everything there is a season and a time for every matter under heaven.
>
> —*Ecclesiastes 3:1*

When is the peak time for suicide? Not, as one might guess, during the dark and gloomy days of winter—though this was long held to be the case—but during the warm, sunny days of spring and summer. In his classic text, *Suicide: An Essay on Comparative Moral Statistics*, Henry Morselli analyzed data from much of Europe and showed a peak incidence of suicide in the two warm seasons, spring and summer, for almost all countries. He looked to temperature as the cause of these seasonal changes, but failed to find a clear-cut connection between environmental temperature and the incidence of suicide. He concluded that "suicide and madness are not influenced so much by the intense heat of the advanced summer season as by the early spring and summer, which seize upon the organism not yet acclimatized and still under the influence of the cold season." Morselli also recognized a second peak in suicide, in the months of October and November, in the annual curves of some countries.

Emil Durkheim, the famous French sociologist, accepted Morselli's figures but rejected his explanation of them. He pointed out that there was a far better correspondence between length of day and incidence of suicide than between temperature and suicide. In his view, this was a strong argument against a physical environmental explanation for the seasonal variation. Instead, he suggested that this trend was due to differences in the amount of social interaction occurring during the long days of summer, as opposed to the short days of winter. Why a greater opportunity for social interactions should predispose people to suicide, rather than protect them against it, is not clear to me, but that was how Durkheim saw it.

The controversy between climatic and sociological explanations for the seasonal variation in suicide was impossible to resolve, in large measure because the information was correlational. Scientists have frequently pointed out that just because two things change together, you cannot assume that one causes the other. Often such associations are the first clue that a cause-and-effect relationship exists, as in the case of smoking and lung cancer, but actual experiments are required before such a relationship can be definitively established. Population studies are therefore only able to provide us with clues about the effects of the seasons (and the environment in general) on human behavior, but not with conclusive answers.

More recent studies of seasonal patterns of suicide continue to point to spring and summer as peak seasons, although in many studies a smaller peak is also apparent in the fall. Dr. Jürgen Aschoff, one of the major figures in studies of biological rhythms in humans, has reviewed patterns of suicide in Europe and Japan for the past century and related the pattern of seasonal change in different locations to patterns of change in climatic variables, such as temperature and daylength. These variables show a minimum seasonal variation just north of the equator along a line that could be considered "the biological equator." Aschoff has found a close correlation between the amplitudes of seasonal rhythms of suicide and of two environmental variables: temperature and the number of hours of sunlight per day. In the Northern Hemisphere these rhythms all reach their maximum amplitude at about 40° north. This does not mean that the actual rate of suicide varies with latitude. Rather, it is the *amplitude* of the seasonal rhythms of suicide—the extent to which the rate of suicide varies with the seasons—that is associated with latitude. Aschoff has pointed out that the amplitude of the seasonal variation in suicide has decreased over the past century, and that this decrease corresponds to the increase in industrialization, which may diminish the impact of the changing seasons on our behavior. This difference in the extent to which we are directly exposed to our physical environment may also explain why urban dwellers have shown less seasonal variation in suicide than those in rural areas—an observation that has been made for at least a century.

Despite the increased sophistication of studies such as those conducted by Aschoff, we still don't know for sure why the rate of suicide varies markedly with the seasons. However, recent studies of the effects of such physical factors as light and heat on mood make physical environmental theories more plausible than ever. I should emphasize that even hard-nosed proponents of physical environmental theories, such as Morselli, recognized that suicide is a complex act, occurring in vulnerable individuals for a multitude of reasons. These researchers did us a service, however, in drawing our attention to the role of physical and climatic influences on the tragic—and often preventable—phenomenon of suicide.

The Connection Between Heat and Violence

I pray thee, good Mercutio, let's retire.
The day is hot, the Capulets abroad,
And if we meet, we shall not scape a brawl,
For now, these hot days, is the mad blood stirring.
—SHAKESPEARE, *Romeo and Juliet*, III:1

The debate about the nature of the relationship between suicide and the seasons that began over 100 years ago was replayed not long ago in scientific journals and the popular press in relation to the association between the seasons and violence. Two leading researchers in the field, Drs. Richard Michael and Doris Zumpe, published a paper in the *American Journal of Psychiatry* in 1983, called "Sexual Violence in the United States and the Role of Season," in which they analyzed seasonal variations in over 50,000 rapes in sixteen locations in the United States. They found a seasonal variation, with peak occurrences in July and August. This corresponded closely to the seasonal variation in assaults, but not to that for robberies, which peaked in November and December, or for murders, which showed no specific pattern. The timing of the maximum incidence of rape closely paralleled that of the maximum temperature values. These researchers suggested that environmental temperature might influence this seasonal variation by its effect on the secretion of certain hormones. Indeed, the male sex hormone, testosterone, has been shown to have a seasonal rhythm in humans, with a peak in the summer months; this hormone is also known to influence aggressive behavior in both humans and animals.

An outcry followed. A strongly worded essay by Stephen J. Gould in Discover magazine pointed out the hazards of confusing correlation and causation, and suggested the "more obvious" association between hot days and the opportunity for violence when people are out and about. This argument is reminiscent of Durkheim's sociological explanations. Two prominent psychiatrists wrote a letter to the editor, criticizing Michael and Zumpe for making "statements that appear to embody misperceptions of the experience of sexual violence and that look narrowly at an enormously complicated interaction between biological, psychosocial, and environmental determinants of human behavior." The researchers replied that they were not disputing the importance of all sorts of factors as determinants of rape, but simply drawing attention to the potential importance of temperature, "a factor that has been ignored by science for one hundred years." Indeed, Morselli wrote about the influence of temperature on the seasonal variation of violent crime in the nineteenth century.

Michael and Zumpe, commenting on the outcry produced by their paper, suggested that this came from "all those who believe passionately that men and women should be in total control of their personal destinies and that, if they are not, then it is society that has perverted them." They addressed some of their critics in a follow-up study on domestic violence, a type of behavior where accessibilty to the victim does not vary seasonally in the same way as in community violence. Once again they found a peak incidence of crisis calls to shelters for battered women in the summer months, corresponding closely to the peak environmental temperatures. Besides the excellent work of these researchers, there is a substantial scientific literature on the influence of temperature on irritability, which may in turn lead to anger, directed at someone who just happens to be in the way.

It has been my experience that criticism and derision frequently attend any suggestion that human emotions and behavior are influenced by our physical world. Such physical influences are often not regarded as plausible explanations for our actions, since we consider ourselves to be reasonable creatures. In the early years of our research on the seasons, we experienced a great deal of derision over SAD and the postulated effect of light on human mood—until our studies were widely replicated by other research groups.

Full Moons, Air Ions, and Evil Winds

> Demoniac frenzy, moping melancholy,
> And moonstruck madness.
> —MILTON, *Paradise Lost*

> The wind's in the east . . . I am always conscious of an uncomfortable sensation now and then when the wind is blowing in the east.
> —CHARLES DICKENS, *Bleak House*

So central is the influence of the moon in the mythology of madness that it would hardly be right to omit a discussion of it from this book. The word "lunacy" derives from this belief. Yet the actual evidence of the moon's influence on human behavior and emotions is rather slim. Dr. Arnold Lieber analyzed the patterns of homicides and aggravated assaults in Dade County, Florida, and showed that they tended to cluster around the time of the full moon. Yet others have failed to replicate this work in other parts of the country. Dr. Charles Mirabile has analyzed medical records at the Institute of Living in Hartford, Connecticut, and has found a small rise in paranoid behavior around the time of the full moon. The behavioral effects of the moon—if indeed they exist—may be due to its light or its gravitational effects on body fluids. I have occasionally come across individuals who say they are strongly influenced by the phases of the moon, but I have never seen this influence convincingly documented in any particular individual. Until someone is able to do so, the age-old beliefs in the powers of the moon over humankind will continue to lack a compelling scientific basis.

The weather has been held to have powerful effects on human functioning since the time of Hippocrates. An entire section of one of his famous works, "On Airs, Waters, and Places," outlines his beliefs on the importance of our physical environment. He emphasized the effects of good and bad winds. In a modern text, Dr. Felix Sulsman writes at length on the effects of weather on humans. He devotes an entire section to the "medical impact of evil winds." Prominent among these are warm winds that come down from the mountains—such as the Santa Ana in California, the *foehn* in Europe, and the Chinook in Canada. These winds are reported to cause irritability, restlessness, lethargy, depression, and general debility. The *foehn* has been associated with increased rates of crime, suicide, and traffic accidents.

I have already discussed the important effects of heat on emotions and behavior. Because these mountain winds generally raise the environmental temperature abruptly by as much as 15–20°C, it is possible that many of their effects may be due to heat alone. However, they do have other meteorological effects as well, including the introduction of positive air ions, and these positively charged particles have been shown experimentally to increase irritability in people.

Just as particles with a positive electrical charge (positive ions) are reputed to have a disturbing effect on the psychological equilibrium of those who cross their path, so particles with a negative electrical charge (negative ions) are reputed to have a calming effect. Such negative air ions are found outdoors more than indoors. Dr. Charmane Eastman of Rush Presbyterian–St. Luke's Medical Center in Chicago has suggested that because people are outdoors more during the summer months, they may be exposed to more negative air ions at those times than in the winter. She is currently exploring the hypothesis that SAD may be related to inadequate exposure to negative air ions during the winter, and evaluating the possible beneficial effects of negative air ions in patients with SAD. Drs. Michael and Jiuan Terman are undertaking similar trials of negative air ions at Columbia University in New York. It is too soon to say whether this approach will offer any benefits for SAD patients.

Those who have studied the effects of weather changes on people observe that some individuals are particularly sensitive to these changes. The famous German poet Goethe wrote, "It is a pity that just the excellent personalities suffer most from the adverse effects of the atmosphere." He numbered himself among that unfortunate but select group. It does indeed seem as though different people react differently to various weather conditions. I have seen a few people who have reported marked feelings of depression or irritability when the weather changes, particularly when a storm is about to hit.

For one man, "Ahmed," a computer scientist in his early forties, the problem was serious enough to induce him to come from Saudi Arabia to Washington, D.C., for a consultation on his problem. He noticed that just before clouds drifted across the sky, he began to feel weak and depressed. His stomach seemed bloated, and his head felt "blown up." When the weather was stable, he would feel even better than normal—exceedingly energetic and enthusiastic about life. Several members of his family reported almost identical weather-related symptoms. Because he had suffered from multiple depressions and mild high periods, I suggested that he be treated with lithium carbonate, which is often very helpful for stabilizing such mood fluctuations.

The effects of weather on vulnerable individuals have been rather neglected area in scientific research. Apart from the specific focus on SAD that I have already discussed, little systematic work has been done on other types of climatic influences. The literature is full of assumptions and old nostrums, culled from the classics. It has been widely claimed that some people are able to predict the weather through effects on their minds and bodies. This phenomenon is also poorly understood, and we are little further along in our understanding of it than the author John Taylor (1580–1653), who wrote:

> Some men 'gainst Raine doe carry in their backs
> Prognosticating Aching Almanacks.
> Some by painful elbow, hip or knee
> Will shrewdly guesse what weathers like to be.

Recent research bears out Hippocrates's view that "Of natures, some are well or ill adapted for summer, and some for winter." Just as some people are adversely affected by the physical environment in winter (the darkness and cold) others have trouble with heat and humidity. Characteristic patterns of depression may result. The symptoms of winter SAD usually include decreased activity, overeating, oversleeping, and weight gain, whereas the symptoms of summer SAD often include loss of appetite and weight, insomnia, and agitation. It seems as though these two patterns represent extreme manifestations of physical changes seen in a large proportion of the population in these two seasons. Somehow, seasonally depressed people seem less well insulated against the effects of extreme changes in climate, and are unable to function adequately in such conditions. The symptoms of depression result. Fortunately, there are many ways in which a depressed person can find relief from these symptoms. The second part of this book describes how this can be accomplished.

PART 2

Treatments

> Everybody talks about the weather; but nobody does
> anything about it.
> —Charles Dudley Warner

There are many ways in which our physical environment can
influence, for better or worse, the way we feel and act. But what can we
do about it? The most exciting discovery in the field of SAD, or winter
depression, is that this type of depression can be helped by light therapy
in most cases. Regular summer depressions, on the other hand, appear
to be influenced more by environmental temperature than by light,
and it is possible that cooling the environment can help a person who
gets depressed during the dog days of summer. Since winter depressions
are more common than summer depressions (at least in the northern
countries), and since we know more about them, most of this section
deals with how best to handle the gray days of winter.

The development of the best treatments for emotional conditions
has been greatly slowed down by professionals who are sure that their
particular theory is the only one that will really cure a problem. Such
an approach closes a therapist's mind toward other possible avenues of
treatment. Many modern therapists have learned to take a more
eclectic approach to treatment and are showing a greater willingness to
combine different types of treatment. Of course, in order to do so, a
therapist has to be either skilled in many different types of treatment,
or willing to refer a patient to somebody else for treatment that he or
she is not qualified to administer. In practice, this ideal is often not
met. The therapist may be ignorant of new developments in one area
or another, or may be skeptical of the value of some new treatment,
even though he or she has not really examined the evidence for and
against it. This is the therapist's problem, but it also becomes the
patient's problem in that the patient may be delayed in, or prevented

from, getting the necessary treatment. This problem is especially likely to occur with newly described conditions, such as SAD, and with newly developed treatments, such as light therapy.

In my experience, a patient can usually tell when a therapist is being defensive about a new type of treatment. The therapist may offer critical or discouraging comments without being able to substantiate them with good reasons. Or the therapist may "interpret" the wish to seek other treatments as a patient's "resistance" to looking into the true causes of his or her problems. Patients have the right to have their questions about new types of treatments dealt with on the questions' own merits. These inquiries should be taken seriously by the therapist, who should ask the most relevant questions: Is this treatment likely to be helpful for a particular patient, and what harm, if any, is associated with it?

One patient I recall, a physician himself, was in traditional psychoanalysis. When he became interested in exploring the possibility of light therapy for himself, his analyst "interpreted" this wish as an attempt to avoid dealing with his underlying unconscious conflicts. Nonetheless, he looked into light therapy and decided to enter the research program at the NIMH. His analyst took a traditional hard-line approach toward the decision and gave him an ultimatum: light therapy or analysis, not both. The patient chose light therapy and has done very well with it. However, the ultimatum induced him to stop his analysis abruptly, which was less than ideal for his general treatment. It is possible for therapists to collaborate successfully in the treatment of a patient, and I have seen many people treated successfully with light therapy in conjunction with other types of therapy, including psychoanalysis.

Any depressed person should obtain the help of a qualified professional, and the person with SAD is no exception. Although it is often easy to diagnose SAD on the basis of a patient's history, there are other conditions that may masquerade as SAD—for example, underactivity of the thyroid, hypoglycemia, chronic viral illnesses, and chronic fatigue syndrome. These problems should be considered and ruled out before SAD is diagnosed. The first treatment tried may not be helpful, and it is important for the patient not to despair, but to try other approaches as well. It is also possible that the treatment is not being carried out correctly. A professional may be able to detect this and make the necessary suggestions for correcting the problem. Side effects may develop, and an expert may be able to help minimize these.

As the slogan of a well-known discount store goes, "An educated consumer is our best customer," and this applies no less to getting the best type of health care than it does to the purchase of clothing. One of the chief goals of this book is to provide the sort of education that will ensure that those who have difficulties with the seasons get the best type of assistance for their problems. What follows is a comprehensive picture of the treatment choices available to individuals with seasonal difficulties. I hope that it proves helpful not only to them, but also to their families and friends.

CHAPTER 6

Light therapy

Light therapy is a relatively new type of treatment for depression, and we are still learning how best to use it. In fact, there have been substantial changes in our understanding of light therapy even in the few years since the earlier version of this book, *Seasons of the Mind*, was published. In this chapter I present my latest views on light therapy, fully recognizing that they will need to be updated from time to time. This chapter is divided into three parts: basic principles and considerations involved in administering light therapy; the practical aspects of treatment; and the latest research developments, which may well guide future directions in treatment.

Light Therapy: Basic Principles and Considerations

"*Mehr licht*," exclaimed the poet Goethe as he lay dying—"more light." And with those words he summed up the chief principle involved in successful light therapy. Patients with SAD develop their symptoms during the winter or when deprived of light in any situation. According to recent research by Dr. Dan Oren and colleagues at the NIMH, SAD patients are exposed to no less light during the winter than their nonseasonal counterparts; for whatever reason, they just need more of it.

What Type of Light Is Best?

Providing more light was the challenge we faced when we first treated Herb Kern in the early 1980s. In order to do so, we used a metal light box with several fluorescent tubes in it, which looked rather like a ceiling fixture, placed on its side on a table in an upright position. The fixture contained fluorescent lamps (as opposed to incandescent light bulbs) and a diffusing screen in order to spread the light out over a large surface. It has been shown that light diffused in this way is safer for the eyes than light that emanates from a small source, such as the filament of an ordinary light bulb or halogen lamp.

Most light therapy studies have used fluorescent lights, so there is much more information about their effectiveness, compared to that of incandescent lights. More important, though, is the issue of safety, where fluorescents are clearly superior. Fixtures containing unshielded incandescent lights have been manufactured and marketed. I would caution you against their use, as they are untested with regard to both their effectiveness and their safety. It may be possible to derive benefit from incandescent lights, but only if the light is indirect—for example if it is bounced off a surface and not stared at directly (see "Other Innovations: Light Rooms and Indirect Light," on pages 128–129).

Some studies have examined what colors of light are important for light's antidepressant effects. Dr. Dan Oren and colleagues at the NIMH showed that green light, to which the eyes are most sensitive, is more effective than red light. Dr. George Brainard at Jefferson Medical College and colleagues at the NIMH have shown that white light is more effective than either blue or red light. Most research has been done with white fluorescent lamps, and most standard fixtures contain them. These lamps go under a number of trade names and there is no evidence that one type is superior to another.

In our early studies we used lights that imitated the balance of colors found in sunlight—so-called "full-spectrum light." Researchers have found no evidence that such light is any better than ordinary white fluorescent light. In fact, since the manufacturers of "full-spectrum" lights were trying to replicate the pattern of colors (or wavelengths) found in sunlight, the lamps were designed to emit more ultraviolet rays than regular fluorescents. There is no evidence that ultraviolet rays are necessary or even beneficial in the treatment of SAD, and their potentially harmful effects to both skin and eyes are a distinct disadvantage. Several manufacturers have recognized this fact and sell fixtures with special screens that filter out almost all ultraviolet rays, which are given off even by ordinary fluorescent light bulbs. Ultraviolet rays can also be reduced by using certain types of fluorescent lamps. Be sure that any fixture you purchase contains such ultraviolet-reducing features.

Where Is the Light Acting?

As you may have noted, I have emphasized the importance of the amount of light that reaches the eyes. "Why the eyes and not the skin?"

you may ask. This is a question Dr. Thomas Wehr and I asked in the early stages of our research in light therapy. Using fluorescent light fixtures, we treated SAD patients in two separate conditions. In one condition we exposed their skin to the light, and in the other condition we exposed their eyes to the light. Response to the eye exposure proved to be far superior, leading us to conclude that the antidepressant effects of light therapy in SAD patients are probably mediated by the eyes rather than by the skin. This finding has important implications for treatment. On the one hand, it means that when you are receiving light treatment, you need to be aware of where the light is in relation to your eyes. On the other hand, it means that treatments that are geared primarily to the skin are unlikely to benefit patients with SAD. Such treatments are routinely dispensed in tanning salons, which are not recommended at this time for the treatment of SAD. Not only is there no good evidence that they work, but the lights used in such salons contain significant amounts of ultraviolet rays, which can be damaging to both the skin and the eyes.

Clinical and research experience indicates that you can derive a great deal of benefit from light therapy simply by sitting in front of the light fixture at the appropriate distance with your eyes open. It is not necessary to stare continuously at the light, though it may be helpful—and is quite safe—to do so from time to time. The fact that light therapy works even if you do not stare directly at the light source suggests that the entire retina takes part in the response to light therapy and not just the central (most visually sensitive) area. The peripheral part of your retina, which you use for spotting things in the periphery of your field of vision, is rich in receptors that are able to trap light. These receptors may be important for mediating light's antidepressant effects.

How Much Light Is Desirable?

As you may recall, even in our earliest experiments with light, we hypothesized that the amount of light reaching the eyes (which I refer to here as the "intensity") was an important factor in achieving an antidepressant effect. This has indeed proven to be the case, at least as far as light boxes are concerned. Light intensity is measured in units called "lux." A bedroom illuminated by a single bedside lamp would have a light level of about 100 lux. Ordinary indoor lighting levels are about 300 to 500 lux, whereas a well-lit office interior might give light measurements of 500 to 1000 lux. The original light box, which we used with Herb Kern, emitted 2500 lux—about five times as much as he would have received under ordinary circumstances during the

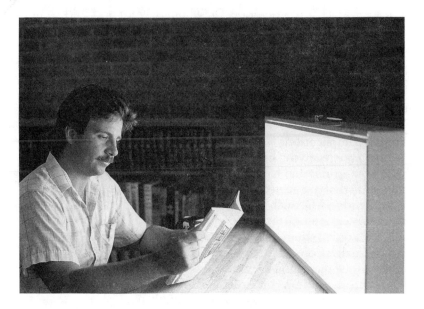

Figure 3. Standard 2500-lux light box. Contains fluorescent tubes that give off approximately 5 times as much light as regular indoor lighting.

winter months from regular room lighting. Modern versions of this earlier box continue to be available (see Figure 3). In the early NIMH studies, we found that treating patients with 2500 lux of light was more effective than treating them with 100 to 300 lux.

One of the problems with these earlier treatments, however, was that patients frequently had to use their light boxes for several hours each day—a commitment of time that many found unacceptable. To overcome this difficulty, Drs. Michael and Jiuan Terman at Columbia University developed a light box that delivered 10,000 lux of light to the eye (see Figure 4). The advantage of this box was that it produced significant antidepressant effects in a much shorter time—as little as thirty minutes in some cases.

The knowledge that light of high intensity is antidepressant can be used to obtain light therapy naturalistically. For example, gazing up at the sky, even on a winter day, may deliver several thousand lux of light to the eyes. *Be sure never to stare directly at the sun, however, even during the winter.* The intensity of light entering the eyes is substantially modified by the surfaces off which the light is reflected. Grass, trees, and shrubbery, for example, may reduce the intensity of outdoor light entering the eyes by as much as 90 percent. Snowy landscapes, on the

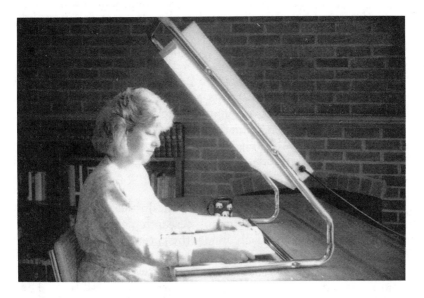

Figure 4. Research findings show that the smaller, slanted 10,000-lux light box is more efficient than the standard box.

other hand, are often dazzlingly bright, delivering much more light to the eyes than you would obtain even from the brightest of light boxes.

The amount of light to which you are exposed depends not only on the intensity of the light source, but also on the duration of exposure. For example, two hours of treatment with 2500 lux per day may have an antidepressant effect equivalent to that of thirty minutes per day at 10,000 lux. Although the high-intensity light boxes allow for shorter durations of treatment, it is not possible to predict exactly how long your treatments will need to be on the basis of your previous experience with the lower-intensity boxes. In practice, you generally have to rely upon a system of trial and error, which I outline more fully later in this chapter (see "Time of Day and Duration of Treatment," p. 119–120).

At What Time of Day Should You Get Your Light Therapy?

Whether there is a "best" time of day for treatment has been one of the most controversial questions in light therapy for SAD. The bottom line—as far as we can tell at this time—is that for most people it probably doesn't matter when during the day light therapy is administered. The controversy persists because the results of research on the question are somewhat contradictory. Our early NIMH experience suggested that it probably did not matter when light therapy was given. Treatment in the evening—or even in the middle of the day—seemed to be as effective as treatment in the morning.

Well-conducted studies by Drs. Alfred J. Lewy and Robert Sack in Oregon, however, as well as those by Dr. David Avery and colleagues in Seattle, suggested that patients responded much better to light treatments when these were given in the morning than in the evening. Avery found that those SAD patients who tended to oversleep in the morning did particularly well with morning light treatments. These researchers used the standard "crossover" design in their studies—a design in which patients are treated first with one type of treatment and later with a second treatment condition.

In a more recent study, Dr. Anna Wirz-Justice and colleagues in Basel, Switzerland used a different research design. Known as a "parallel design," this approach divides the patient population into two or more groups, and one of each of the treatment conditions to be studied is administered to each group. In other words, the same patients are not crossed over to the alternate treatment condition. These researchers found no difference between light treatments administered in the morning and those given in the afternoon or evening.

How can one reconcile the contradictory findings between different research groups with regard to the importance of timing in the light treatment of SAD? The Termans at Columbia University have helped to resolve this question. They explored the possibility that the order in which light treatments were presented in a crossover study might influence outcome. They tested this theory by studying patients in whom morning and evening treatments were presented in different sequences. Sure enough, they found that the sequence mattered. All treatments in all sequences worked equally well—with one exception. When evening light was presented to people who had previously been treated with morning light, it did not work as well as morning or evening light treatment when given in any of the other sequences. This may explain why the crossover studies from Oregon and Seattle found evening light to be inferior to morning light, whereas the parallel study from Basel found no difference between conditions.

The explanation above is confounded, however, by another large study by Dr. Ybe Meesters and colleagues in The Netherlands, who treated patients with light in the morning, afternoon, and evening in various sequences. Like the Swiss researchers, they found no differences between treatments given at different times of day.

In practice, it is unlikely that a therapist would prescribe—or a patient would use—light therapy in the unusual sequence prescribed in crossover studies. In practice, I would advise you against being rigid about when you get your light treatments. It is much more important for you to be able to fit your light treatments into your schedule than to get the timing exactly right; overconcern about timing may cause you to skip treatments and become depressed again. I would encourage you to try different treatment times until you find those that work best for you and fit best into your schedule. Oren and his colleagues followed up a group of patients who had been involved in light treatment research at the NIMH and found that about half of all patients used light treatment in both the morning and the evening, while the other half were equally divided between those who used it only in the morning and those who used it only in the evening.

Some people find that when they use light therapy very late at night, it prevents them from getting to sleep. On the other hand, recent research by the Termans shows that for many people, light treatment very late at night is quite effective and has no detrimental effect on the quality or timing of their sleep. In conclusion, though different times may work best or be more convenient for different people, there are no hard and fast rules as to when light treatment should be administered for SAD patients in general. Therefore, feel free to try light treatment at whatever time of day is most convenient for you, but be ready to experiment with different times if the first schedule is not satisfactory. It is probably best, however, to try a given light treatment schedule for a week before concluding that it is not working and shifting to another schedule.

How Long Does Light Treatment Take to Work?

It is very reasonable for someone who undertakes a course of treatment to want to know how long he or she needs to persist with it before expecting some sort of result. For light treatment, the time course to response is quite variable. Some people may experience improved mood and energy even after a single session, though this is unusual. For most, it takes two to four days for a sustained sense of improved well-being to set in. The latest research shows, however, that it may take several weeks for some people to register the full beneficial effects of light therapy.

It is curious how some people experience an immediate lift—a feeling of elation or energy or calm—when they sit in front of a light box, while others do not. It may be that those people who experience this immediate positive effect of bright light are the same ones who experience "light hunger" during the winter and have learned to seek out bright places. On the other hand, those who respond more slowly to light therapy—over the course of days or weeks—may not have learned to associate the way they feel with the brightness of their surroundings. This last group may seclude themselves when they feel depressed and rest in darkened rooms, thereby inadvertently making their symptoms worse.

When I think of those patients of mine who have experienced an immediate response to light therapy, the man who comes first to mind is a car salesman in his early thirties. He had suffered winter depressions for several years, and had used cocaine in an attempt to increase his energy level and remain functional at his work during the difficult winter months. It is hard to imagine a job more difficult for a depressed person than that of a salesman, whose success depends upon his being upbeat and persuasive. As you might imagine, the cocaine had made matters worse. He became increasingly addicted and experienced many of the problems associated with this dangerous drug. He had quit cocaine a few years previously with great difficulty. Now, however, confronted once again with a severe winter depression and unable to function at work, he was considering restarting his cocaine use unless I could find something else to help his depression.

As he began to tell me his story, he was so slowed down and listless that it was hard to imagine him capable of making any sales—or functioning at all in his present state of mind. I wondered whether he might feel better if I turned on the light box in my office during the consultation and directed it toward him. I did so, and within half an hour I noted a marked difference. The pace of his speech picked up, animation returned to his face and body gestures, and enthusiasm came back to his voice. At that moment, it became clear to me what a successful salesman he could be when he was feeling well. He used light successfully throughout the winter and did not even consider returning to cocaine.

Such rapid responses are rather unusual, so don't be disappointed if you experience no immediate effects from the light. *You should therefore not give up on light treatment until you have used it consistently for at least two weeks.* Most people who will benefit from light show some favorable response to treatment within the first week or two—and most research studies performed to date have not treated patients for longer than this. More recently, however, there have been some studies in which patients have been treated for four weeks, and researchers have observed that, in general, a patient's mood continues to improve throughout the duration of study. Given these findings, it may be worth persisting with light therapy even if there has been no marked response within the first few weeks.

What Happens If You Stop Light Therapy?

Since light therapy may involve a certain amount of inconvenience—remembering to do it, sitting in one place, or carving the time out of a busy schedule—it is important for people to know what happens if they stop treatment for a day or two, or altogether. Will they relapse or will the benefits persist? The effects of discontinuing light therapy are quite variable, depending on the individual and the time of year. Some people have feelings of withdrawal from light treatment as soon as they turn the box off. I recommend that these people taper off their exposure gradually toward the end of a treatment session. More typically, relapse is seen within a week or two of discontinuing treatment, most usually by the third or fourth day. Occasionally, however, improvement persists after treatment is stopped, at times for weeks or even the entire duration of the winter. Controversial new research by Meesters and colleagues in The Netherlands suggests that long-standing remissions, even after light treatments have been discontinued, may occur especially if symptoms are treated at the beginning of the winter. In my experience, however, long-standing remissions are the exception rather than the rule—unless you continue to supplement your environmental light exposure in some other way, such as by walking outdoors every day.

The implications of different patterns of relapse are twofold. If you relapse when you stop using your lights, you should be diligent in your light use. Failure to do so will result in a spotty or incomplete treatment response. On the other hand, if you are in that fortunate group who derive long-standing benefit from treatment of relatively short duration, you may be able to use this knowledge to stay well for extended periods without the inconvenience of having to continue your daily treatments. Only trial and error will identify which category you fall into, but it is worth finding out because it will inform you as to how frequently you need treatment.

The effects of discontinuing light treatment also depend on when you do so during the course of the season. For example, you may be able to discontinue treatment with impunity during the spring, when the daylight hours are expanding, but you may need treatments every day in the midst of winter. Spring weather is notoriously erratic, though, so be watchful for cloudy spells that may bring on a relapse of your symptoms, and be prepared to turn your light box on again if necessary.

Ultimately, during the summer, most people with SAD are able to stop light therapy. However, a minority of patients continue to need light treatment even then, either because they continue to be light-deprived or because they have an extreme need for light.

What Can You Expect from Effective Light Treatment?

The first sensations you may experience in response to light therapy may be physical—a sense of lightening of the body, calm, or increased energy. There may be a feeling of "butterflies" in the stomach or "pins and needles" in the hands. In the days that follow, you may feel as though some fundamental problem is being corrected. Ideally, the symptoms of SAD should disappear, one by one. In some people, this effect takes hold completely and the results may seem like a miracle. In others, the result is less complete; treatment may help, but some difficulties may remain. In a minority of people, the light treatment may not work at all. The good news is that over 80 percent of people with SAD or the winter blues may expect to benefit from light therapy, although it is unusual for all winter difficulties to disappear.

If the light therapy works, you should begin to feel more energetic. Suddenly, chores and daily activities no longer feel like drudgery. Along with a physical sense of lightness, the burden of living, of carrying your body around from place to place, seems to lift, and the overwhelming need to sleep subsides. Suddenly, you feel less driven by cravings for sweets and starches. Cakes and candy bars become resistible. Even dieting seems possible again! Thinking becomes more efficient. No longer does your mind creak along like an old machine in need of oiling. Your computer is up and running again. Computations and calculations are possible, and new ideas spring readily to mind. You think of tackling problems in new ways. Exercise becomes less onerous—no longer does that trip to the gym, walk, jog, aerobics class, or exercycle session seem like a mountainous obstacle. There is once again a wish to communicate: to call friends, write notes, and arrange trips to the movies, a ball game, or the theater. Sex seems not only possible, but even desirable. In short, you feel human again.

In the section of this chapter devoted to practical considerations, I will show you how you can monitor the effects of light on your own symptoms and determine the degree to which it has taken care of the problem (see Appendix 1, pages 311–313).

Are There Side Effects of Light Treament?

In my experience with hundreds of patients, light therapy is generally very well tolerated, and side effects, when they occur, are generally mild. It is unusual for someone to be unable to use light altogether because of side effects, though there are some people in whom these may be a problem. The side effects I have encountered most commonly in my patients are as follows:

1. Headaches
2. Eyestrain
3. Irritability
4. Overactivity
5. Insomnia
6. Fatigue
7. Dryness of the eyes
8. Dryness of nasal passages and sinuses
9. Sunburn-type skin reaction

If headache or eyestrain is a problem, I suggest restarting treatment with a shorter duration of exposure—for example, fifteen minutes per day—and then building up gradually over a week or two to the more usual exposure durations. The problem can also be handled by sitting slightly farther away from the light source until the symptoms subside. Generally, it is possible to move closer to the light box again after several days without having these side effects recur.

People who become irritable or overactive during light therapy usually compare these feelings to the way they feel during the summer. On occasion, light therapy may induce a hypomanic episode, with all its attendant problems, such as I described in Chapter 4. This problem responds well to decreased exposure.

Insomnia may occur when the lights are used late at night. Some people complain that light treatment makes them feel too energized and "wired" to go to sleep. The best way to handle this problem is to shift the treatment to an earlier time of day, either in the morning hours, earlier in the evening, or even during the day.

Fatigue may occur after several days of light therapy, especially if the amount or timing of sleep has been changed in order to accommodate treatment. This problem is usually transient. It may require shifting the time of treatment to allow you to get enough sleep.

The heat generated by the light box can dry out the surrounding air, which may cause dryness of the eyes, nasal passages, or sinuses. In contact lens wearers, dry eyes may be more than an irritant, and may actually result in abrasions of the cornea. Artificial tears may be helpful in combating this problem, as may a humidifier placed in the vicinity of the light box. Dryness of the nasal passages and sinuses may also be relieved by the humidifier, as well as by drinking hot beverages.

Skin reddening of the type found in sunburn may occur, especially in those with fair, sun-sensitive skin or in those taking certain photosensitizing medications. Such reddening is evidence that, despite all attempts at removing ultraviolet rays, some of them penetrate the screen and reach the skin. If this is a problem, it can be treated with sun-blocking creams.

Some people dislike fluorescent lights, which they say cause them to feel anxious, irritable, or "wired." These people are understandably concerned when fluorescent light fixtures are recommended to them as a treatment. In my experience, however, SAD patients rarely object to the quality of the light emanating from standard light treatment fixtures; on the contrary, they generally find it to be relieving, soothing, or invigorating. Modern light fixtures contain special "ballasts," structures that minimize the irritating flicker that many associate with fluorescent lights. I have been asked by people with seizure disorders whether light therapy might provoke a seizure. There is no reason to believe this to be a risk when treatment is administered as prescribed in this book.

Pregnant women have wondered whether there are any adverse effects of light therapy on a growing fetus. Although relatively few pregnant women have been treated with light therapy (given the newness of the treatment), we have no reason to believe that light therapy would harm a fetus. It has been a pleasure to see the few pregnant women whom I have treated with light therapy during the winter get through their pregnancies without feeling depressed, and give birth to healthy babies. When it comes to nursing, I would not recommend exposing a baby's eyes directly to the light at close quarters, since the impact of the light on newborn babies is unknown at this time. There is no reason, though, why a mother should not nurse in front of the light, provided the baby's face is turned away from it.

Are Precautions Needed for Long-Term Usage?

"Does light therapy have any long-term side effects? Is it harmful to the eyes? What steps or precautions should be taken in this regard?" These are among the questions I hear most frequently from those who have benefited from light therapy and want to continue to use it year after year, but who are concerned as to whether such long-term usage may be harmful in any way. We are limited in our ability to answer these questions, since light therapy has only been around for the past fifteen years, and widely used for the past ten years. The good news is that so far there have been no reports of any cases of long-term side effects, particularly adverse effects to the eyes. Drs. Paul Schwartz and Charlotte Brown recently surveyed over fifty patients from the early NIMH studies, and none of them reported having suffered any eye problems.

Dr. Chris Gorman and colleagues in Calgary, Alberta, Canada performed eye examinations on seventy-one patients treated annually with light therapy for five years and they found no evidence of retinal damage in any of their patients.

The absence to date of any reported cases of eye problems related to light therapy is encouraging and is in keeping with our expectations, given the amount of light used in standard treatments. Even the higher-intensity (10,000-lux) light boxes give out no more light than you would receive from the sky just after sunrise. The light levels given off by conventional light boxes fall well within specified safety levels. Even so, researchers have questioned whether there may be special aspects of light therapy that put patients' eyes at greater risk than they would be exposed to simply by looking up at the sky. They have argued, for example, that in reality people do not generally face the sky for prolonged periods. When they are outdoors, they move their heads and eyes around, and in the process may be protecting their eyes from overexposure to light. People receiving light treatment, on the other hand, sit in a relatively constant position in relation to the light box, even though they do not stare at it. Some have argued that exposure to bright outdoor light over the course of many years may speed up degenerative processes in the retina. Others don't share this concern, which they say is not supported by the bulk of available evidence.

Aside from the theoretical possibility that light therapy may be harmful to the eyes in general, it is possible that the eyes of certain people may be particularly vulnerable to the effects of light. This high-risk category might include people with retinal diseases, such as macular degeneration or retinitis pigmentosa. It might also include people who are on certain medications that sensitize the retina to the effects of light. It would be prudent for individuals with retinal problems, and those on medications that may make them more vulnerable to the effects of light, to consult with and be monitored regularly by an ophthalmologist or optometrist. More details about what such a professional might want to look for, and what medications might sensitize the eyes to light, are provided later in Table 4 (page 115) and Appendix 2 (pages 315–318).

In summary, there is no evidence that standard light therapy, when properly administered, is harmful to the eyes. Researchers have not ruled out the possibility, however, that some people might be vulnerable to harmful effects and are continuing to look into the question. In the meanwhile, some element of vigilance may be useful, and specific details about what to look out for are provided below in the section on practical considerations.

Can We Predict Who Is Most Likely to Respond to Light Treatment?

Although it is not possible to predict exactly who is most likely to respond to treatment with bright light, we have some general clues that help us make educated guesses about this. If you have a history of being less depressed in the winter when you are exposed to more light in a natural context, that is a good indicator that you are likely to respond favorably. For example, have your symptoms improved when you have traveled toward the equator in the winter? Have you felt better when working or living in bright rooms, compared to dim ones? Have you been less depressed when you have lived closer to the equator? If the answer to any of these questions is "yes," this would predict a favorable response.

Besides these clues, there are certain depressive symptoms that predict a favorable response to light therapy. These include oversleeping, overeating, carbohydrate craving, and weight gain. Oversleeping in particular stands out as a solid predictor. Eating more sweet foods in the afternoon also appears to be an excellent predictor of a favorable response according to Dr. Anna Wirz-Justice and colleagues. In my experience, severely depressed people who lose sleep, eat less, and lose weight during their winter depressions tend to do least well with light therapy. Nevertheless, if you have a history of seasonal or light-sensitive depressions, it is certainly worth trying light treatment, regardless of the clinical picture of the depression, because it is not possible to predict exactly who will and who will not respond.

Practical Considerations in Administering Light Therapy

The purpose of this section is to take you, step by step, through the practical issues involved in light therapy.

Preliminary Steps

Evaluating and Monitoring Your Own Symptoms

Before undertaking any treatment study, it is usual for researchers to estimate the degree and nature of a patient's depression. Initially, this is done to establish a baseline against which subsequent treatment efforts can be evaluated. Then, as each week of treatment passes, it can be used as a way of monitoring how effective the treatment is, which symptoms respond best to treatment, and which symptoms best predict overall improvement. I suggest that before you start light treatment, you complete the simple self-rating mood scale given in Appendix 1 (pages 311–313) to evaluate how depressed you are at baseline. Then, after each week, repeat the scale to help you evaluate whether you are improving, and, if so, by how much.

The Role of a Professional

If you undertake light treatment for SAD, your use of it should be supervised by a physician or other qualified therapist. There are many reasons for this recommendation. It is important that the diagnosis be confirmed by a qualified person; a careful history should be taken and a physical examination performed. Professional input may also be very helpful in monitoring your mood. Light therapy may not work, and a professional can recommend or prescribe alternative or supplementary treatments. Above all, an informed perspective, encouragement, and support can be invaluable in guiding you through the ordeal of depression. Guidelines as to when a professional should be involved are provided in Chapter 3, pages 37–38.

Having Your Eyes Checked

Several professionals, most notably the Columbia University group, have recommended adding an eye examination to the history and general physical examination that all patients should be given before starting light therapy. The eye check-up routinely performed by this group for users of light therapy is shown in Appendix 2. It should take an ophthalmologist or optometrist no longer than twenty minutes to perform the various tasks described in the list. Either type of professional should be well qualified to complete the form, and an optometrist is likely to charge less. *If there is any possibility that you may have a retinal problem, however, an ophthalmologist should be involved in deciding whether light therapy is justified and, if such a decision is made, in monitoring visual functioning over the course of treatment.*

 I should note that many patients with SAD have been treated without undergoing the visual tests outlined in Appendix 2 without suffering any eye damage. In addition, there are no research findings yet as to how helpful such an evaluation might be. For these reasons, I hesitate to state that everyone who undertakes light therapy must have such an evaluation. Nonetheless, it is a simple and relatively inexpensive precaution; it may be helpful in identifying any eye problems; and it may be valuable as a baseline if any eye problems should develop down the line, whatever their cause may be. For all of these reasons, the Columbia eye check-up for users of light therapy seems like a useful addition to the other safeguards that minimize the chance of developing any eye problems in the course of light therapy.

Once light therapy has been started, the question arises as to whether follow-up eye check-ups should be performed, and, if so, how frequently. Once again, there are no hard and fast rules. One ophthalmologist and researcher in this field, Dr. Charlotte Remé in Zurich, Switzerland, suggests that for younger people (under age forty-five), check-ups every other year may be sufficient; for those over forty-five, annual check-ups may be more appropriate. In those who have visual difficulties or are on medications that may sensitize the eye to the effects of light, annual (or even more frequent) check-ups may be desirable. I should emphasize that these guidelines are very broad, because this is an area where there is a shortage of research findings to inform our clinical guidelines. If there is any evidence that you may have some eye problem, I would strongly recommend that an ophthalmologist be involved from the outset and on a continuing basis.

Some drugs are known to be "photosensitizers"; that is, they have the capacity to enhance the effects of light with potentially harmful consequences. In general, the light responsible for photosensitizing reactions is ultraviolet. As I have already noted, the light sources used for light therapy screen out most ultraviolet rays. Whether the ultraviolet rays that get through the various screens—or the other light wavelength—are capable of doing any harm to the eye, even for people on photosensitizing drugs, is a matter of pure speculation at this time. An additional factor that needs to be taken into account is that as the lens of the eye ages, it becomes yellow and screens out most ultraviolet light entering the eye. Any potential risk of ultraviolet light is therefore of greatest concern in children and adolescents, and of decreasing concern as patients get older. Again, I would hesitate to discourage anyone from undertaking light therapy simply because he or she happens to be on one of these photosensitizing drugs. To do so would be to deny someone the opportunity to try a potentially helpful treatment because of a theoretical risk, the potential danger of which we are unable to estimate at this time. This is particularly important, since these photosensitizing drugs include some antidepressants and lithium—drugs frequently prescribed for depression. A list of potential photosensitizing agents is given below in Table 4.

Although it is worth being especially cautious where the eyes are concerned, I want to emphasize that many people have been treated safely

Table 4. Medications That May Theoretically Increase the Possibility of Light Therapy's Having a Harmful Effect on the Eyes

Drug	Its purpose
Phenothiazine	Antipsychotic
(e.g., Thorazine, Stelazine)	Antidepressant
Imipramine	Antitumor
Porphyrins	Antimalarial
Chloroquine	Antihypertensive, diuretic
Hydrochlorothiazine	(water pill)
Lithium	Mood stabilizer

Note. Being on one of these medications does not mean that you cannot or even should not use light therapy. Rather, it may mean that you should have your eyes more carefully monitored by your doctor. (From M. Terman, C. E. Remé, B. Rafferty, P. F. Gallin, and J. S. Terman, 1990. Reprinted by permission.)

and effectively with a combination of light therapy and antidepressant medications.

In summary, if you have any eye problems or are on any potentially photosensitizing medications, you should be aware that these constitute risk factors (though the degree of risk will vary, depending on your clinical situation). It is therefore necessary that these risk factors be identified by, or communicated to, the person who will be administering the light therapy. If you are a person at increased risk, it is wise for an ophthalmologist to be involved early in the treatment process. The professional(s) involved, in consultation with you will need to decide whether the potential benefits of light therapy outweigh the theoretical risks of eye injury. If a decision is made to start therapy, it should be monitored at appropriate intervals.

Time and further research will clarify the extent to which combining light with photosensitizing drugs constitutes a hazard. In the meanwhile, patients on these drugs should be aware that many thousands of people on the very same drugs have been walking outdoors, exposed to light many times as bright as that emanating from a light box, without suffering any eye-related problems as a consequence.

Precautions for Those with Sun-Sensitive Skin

As I have mentioned above, some ultraviolet rays get through the diffusing screen; although these cause no problem for most people, they may lead to problems in those with sun-sensitive skin. This includes people with conditions such as lupus (more properly known as systemic lupus erythematosis), those who have a tendency to develop skin cancer, and those on photosensitizing medications (see previous page). If you fall into one of these categories, you should consult with your physician and consider using a sun block, as you might do when walking outdoors on a sunny day. I have come across several patients who have both lupus and SAD, and have benefited from light therapy without suffering any skin problems. A sun block may not always be necessary, even for people with sun-sensitive skin; a process of trial and error may be helpful in determining whether to use it or not.

The Nuts and Bolts of Light Therapy

Obtaining a Light Box

Light therapy has usually been administered by means of a light box, a descendent of the original light box that we used to treat Herb Kern. The essential elements of that original box have been retained: a metal box, fluorescent lights, a shiny backing that reflects the light into the room, and a diffusing screen to spread the light evenly over the front of the box and cut down the ultraviolet output. Newer models are vast improvements over the initial light box in several ways. They are sleek and trim, look like pieces of furniture, and are easy to carry. One model weighs as little as nine pounds. By contrast, the initial model was an ungainly clunker that weighed fifty-five pounds. But the biggest advance in light box technology was developed by Dr. Michael Terman at Columbia University.

By slanting the light box toward the eye, Terman increased the intensity of light reaching the eye from 2500 to 10,000 lux. He and his colleagues showed that with an increased level of light delivery to the eyes, it was possible to substantially decrease the duration of light treatment necessary for an effective antidepressant response. Despite the higher intensity of the tilted fixture, it may not appear to be brighter than the conventional fixture, because the light reaches the eye more indirectly and causes less glare. Both the upright (2500-lux) and slanted (10,000-lux) fixtures are shown above in Figures 3 and 4. There have been no documented eye problems in people who have used these intensities, which fall well within published safety specifications. Although the intensity of the 10,000-lux fixtures is considerably higher than that of ordinary indoor lighting, it is far lower than that of outdoor sunlight. For example, 10,000 lux is the amount of light that would reach your eyes outdoors under clear skies about half an hour after sunrise. Of course, you would receive much more light (approximately 100,000 lux) on a sunny day at the beach.

Given its advantage of greater efficiency, I recommend that most people begin treatment with the slanted light box. Some of these boxes have the additional advantage of having a three-way switch, which allows the user to turn it on by degrees at the beginning of the treatment session and off by degrees at the end. This is an advantage for those who find it uncomfortable to turn the light on at its full intensity right away, and for those who feel a sense of being let down at the end of the session when the light is turned off too abruptly. This may be especially important for the early morning sessions, when it is still dark outdoors. One patient, for example, has observed a sudden plunge in mood when he switches off his lights abruptly.

If the slanted box is more efficient, why would anyone use the upright version? It has a few advantages. Some of the upright boxes have surface areas that are larger than those of the standard slanted versions. This allows the user to move around a bit and still be exposed to reasonably high light intensities. Those who like to exercise on a stationary bicycle or a ski machine may find it easier to do so in front of an upright box, which they may attach to the wall. Finally, an upright box takes up less table space and may be preferable where tabletop or desktop space is at a premium. Some boxes are constructed in such a way that they can be used in either a tilted or an upright position.

Suitable light fixtures, lamps included, currently cost approximately $350 to $500. This may sound like a lot of money, and many handy individuals have considered making their own fixtures. In my experience, this has not worked out well for most people. Ordinary fixtures in hardware stores are not usually wired for the right number of lamps, and therefore do not put out enough light. Industrial fixtures, which may be designed for the right number of lamps, may need to be electrically wired. This generally requires an electrician, since amateur wiring can be hazardous. In the case of a slanted fixture, securing the box at the correct angle can be difficult.

Incorrect fixtures can also put out light that is too bright. One patient, an engineer who built his own fixture and supervised his own treatment, ended up with a burn on the surface of his eye. Fortunately, this has not been reported with properly supervised light therapy. Finally, homemade fixtures, if they are made correctly, can cost almost as much as the custom-built ones.

If you do decide to build your own box, here are a few words of advice: Build it in the summer, when you are not depressed. Build it exactly according to specifications, and be sure to wire it correctly.

Some lighting companies offer a rental program, thereby allowing the user to try the lights out for a few weeks at a weekly rental fee, which may be offset against the purchase price if the user decides to buy it. This is an excellent idea, since most people should have some sense of whether they are going to benefit from the box within the first few weeks. If you sign up for such a plan, do be sure to use the lights diligently during the rental period; otherwise the rental time will be up, and you still won't really know whether you are a light responder or not.

Setting Up the Lights

It is important to position yourself correctly in relation to the lights. Consult Figures 3 and 4 above to get a good idea of how to do this. If you are using the 2500-lux fixture, your face should be directed toward the light. For this reason, the light should be placed at eye level—for example, on a desk, table, or other flat surface.

If you are using the slanted fixture, the front of the frame should be lined up with the edge of the desk or table at which you are sitting. You need to be able to get your legs underneath the table or else you will not be close enough to the light source. The light is designed so that your eyes will be exposed to sufficient light if you look down toward the surface of the desk or table, rather than directly at the light.

Although it is very important that your eyes be open during treatment sessions, it is not necessary to stare at the light or even to glance at it on a regular basis, though it is quite safe to do so. Many people have used the time in front of the lights for reading, craftwork, chores, or watching TV.

Distance from the Lights

It is important to sit at just the right distance from the light, because the actual amount that reaches your eyes depends on how far away from it your eyes are. If you are using the 2500-lux fixture, you should sit no farther than three feet away from the front of the box while you are receiving your light treatment. Of course, at other times of the day, you may choose to use the light box as a source of room lighting and ignore the question of distance. If you are using a 2500-lux fixture and find it is not turning out to be as effective or efficient as you hoped it would, the intensity of the light you receive—and perhaps the effectiveness of the treatment—can be increased by sitting a little closer to the light than three feet. There is no reason to believe that this would be harmful, provided you do not stare at the light for long intervals.

If you are using the slanted fixture, it is important that your forehead be just below the upper portion of the light box, which is tilted toward you. If your head is farther back, the amount of light you receive will fall below the required level. On the other hand, if you lean too far forward, your head will cast a shadow on the desk surface, which will also reduce the light level.

Time of Day and Duration of Treatment

The actual amount of light needed varies from person to person, at different latitudes, and at different times of the year. For example, in the early fall, as people begin to feel the winter syndrome setting in, it may be enough to use the lights for fifteen minutes in the morning. As the days get shorter and darker, more light is generally required. A typical person with SAD in the northern United States may start light treatment in mid-September with fifteen minutes (of the 10,000-lux fixture) in the morning, and increase it to thirty minutes in October and November (divided between morning and evening). In December, an extra fifteen minutes may be added in the evening, and in January and February, a total of one and a half hours or more may be necessary. By late February and early March it is usually possible to decrease the length of time gradually until around mid-April, when it may be possible to stop using the lights altogether.

If you begin treatment in the middle of the winter and are already feeling moderately to markedly depressed, it would be reasonable to start with about forty-five to sixty minutes of light per day, divided between the morning and the evening. If that proves to be too much or too little for you, you can easily alter the timing and duration after a week of treatment. For example, if it appears to be working well and you find that the initial dosage of forty-five minutes per day is inconvenient, or if you experience side-effects, you can reduce it to the minimum effective dose, which may be as little as twenty minutes per day.

As I have mentioned above, there is some controversy over the optimal timing of treatment. In my experience, *the most important consideration is that treatment should be administered at a convenient time,* because if you are not able to fit the treatments conveniently into your day, you are less likely to do them regularly and to benefit from them.

Fortunately, for many people, light treatment seems to work well no matter what time of day it is administered. Feel free to break up treatment sessions or to divide your treatment time between the morning and the evening; alternatively, you may get all the light you need during the daytime while you are at work. Although some people find that a single light therapy session in the morning keeps them going all day, others need an extra dose of light later on to prevent an afternoon or evening slump in energy.

Obviously, *the only way you can find the routine that works best for you is by trial and error.* For example, if you should start by using thirty minutes of light in the evening because that is the most convenient time for you, and you find that this isn't working well, it would be advisable to switch at least some of the treatment time to the morning before concluding that light treatment is not helpful. Or if you start with light treatment in the morning, but find you don't have the time and are missing your daily treatment sessions, switch to a more convenient time before giving up.

One of the most important factors determining the amount of light needed for a particular individual at a particular time of year is the amount of environmental light available, rather than the season. For example, an overcast spell of several days may cause SAD symptoms, even if it occurs in the summer. Several of my colleagues have light boxes in their offices, and when the weather turns gloomy, they switch them on—almost as though they have heard a "SAD warning" announced on the radio. Some people with windowless offices, who work long days without sunlight, may be perennially light-deprived and chronically fatigued and depressed. Not surprisingly, some of these folks use their light boxes all year round—even in the summertime.

Consistency of Treatment

For most people, in order for treatment to remain effective, it must be continued as long as there is a shortage of environmental light. For example, if you usually feel the symptoms of SAD between November and March, it is likely that you will have to use the lights on a daily or almost daily basis during those months. It is possible to skip a day here or there without suffering a relapse of symptoms, but many people find that if they skip more than one day, they feel their SAD symptoms creeping—or crashing—back again. As the days become longer and brighter, it is possible to decrease the duration of light treatment and skip more days without adverse consequences. Watch out for the spring, however, when the weather tends to be erratic. Bright sunny days alternate with cloudy and rainy ones. You may think that the problems are over for the season and then—crash!—back they come. So keep an eye on the sky before you pack your lights away. As I have mentioned above, some people who need light treatment at first may be able to stop treatment after their symptoms have subsided. At this time, we are unable to predict who those people will be and under what circumstances such a lucky outcome may be expected. My guess is that such good fortune will prove to be the exception rather than the rule, and that in most cases, as long as the days are dark, symptoms will return sooner or later to a greater or lesser degree.

Troubleshooting

The effects of light treatment are usually apparent within four days. What should you do if this does not occur? First, make sure you are using the equipment correctly. Do you have the right sort of fixture? Have you placed it at eye level, and are you sitting at the right distance from the fixture? Have you been using the lights for long enough each day? It may be helpful to shift the treatment to a different time of day. If the therapy is still not helping or is only partially helpful, be sure to ask the professional(s) you are consulting about this. *Above all, don't give up too soon, because a significant improvement may take at least two weeks to occur.*

What should you do if therapy is helpful for a while but becomes less effective over time? Although this may occur, it is rarely because the benefit of the light has been lost. If your mood declines after an initial response, this may be due to several identifiable causes: a change in your life circumstances, decreased environmental light, inconsistency of light treatment, or decreased intensity of the fluorescent lamps. You should consider each of these possibilities.

First, has your life become more stressful in any way? For example, has anything changed at work or in your relationships? If so, it is important to attend to the stresses in your life so that you can alleviate their effects on your mood.

Second, has it become darker outside? Light treatment that is completely effective in November and December may become only partially effective in the darker days of January and February. Although the days are getting longer in those months, they are also often cloudier, so there is less light available. In order to combat this climatic change, you may need to increase the amount of light or add some other type of treatment.

Third, have you been using the lights consistently, or have you slacked off, skipped days, or cut your treatments short? Are you using the lights properly—for example, are you facing the fixture so that your eyes are exposed to sufficient light?

Finally, how old are the fluorescent lamps in your fixture? After one season of use, the amount of light given off by the lamps may decrease enough to diminish their effectiveness. If you feel you are responding less well to treatment than you were previously, and the lamps in your fixture are more than two years old, consider replacing them.

How to Handle Others' Reactions to Your Light Therapy

Bringing a large box that its intense light into an indoor environment is certain to have some impact on those around you. Those patients who have used the light in work or home settings have found that some people are drawn to it and find it pleasant, while others dislike it and find it irritating.

Many patients are concerned that bringing a light box into the workplace will label them as disturbed or peculiar in some way. Reactions of colleagues and employers vary quite a bit in this regard. In most cases, it is possible to get a general sense of how accepting the people at work will be and whether it is advisable to use the lights in that setting. Supervisors and coworkers at a graphic design company or a mental health center may be more understanding and accepting of lights than workers at the CIA or the Pentagon—settings where it may be imprudent to bring a box in to work. Most people, however, have been surprised at how accepting their colleagues are toward the light box and the underlying condition that its presence implies. Perhaps it is because most people understand that seasons can affect behavior in animals, and the majority of the population experiences some seasonal changes, albeit to a milder degree.

Questions about the lights are best handled in a matter-of-fact way, though one college student I know chose humor instead. When asked by his roommates why he used the lights, he replied that experiments had shown that bright light maintained rats in a constant state of sexual arousal. That usually put an end to the questioning.

Many people have commented that their pets seem to react favorably to the lights. I have been told that cats in particular seem drawn to them and sit mesmerized in front of them. The best pet story I have heard concerned a cat and a parakeet. The parakeet was able to open his own cage. Ordinarily, when the cat encountered the bird he would give chase, and the parakeet would make a dash for his cage and slam the door shut behind himself. However, when the bright lights were turned on, the parakeet emerged from his cage and strutted in front of them, despite the dangerous proximity of the cat. The cat, for his part, appeared so entranced by the lights that he showed no interest in pursuing the parakeet. (Perhaps we should try out the lights on the proverbial lion and the lamb!)

Of greater interest than the reaction of pets to the light fixtures is the reaction of insurance companies. Many people I know have tried to get reimbursed for their light boxes, and some have succeeded. Clearly, the expense of the light box is medically justifiable, and I have little doubt that insurance companies will come to acknowledge this in time. Meanwhile, it may still be worth having your physician write a letter to your insurance company to substantiate your claim. One that I have used in the past, with variable success, is shown below.

Sample for Insurance Reimbursement

To whom it may concern:

This is to certify that Ms. Jane Smith has been a patient of mine since June 1985. I have treated her for recurrent major depressions (DSM-III-R 296.3), with a seasonal pattern. This condition, also known as Seasonal Affective Disorder (SAD), has been shown in many studies in the United States and elsewhere in the world to respond to treatment with bright environmental light (light therapy). Light therapy is no longer considered experimental, but is a mainstream type of psychiatric treatment, described in the *Task Force Report of the American Psychiatric Association: Treatment of Psychiatric Disorders*, Vol. 3, pages 1890–1896, APA Press, 1989. In order to administer light therapy adequately, a light box, such as the one described on the attached invoice, is required.

Although a light box is an expensive piece of equipment, the experience of clinicians who have used it for many patients indicates that it saves a great deal of money in the long run, by reducing the number of doctors' visits and laboratory investigations of persistent symptoms, as well as the indirect costs of lost productivity. I contend that in Ms. Smith's case the use of such a light fixture should be regarded not only as a medical necessity, to be used in preference to (or in addition to) other forms of treatment, but also as a means of reducing her overall medical costs.

The Cutting Edge: Future Directions in Light Therapy

Simulating Dawn's Early Light

> In winter I get up at night,
> And dress by yellow candle-light.
> In summer, quite the other way,
> I have to go to bed by day.
> —ROBERT LOUIS STEVENSON

Why is it that on a summer day you can bound out of bed ready to get going, eagerly anticipating an enjoyable day, whereas on a dreary winter day your body feels like lead and you could go on sleeping for hours if only the world would let you? How does your body know what it's like outdoors when you haven't had a chance to look out of the window or even hear a weather report? This is a question that Dr. Michael Terman has addressed; in doing so, he has opened up one of the most exciting new directions in light therapy. Drawing from his basic research on biological rhythms in animals, Terman realized that the transition times between night and day—namely, dawn and dusk—have a very important influence on the animal's daily rhythms. At those times the eyes may be especially sensitive to environmental light. Terman hypothesized that humans might also be particularly sensitive to light at dawn—so sensitive that they might respond to the effects of even relatively low levels of environmental light transmitted through the closed eyelids.

To test this hypothesis, Terman developed a computerized dawn simulator, which could be programmed to turn on the light in the room at a predesignated time and to increase the intensity of the light gradually until, after a certain amount of time, the maximum intensity of the light was reached. This idea has since been taken up by certain lighting manufacturers, who have developed extremely handy electronic devices—small enough to fit in the palm of your hand—which can be programmed to create a dawn of specified onset and duration (see Figure 5, below). Various light sources for this artificial dawn have been developed, the simplest of which is a bedside lamp, which can be selected for intensity and quality of light and positioned at a suitable distance from your head. Dr. Michael Terman in New York and Dr. David Avery in Seattle, Washington, have studied the effects of dawn simulation in SAD patients and have found it to be effective both in reducing symptoms and in helping patients wake up more easily in the morning. According to Avery, patients who tend to have difficulty waking up during the winter tend to respond especially well to this treatment. Avery, who has now replicated his and Terman's original

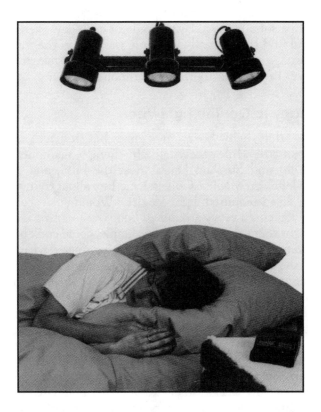

Figure 5. A dawn simulator. Photograph courtesy of Pi Square Inc.

findings, recommends a dawn of one and a half to two hours, with the room starting off in complete darkness and reaching an intensity of about 250 lux, as measured at the eyes. This is approximately the amount of light to which your eyes would be exposed if they were a few feet away from the shade of your bedside lamp.

One question that has not been properly studied is whether it would be just as effective—or almost as effective—to have your bedside lamp on a timer, set to turn the lamp on one and a half to two hours before you plan to wake up in the morning. One uncontrolled study by Dr. Frederick Jacobsen found that such a set-up helped patients who slept excessively to curtail their sleep duration. If this simpler arrangement is effective, it would save patients money, because dawn simulators currently cost about $200. It may be worth trying the simpler and less expensive remedy (the light on a timer) first; if it turns out to be highly effective, you may find it unnecessary to buy the dawn simulator. I personally use a dawn simulator each day, even during the summer, and find that it really helps me wake up in the morning. An added advantage of the device is its portability, and I take it along with me whenever I travel during the winter months.

Light Therapy to Go: The Light Visor

Recognizing that light boxes are somewhat restrictive, requiring patients to sit still while receiving light therapy, my colleagues (Drs. Thomas Wehr and Stephen Leighton at the NIH, and Dr. George Brainard at Jefferson Medical College) and I set about trying to develop a portable, head-mounted light device. Wouldn't it be great, we thought, if you could move around and do your morning chores while receiving light therapy? A parent, for example, could cook breakfast for the kids and get them off to school while being treated with light. This idea led to the development of the Light Visor, a device shaped like a baseball cap and worn on the head, with the light-containing visor portion suspended above and in front of the eyes (see Figure 6).

The Light Visor has by now gone through many different designs and, along the way, has been tested at multiple centers on over 200 patients with SAD. The results of these studies are open to different interpretations. On the plus side, a high percentage of patients reported improvement after using the Light Visor for thirty to sixty minutes per day for one or two weeks; some went on to purchase Light Visors themselves. In over fifty percent of patients, symptoms resolved almost completely. The problem in interpreting the Light Visor results arose because there was no difference in the degree of improvement observed when patients were treated with visors of widely differing intensities (ranging from 30 lux to 6000 lux). This finding stands in sharp contrast to studies of light therapy with light boxes, where higher response rates have been found with higher intensities of light.

In trying to understand the results of the Light Visor studies, researchers have suggested two different explanations. On the one hand, it is possible that the Light Visor is no more than a placebo—in other words, all its beneficial effects may be the results of the patients' expectations of improvement with treatment, or nonspecific responses to the support, encouragement, and involvement of the researchers. On the other hand, it is possible that when light treatment is administered from a light source that is quite near to the eye—as with the Light Visor—then we may have more options for regulating the amount of light that enters the eyes than we would have with light from a more distant source, like the light box. For example, very bright

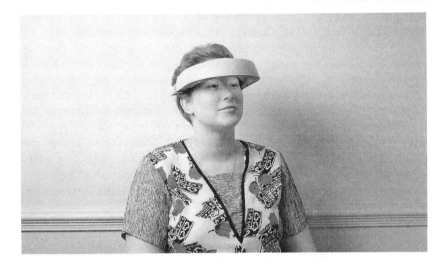

Figure 6. The Light Visor.

light may cause us to squint, thereby limiting the amount of light reaching the eyes; or very dim light may cause our pupils to expand and allow more of the available light to enter. These different types of reactions may lead to similar treatment responses with widely different Visor intensities.

Although we have had more clinical experience with the light box than with the Light Visor, if it is important for you to be able to obtain your light therapy while moving around or traveling, the Visor is certainly worth a try. Once again, I recommend that if you plan to try the Light Visor, you seek out distributors that have a rental program or offer a money-back guarantee if it does not prove helpful.

Early Light Treatment to Prevent SAD

Dr. Ybe Meesters and colleagues in The Netherlands introduced into the literature the provocative idea that light treatment administered for a brief period early in the winter may have continued antidepressant value for the rest of the winter, even after treatment is discontinued. These researchers reported that in a small number of SAD patients, treatment with merely five days of light therapy, when patients first noted moderate symptoms of winter depression, was followed by low depression levels for the rest of the winter. One of my ex-patients actually called me from The Netherlands to convey her excitement and feelings of optimism at having enjoyed a depression-free winter, which she attributed to this experimental treatment.

Although these preliminary results are intriguing and there is certainly no harm in trying this approach, it is still quite experimental. The Termans at Columbia University were unable to replicate these findings; within several weeks of discontinuing treatment, most of their patients relapsed. I have certainly seen many patients for whom early treatment in the winter was no protection against becoming depressed later on. The discrepancy in findings and observations about the prophylactic value of early light treatment is therefore a mystery waiting to be resolved. Given the rapid growth of the field of light therapy, I am confident that it will be resolved before the next edition of this book is published.

Other Innovations: Light Rooms and Indirect Light

Several researchers have explored the possibility of making a whole room so bright that a person could wander around in it and be exposed to therapeutic levels of light without having to gaze in any particular direction. My wife and I have actually done this with our own bedroom, to which we frequently retreat on dark winter days and nights to absorb the rays without the constraints of sitting in one place. I can easily imagine the "light bedroom" of the future, computerized to start getting light at a preprogrammed time and gradually becoming brighter and brighter until it's time to wake up. This same room would be very bright in the evening and would gradually become dimmer, simulating the effects of dusk. Such a room could be decorated with dioramas of glass or plastic, showing scenes of lakes or forests. Imagine that as the room becomes brighter in the morning, a sun can be seen cresting over the horizon on the lake; birds begin to chirp, and deer wander through the forests. Computerized dioramas such as these exist already, though they are prohibitively expensive for most people. As technology advances, they may become commonplace, and we may find the artificial type of light therapy we receive today gradually merging into a type of naturalistic light treatment that enriches and blends in seamlessly with the rest of our lives.

To return to the present, however, I would like to direct you to a more pedestrian—though extremely useful—strategy for bringing more light into your environment: the use of indirect light. For the light therapy that I have discussed thus far, I have recommended the use of fluorescent lights. There is no reason, however, to believe that regular, incandescent, or halogen lamps would not be effective in the treatment of SAD. The problem with these types of lamps is that they give off a great deal of light from small, very bright filaments. *Staring directly at these filaments could certainly harm the eyes.* On the other hand, if the light is reflected off a large surface, the *indirect* light should be quite safe to look at. This effect could be obtained for example, by shining a halogen lamp against a white wall, or having the light of a bright hanging incandescent lamp bounce off a white tablecloth. Such strategies have been successful for some patients I have known.

An advantage of using incandescent lights is that they are cheap. Nonetheless, there are certainly major disadvantages in doing so. Chief among these is the possibility that you might inadvertently gaze at the light source and damage your eyes. In addition, unless you obtain a good light meter and take light measurements, you will not know how much light is reaching your eyes, and thus whether your homemade set-up is falling within the therapeutic range. In addition, we do not have the wealth of clinical experience and scientific literature for incandescent lamps that we have for fluorescents. Finally, incandescent lights generate more heat than fluorescent lights and consume more energy for the amount of light generated. Given these disadvantages, I would recommend that professionally made fluorescent devices be used as a first choice, and that indirect light from incandescent or halogen lamps be used merely to enhance your general indoor lighting, which may be beneficial in itself. I will discuss further the value of increasing environmental light in the next chapter.

Conclusion: Creating a Light Therapy Program That Works for You

I have outlined several approaches to light therapy, but they need to be synthesized into a comprehensive program and this program needs to be integrated into a general program for dealing with the symptoms of SAD. In Chapters 7, 8, and 9, I describe other ways of treating SAD; in Chapter 10, I provide some examples of how the different treatments can be integrated into an overall treatment program. In creating a light therapy program that works for you, you often need to draw upon your own creativity, as did one reader of the earlier version of this book, who wrote me from Albuquerque, New Mexico:

I would like to see [you discuss] how important it is to work with the lights in order to fine-tune them to one's own needs (which can be very unique). Thanks to light therapy, in 1993 I had my first depression-free winter in 10 years. *BUT*—the light box did not work by itself!! It *did* work in the early fall, when the sun was still coming up pretty early. But when the mornings were dark, the box ceased working—no matter how long I used it, or at what time. I carefully read all the various books—to no avail.

Almost hopeless, I asked *myself* what was wrong, and realized that what I craved was to be submerged in light—like I was sitting on a beach. Sitting in relative darkness, with regular home lighting, focusing on a single strong light source (the light box), didn't feel "right" to me. I followed my instincts [and] set up my light box in my bedroom, along with all my old homemade light boxes (a total of eight four-foot-long fluorescents), which had worked moderately well in past winters (if I used them for four hours a day!). I submerged myself in light in the mornings—and that's what turned the switch on again. And it stayed on consistently through the winter. (How do I know I have gotten my dose? My hands tingle! it's like the circuit is connected.)

She adds the following comments about doctors who have been dismissive of her symptoms or have given her casual advice that has not gone far enough in addressing the seriousness of her winter problems:

Soon I hope the doctors in this area will stop saying, "You can't have SAD in Albuquerque—it's sunny here." Don't they read?

And:

Beware of doctors who claim that "going out for an hour a day," adding more light bulbs in home fixtures, etc., is all you need. This is what I was told by various psychiatrists—of course, it didn't work, and I discovered what I need to do only through my own reading and my . . . support group.

This reader has discovered the critical importance of taking some responsibility for her own treatment and not relying entirely on her doctors. I strongly endorse the idea that patients should educate themselves about their illness and its treatments and apply their thoughts and creativity to helping themselves in addition to consulting professionals. It is in the service of that idea that I have written this book. In addition, I have provided information about other sources from which you can learn more about SAD and light therapy, as well as support groups you can join, in the "Resources" section at the end of the book.

CHAPTER 7

Beyond light therapy: Other ways to help yourself

Although most people with SAD can benefit from light therapy, this is often not a complete solution to the problem. Some difficulties may persist, albeit to a lesser degree. While many people find that light therapy has made an enormous difference in the way they feel, they still don't feel as well in the winter as they do in the summer. Luckily, there are many other ways in which people can help themselves or be helped through winter depression—or indeed, depression at any time of the year.

Understanding SAD: The First Step

One of the most useful things that the definition of SAD has accomplished is that it provides people who suffer from the condition with a new way of understanding their difficulties. This understanding has developed only relatively recently, so people who have suffered from the condition have long been misunderstood, and have also failed to understand their own difficulties. Classical depressions—the kind that physicians have traditionally recognized as coming from within, and have thus termed "endogenous"—have typically been associated with loss of appetite, weight loss, and insomnia. People who suffer from this condition are often completely incapacitated, may have seriously considered taking their own lives, and often require hospitalization. In contrast to this dramatic picture of classical depression, patients with SAD are usually less severely affected and are able to continue functioning to some degree at work or at home (although much less effectively than they do at other times of the year), and they rarely need hospitalization. In addition, the pattern of eating and sleeping in

131

SAD patients is frequently different from that seen in the types of depression more easily recognized by physicians. Patients with SAD often tend to eat more, crave carbohydrates, and gain weight during the winter. Their energy level is very low, and they often feel fatigued, physically heavy, and weighed down. They withdraw and want to be left alone.

Since the pattern of symptoms in SAD is as much physical as psychological, patients with this problem often seek help from family practitioners and internists, rather than psychiatrists or therapists. They have frequently been examined and tested for various medical conditions: underactivity of the thyroid, hypoglycemia, or chronic viral infections such as the Epstein–Barr virus. When these investigations come back negative, as they generally do, a physician may not make the diagnosis of SAD or recognize that there is a clear course of treatment to suggest. The physician may honestly declare that he or she does not know what is wrong, or imply that a patient is exaggerating the problem. The patient can easily be left with the impression that because the tests have come back negative, the problem is not real, but imaginary. He or she may feel responsible for the predicament. After all, if the doctor can't help, it's up to the patient to find the solution. *It is important to remember that at present, there is no laboratory test for SAD. The diagnosis is made on the basis of history alone.*

Before the recognition of SAD, psychiatrists also often had trouble understanding what was going on. These patients were not, after all, incapacitated by depression; they could continue to work and function to some degree. Psychiatrists generally concluded that the problem must therefore be "neurotic"—a result of psychological conflicts or of difficulties in adjusting to life stress.

Many of my patients have told me how guilty they have felt about their inability to perform at their usual level, to meet the demands they make on themselves (or those others make) during the winter months. Attempts to explain this disability on the basis of psychological factors—childhood traumas, conflicts, anniversary reactions—have been ineffective, and patients have often viewed their inability to benefit from such treatments as just one more failure. The understanding that seasonal problems are an unusual or exaggerated response to physical and climatic changes makes intuitive sense. After all, plants and animals change with the seasons, so why should humans be different? This idea often relieves my patients from feelings of guilt and responsibility for their symptoms; it makes their seasonal changes in mood and behavior understandable, and therefore easier to deal with.

The explanation that the exaggerated response to the seasons, and the symptoms that result from it, are results of a disturbance in brain chemistry is an example of the "medical model." According to this model, disturbances of brain function are regarded as comparable to those of any other organ—for example, the pancreas in diabetes. Just as the diabetic does not produce enough insulin, the patient with SAD does not produce the correct chemical response when there is inadequate environmental light. And just as an injection of artificial insulin can control the symptoms of diabetes, so bright light can control the symptoms of SAD. The result of the medical model is that the symptoms of depression are no longer seen as character flaws for which a sufferer is somehow responsible, but rather, as the afflictions that they really are. Many people have told me that, before their diagnosis of SAD was made, they felt lazy, bad, or immature. Just knowing that they have an illness with a name and an explanation, and for which effective treatments exist, is already therapeutic.

There is also considerable comfort in knowing you have control over your life, despite the symptoms of SAD. The availability of light and many other ways to combat symptoms make you feel less like a victim of fate and allow you to take charge of things. People who have been accustomed to functioning at low levels during the winter can now plan for year-round productivity. In some instances, this allows people to make certain long-term plans—for example, to go to graduate school or start a new business—that would formerly have been unthinkable.

In summary, the benefits of recognizing that one may be suffering from SAD, and that light can have antidepressant effects, go well beyond the immediate relief of symptoms. They alter the way a person thinks about the problem, its future outlook, and the options available, and can therefore be a liberating experience that continues to deliver new rewards over time.

Taking SAD Seriously

It is one thing to understand intellectually that you have SAD, but another to acknowledge the degree to which it is interfering with your life—your capacity to enjoy yourself or to be productive. I have seen several patients suffer unnecessarily for several winters after being diagnosed with SAD, simply because they have had trouble accepting it. One woman, for example, who had a tendency to neglect her own well-being, did not sit in front of her lights on a regular basis for two winters until she came to accept, as part of her ongoing psychotherapy, that she had trouble attending to her medical needs. After she came to terms with her condition and its impact on her life, she had her best winter ever.

Sometimes taking SAD seriously means making significant life changes in order to ease the difficulties of everyday living during the winter. The treatment of one of my SAD patients was made far more difficult by the fact that she had to spend many hours in her car each day commuting to and from work and carpooling her children. This added enormously to the daily stresses of her life, and prevented her from being able to exercise regularly and get sufficient light exposure. When we analyzed her life circumstances, it became clear that if she could move closer to her work and her children's social and recreational network, life would become far more manageable. By taking her problem seriously and conveying this understanding to her husband, she has managed to persuade him to put their much-loved home on the market and move. I have little doubt that this life change will pay off richly for the patient and her family in the coming winters. The story of another SAD patient, "Sara," who is profiled in Chapter 10, also shows the value (and, indeed, necessity) of taking SAD symptoms seriously and acting accordingly.

Changing the Environment

More Light

The benefit of increasing environmental light can be obtained not only from formal therapy in front of a light box, but whenever your environment is brighter. Some people have several light boxes in the house, which gives them more exposure to light without the feeling of being trapped in one location. It is not always critical for the extra light to come from special boxes. Enhancing light levels in your home or in the workplace may be helpful, even if this is accomplished by installing more lights on the ceiling or placing more lamps in the room.

Modifications of the home to increase indoor light levels may be as simple as trimming hedges around the windows or low-lying branches of trees near the house, or as elaborate as constructing skylights. One useful new product is the "Sunlight Pipe," which is a shiny aluminum tube extending from the outside of the roof to just below the ceiling. Like a skylight, it transmits natural light into the house. Not only is the extra indoor light welcome, but there is the added advantage of feeling connected to the passage of the sun across the sky and even to the moonlight when the moon is full (see the "Resources" section at the end of this book for more details). Using bright colors and surfaces can also be effective. Many of my SAD patients have found attractive ways of accomplishing this. Dark wood paneling can be replaced with light-colored wallpaper. Splashes of yellow and orange on curtains and cushions seem to be popular with some of my SAD patients, while others choose white or off-white carpeting and furnishings. SAD patients who buy new homes should pay attention to the size of the windows and the directions in which the rooms face.

Exposure to natural light can be both enjoyable and therapeutic. This applies to lunchtime walks on sunny winter days or sunlight reflected from snow. Dr. Anna Wirz-Justice in Switzerland actually studied the value of exposure to natural light systematically and found that morning walks were highly beneficial for her SAD patients. Many people have told me that the light reflected from snow is one of the reasons they enjoy skiing. Some people have chosen to work the evening shift so that they can enjoy as much outdoor sunshine as possible during the day. At the other extreme, according to one Hawaiian psychiatrist, are SAD patients who develop symptoms because they *don't* venture out into the sunlight, even though it is abundantly available for most of the year. This psychiatrist has found that simply encouraging patients to get outdoors during the day can provide them with sufficient light to control their depressive symptoms.

Once you pay attention to the amount and quality of your environmental light, you will come up with all kinds of ways to enhance it, which will help you feel more comfortable and cheerful.

The Value of Warmth

Many patients have told me that warmth, in conjunction with light, seems to be helpful in combating the symptoms of SAD. They have reported feeling better in winter when they turn up the thermostat, use electric blankets, and drink warm beverages. Although this strategy lacks scientific backing, it may help and can't hurt. Among animals, environmental temperature is an important influence on seasonal rhythms, and often operates in conjunction with environmental light.

Winter Vacations

Bright light and warm temperatures can be pleasantly combined in the form of a winter vacation in the south. Many of my patients have learned that if they have a choice, it's better to take vacations in the winter than in the summer. Two weeks in a sunny climate in January can effectively interrupt the worst stretch of the winter. I am reminded of a television commercial in which a somber-looking man stands on the beach in Jamaica on the first day of his vacation, looks a little more cheerful on the second day, and is positively blissful by the third day. For the SAD sufferer, this is truth in advertising! People seem to feel better in this natural sunlight than they do up north, even with light therapy. As an alternative to popular seaside resorts, some of my patients have undertaken adventurous trips—to Antarctica (where the days are very long when it's winter in the Northern Hemisphere) or the Galapagos Islands, for example, with similarly beneficial results. Unfortunately, the beneficial results are usually short-lived; after a patient returns from vacation, the regimen of light therapy must usually be resumed. Some people find that the sudden exposure to intense sunlight in the middle of winter can make them feel overstimulated, as they are in summer. It is important to watch out for this possibility and monitor exposure to sunlight accordingly.

Relocation

Several of my patients have chosen a more dramatic solution than those outlined above—to move permanently to places with sunnier climates. Again, an example of such a patient is Sara, whose problems with SAD are discussed in Chapter 10. Generally, patients who have relocated have been pleased with these moves. They feel more energetic, and their energy level is more evenly distributed year round. Of course, there are many factors other than climate that have to be taken into account when one relocates. One must decide whether relinquishing all the benefits of one's current lifestyle—the proximity of friends and family, job, and cultural amenities—will be repaid by life in a sunnier climate. Clearly, the pros and cons of such a move have to be carefully weighed. If you are considering such a move, you should take the following considerations into account:

- How well can the SAD symptoms be controlled by light therapy and other means?
- Will you really feel better during the winter in the new climate? One way to test this is to visit the place during the winter before making a commitment to move.
- What are the exact weather conditions in the place in question? For example, even though a place may be located in the south, local weather conditions may cause clouds to obscure the sun for much of the winter.
- What is the summer like in the new place, and how do you respond to heat and humidity? Be careful that a move doesn't result in your exchanging one climatic problem for another.

Diet and Exercise

Diet and exercise are important considerations in SAD, not only because they can have a valuable effect on mood control, but also because of their beneficial physical effects. Patients with SAD often put on weight during the winter, as a result of a combination of overeating and being inactive. Although it is easier to lose weight during the summer, there is a tendency to retain pounds with each cycle of the seasons; over the years, this can result in obesity. Researchers have shown that obesity resulting from cyclical increases and decreases in body weight can be particularly bad for one's physical health. Light therapy, in my experience, for all its benefits, often proves disappointing to those who hope that they will automatically shed their excess weight as they begin to feel better. Diet and exercise should therefore be part of the SAD patient's overall health maintenance plan. For SAD patients, there are certain special aspects to consider and certain special advantages to be derived from diet and exercise. These are discussed below.

Exercise

There is growing evidence that regular aerobic exercise has a beneficial effect on mood control in those who suffer from depression in general. In SAD, where the exercise may mean an increase in exposure to bright light—either outdoors, or on a stationary bicycle or ski machine in front of a light box—the antidepressant effect can be even greater. Typically, if exercise alone is chosen as the mode of treatment, people often do not have enough willpower to continue it through the winter months. However, the combination of exercise and light therapy may work better than either treatment alone. Exercise, of course, has the added virtue of reducing weight, or at least preventing the much-dreaded winter weight gain.

Most patients with SAD can derive some benefit from exercise. The most important factor in finding the best regimen for you is to choose an activity you enjoy. This could be brisk walking, swimming, jogging, cycling (moving or stationary), cross-country skiing, or aerobic dancing. If you enjoy it, you are much more likely to stick with it. If you choose the exercise on the basis of its aerobic properties or therapeutic value and don't enjoy it, it's unlikely to work out over the long haul. Finding a friend who also wants to exercise can be a valuable support, and you can bolster each other's motivation during the dark days.

A key to losing weight is raising your metabolic rate—the rate at which you burn calories. One way to accomplish this is by vigorous exercise, especially if it is carried out for a sustained period (for example, twenty minutes or more). An added benefit of this "fat-burning" exercise is that you continue to burn off more calories than usual for some time after you have stopped exercising, as it takes a while for your metabolic rate to settle back down to resting levels. Another way in which exercise can help increase your metabolic weight is by turning fat into muscle, which occurs, for example, with regular weight lifting. Since muscle cells have a higher metabolic rate than fat cells, you can think of your muscles as calorie-burning factories. By increasing your muscle mass, you are therefore increasing the rate at which you burn calories, even when you are at rest.

Diet

Unfortunately, exercise alone is usually inadequate to reverse the weight gain resulting from the ravenous hunger and cravings for sweets and starches that so commonly occur in SAD. There is no getting away from the fact that diet has to be taken into account as well. Although nobody likes to diet, the good news is that there are now at least three promising dietary approaches that can help you keep your weight gain to a minimum during the hungry winter months; in some cases, it may actually be possible for SAD patients to *lose* weight in the winter.

The three type of diets that I believe offer the most promise are as follows:

- High-carbohydrate, reduced-calorie diets
- The Carbohydrate Addict's Diet®
- The Paleolithic Diet: Balancing carbohydrates with protein

Before discussing these diets, I would like to dispense with some popular diets that are quite *unhelpful*, in the experience of most experts who have dealt with obesity associated with carbohydrate craving. These are diets that call for strict limits on carbohydrate consumption. They work for a while because, unless you eat enough carbohydrates, you will not be able to metabolize the other major food types—proteins and fats. In other words, instead of landing on your hips or belly, the calories from dietary protein and fat will be excreted in the urine in the form of substances known as "ketone bodies." The presence of ketone bodies in the system reduces hunger in the short term, making it easier to diet, and the pounds may come off relatively easily and rapidly. In the long term, however, carbohydrate cravings will gain the upper hand, and the dieter will almost always gain back all of the lost weight. An example of this type of carbohydrate-restricted diet is The Scarsdale Diet.

Other diets that severely restrict carbohydrates—and, indeed, all major food groups—are the rapid weight loss programs, which rely on protein powders or other types of dietary supplements as the major source of nutrients. Once again, in most cases the rapidly lost weight is rapidly regained, often with interest. The "yo-yo" pattern of weight change resulting from these diets is both frustrating and unhealthy.

The key to a successful diet is that it must be sustainable over time with relative ease. The three dietary approaches outlined below all qualify in this important regard, at least for some people. Because different approaches may work for different people, it is important that you find the approach that is right *for you*, and that you don't give up on the idea of dieting if the first or second approach doesn't work. Go right on down the line and try the next one. I now discuss each of the approaches that have been found to be helpful by at least some SAD patients.

High-Carbohydrate, Reduced-Calorie Diets

Counting calories is boring; there is no denying that. Yet restricting calories is an effective strategy for many people and is widely endorsed by nutritionists. In the first set of diets provided in the "Resources" section of this book, you will find simple guidelines for this type of dietary approach. The calories in these diets come for the most part from carbohydrates, in accordance with currently recommended nutritional guidelines.

I believe that carbohydrates offer us an important clue to our understanding of the basic biochemical problems in SAD. They may also provide a clue as to how to treat SAD, and particularly the weight gain that so often accompanies the condition. Most people tend to eat more carbohydrates in the winter than in the summer, and show the opposite seasonal pattern for protein intake. In SAD patients this tendency is exaggerated. These patients may actually binge on sweets and starches, which can wreak havoc with any attempt at weight control. My colleagues and I at the NIMH have found that carbohydrate-rich meals actually make SAD patients feel energized, whereas they make non-SAD people feel sedated. Since draggy, low-energy feelings are a major problem for people with SAD, it is easy to understand why many of them gravitate to foods that give them an instant energy boost, especially if they have work to do. Is this energy boost a good or a bad thing? Are carbohydrates a good drug for patients with SAD, or are they harmful? Experts are currently debating these questions, and I present the different sides of the debate here. Although experts may disagree on what is best in this regard, I encourage you to find out for yourself whether a diet rich in carbohydrates is right or wrong *for you.*

In the experience of Dr. Judith Wurtman from MIT, who has worked with many overweight people who crave carbohydrates, high-protein, carbohydrate-restricted diets invariably increase cravings for carbohydrates, which ultimately cause the diet to fail. This has led her to suggest that overweight carbohydrate cravers should be encouraged to eat carbohydrate-rich meals and snacks. The dietary guidelines provided in the first set of menus in the "Resources" section follow some of the principles she outlines. I would also heartily recommend her own books on the topic, listed under "Further Reading" in the "Resources" section, which are full of valuable tips. For example, Wurtman points out that satiety—the awareness that you have had enough to eat—takes a little while to kick in, perhaps twenty to thirty minutes. This may take longer or be less complete if you are a carbohydrate craver. She points out the value of waiting at least thirty minutes after eating a carbohydrate-rich snack before deciding whether you want another one or not. This can be a helpful strategy in forestalling a binge. She also suggests that you eat snacks that are separately wrapped or packaged to avoid the "cookie jar" phenomenon, where your hand is back in the jar again before you have completely swallowed the previous handful.

Judith Wurtman's work has its theoretical basis in the work of her husband, Dr. Richard Wurtman, and their colleague, Dr. John Fernstrom. Fernstrom and Richard Wurtman showed that dietary carbohydrates increase production of a neurotransmitter, serotonin, in the brains of animals by a series of biochemical steps. There is now evidence that this same effect may occur in people. Serotonin is known to play an important role in satiety in animals. It is possible that eating carbohydrate-rich meals increases concentrations of serotonin in the brain and promotes feelings of satiety. In other words, dietary carbohydrates, working through serotonin, may be one important cue telling us when we have had enough to eat.

One controversial element in Judith Wurtman's dietary advice is her recommendation of dietary carbohydrates that release sugar rather readily into the bloodstream, technically known as foods with a "high glycemic index" (see Table 5 on page 142). Wurtman advises carbohydrate cravers to snack on high-glycemic-index carbohydrates, such as candy, cookies, jams and jellies, and soft drinks; in her view, they will be most effective in causing brain serotonin levels to increase and satiety to kick in. Foods such as apples or oranges, which result in a slower absorption of glucose into the bloodstream, are said to have a lower glycemic index, and Wurtman considers these less useful in the control of carbohydrate craving. As you will see below, others disagree with the policy of specifically seeking out high-glycemic-index carbohydrate-rich foods. Although these may work for you, as they have for many of Wurtman's patients, my inclination is to prefer foods that release glucose more slowly into the bloodstream, such as those outlined below and in several of the recipes in the "Resources" section (see Table 5 below for the glycemic index for many foods).

The Carbohydrate Addict's Diet®

Another diet that favors carbohydrates as the major source of calories for overweight carbohydrate cravers is the Carbohydrate Addict's Diet®. It was developed by two researchers and self-acknowledged carbohydrate cravers, Drs. Rachael and Richard Heller of Mount Sinai School of Medicine in New York City. A key insight into the discovery of the Carbohydrate Addict's Diet®, which is also the name of the Hellers' book on the subject (and one that I highly recommend) came from Rachael Heller's own personal experiences. She found that her carbohydrate cravings and hunger were generally decreased during the day to a greater degree if she had skipped breakfast altogether than if she had eaten a carbohydrate-rich breakfast. In fact, this observation inspired one of the questions she asks her patients in order to help them determine whether they are carbohydrate cravers or not: Is it easier to go through to lunch without snacking on those days when you skip breakfast—or have had no more than a cup of coffee—than on those days when you have had a full carbohydrate-rich breakfast consisting of cereal, toast, and fruit? If the answer is yes, chances are that you are a carbohydrate craver. A more complete test to determine whether you are a carbohydrate craver or not is available in the Hellers' book. In my experience, however, most SAD patients do not need to take the test. They know that they crave carbohydrates, and they do.

From their scientific observations, the Hellers concluded that it is very difficult for carbohydrate cravers to eat just a small amount of a carbohydrate-rich food, whether in the form of a snack or as part of a meal. Unlike other people, who are satisfied by measured quantities of carbohydrates, a carbohydrate craver is, according to the Hellers, an addict—someone whose addiction is stimulated and kindled by the substance to which he or she is addicted. This observation has led them to recommend that their patients eat low levels of carbohydrate-rich foods *for most of the day*, but that they allow themselves one Reward

Table 5. Glycemic Index: The Area Under the Blood Glucose Curve for Each Food Expressed as a Percentage of the Area After Taking the Same Amount of Carbohydrate as Glucose[a]

100%	50 to 59%	30 to 39%
Glucose	Buckwheat	Butter beans
	Spaghetti (white)	Haricot beans
80 to 90%	Sweet corn	Blackeyed peas
Corn flakes	All-Bran	Chick peas
Carrots	Digestive biscuits	Apples (golden
Parsnips	Oatmeal biscuits	delicious)
Potatoes (instant, mashed)	Peas (frozen)	Ice cream
Maltose	Yams	Milk (skim)
Honey	Sucrose	Milk (whole)
70 to 79%	Potato chips	Yogurt
Bread (whole wheat)		Tomato soup
Millet	40 to 49%	
Rice (white)	Spaghetti (whole wheat)	20 to 29%
Potatoes (new)	Oatmeal	Kidney beans
Turnips	Potatoes (sweet)	Lentils
	Beans (canned navy)	Fructose
60 to 69%	Peas (dried)	
Bread (white)	Oranges	10 to 19%
Rice (brown)	Orange juice	Soy beans
Muesli		Soy beans (canned)
Shredded wheat		Peanuts
Ryvita		
Water biscuits		
Beets		
Bananas		
Raisins		
Mars bar		

[a]Data from normal individuals. It should be noted that those with diabetes, especially if it is uncontrolled, would have plasma glucose responses that were both quantitatively and qualitatively different.
Source. Jenkins, DJA: Lente carbohydrate: a newer approach to the dietary management of diabetes. *Diabetes Care* 5:634–641, 1982. Reprinted by permission.

Meal®, in which they are permitted to eat as many carbohydrate-rich foods as they like, provided these are eaten within the space of an hour and along with other types of foods. For the other meals and snacks, these researchers recommend that carbohydrate cravers specifically restrict their consumption of high-glycemic-index carbohydrates, which, in their experience, promote craving and bingeing.

As you can see, the Hellers agree with Judith Wurtman that carbohydrate cravers (or addicts) should be permitted to indulge their cravings to some degree. These researchers all recognize the comfort that carbohydrate cravers derive from knowing that their next carbohydrate-rich meal or snack is never too far away. These researchers differ, however, in their recommendations as to the distribution of carbohydrates throughout the day. Wurtman advocates regular carbohydrate snacking, whereas the Hellers believe that this pattern of eating fuels the addiction and makes dieting more difficult.

The researchers also differ in their recommendations about what type of carbohydrates to recommend. As noted above, Wurtman advocates snacking on high-glycemic-index foods, such as candies or cookies, to promote serotonin synthesis in the brain and resulting feelings of satiety. The Hellers, working from a different theoretical basis, point to the facts that carbohydrates cause the secretion of insulin from the pancreas and that insulin secretion is responsible for lowering blood sugar levels. Foods with a high glycemic index will result in a more rapid release of insulin and a correspondingly sharper drop in blood sugar levels. The Hellers have suggested that this drop in blood sugar level is responsible for further carbohydrate cravings, which represent an attempt to restore blood sugar levels to normal. The Hellers hypothesize that carbohydrate cravers may have different patterns of insulin secretion in response to eating carbohydrate-rich foods than those who don't crave carbohydrates. Snacking on high-glycemic-index carbohydrate-rich snacks during the day will result in excessive insulin secretion, according to the Hellers, and this in turn will lead to craving and bingeing that will undermine the diet. Specific details about the Carbohydrate Addict's Diet® are provided in the "Resources" section. In light of the opposing views about carbohydrates and snacking, I would encourage you to evaluate for yourself which of these contradictory strategies works *for you.*

The Paleolithic Diet: Balancing Carbohydrates with Protein

A diet based on a higher percentage of protein and a lower percentage of carbohydrate than in the first two diets I have discussed, has been suggested by Dr. Barry Sears of Bio/Syn, in Marblehead, Massachusetts. I have called this the Paleolithic Diet because the proportions of carbohydrate, protein, and fat in this diet resemble those thought to have been present in the diet of primitive humans. According to Drs. S. Boyd Eaton and Melvin Konner of Emory University in Atlanta, who published their findings in the *New England Journal of Medicine,* the Paleolithic Diet differs from the diet recommended by the U.S. Senate Select Committee, in that it is lower in carbohydrate and fat and higher in protein. The first two diets discussed above are much closer in the relative proportions of their major nutrients to those recommended by the Select Committee.

Sears's diet was brought to my attention by a fellow psychiatrist,

Dr. Michael Norden from Seattle, Washington, who has successfully treated several SAD patients with a diet based on Sears's ideas. As Norden puts it, "We must get away from a 'Let them eat cake' philosophy." He believes, as do the Hellers, that although carbohydrate-rich foods provide SAD patients with an immediate boost, they pay for this boost later on with enhanced feelings of fatigue and renewed cravings. These cravings are reduced, in Norden's experience, by reducing the levels of dietary carbohydrates and balancing them out with protein—in other words, providing a higher proportion of protein to carbohydrate in all meals. If you want to try a diet that resembles that of your Paleolithic forebears and is in line with Norden's successful experiences you might like to try the third series of diets provided in the "Resources" section. These were created by Bette Flax, a dietician with whom I have collaborated in trying to help patients keep their cravings in check.

Sears and the Hellers agree in certain respects and disagree in others. Both regard the excessive stimulation of insulin secretion by carbohydrates as potentially undermining of attempts at weight loss. They also point out that there is a balance between insulin, a hormone responsible for storing glucose in the body, and glucagon, a hormone responsible for breaking down glucose stores and releasing glucose into the bloodstream. Sears has drawn attention to the results of studies showing that the proportions of carbohydrate to protein in the diet can influence the ratio of insulin to glucagon in the blood, and that this in turn can influence how hungry you are (and how difficult it will therefore be for you to diet).

Sears disagrees with the Hellers that a Reward Meal® is a good idea, and considers a day that ends in such a carbohydrate-rich feast as "two steps forward and one step back." He also advises against high-glycemic-index carbohydrates, which are encouraged by the Hellers in their Reward Meal® and by Judith Wurtman in her snacks. Norden concedes that it is not realistic to expect that SAD patients on Sears's diet will not want to "cheat" by eating carbohydrate-rich foods from time to time. Perhaps what both Wurtman and the Hellers have done, in their different ways, is to recognize that for carbohydrate cravers or addicts, such "cheating" has to be accepted as inevitable and that it should be incorporated as an integral part of the diet (either in the form of carbohydrate-rich snacks or a Reward Meal®), rather than be regarded as a failure in compliance. In my experience, this is wise advice not only nutritionally, but also in relieving the dieter's chronic feelings of guilt at repeated "failures." In developed countries such as ours, many of us are blessed—and cursed—with too many good things to eat. Cravings abound, and abstention is probably unrealistic.

Whichever of the three dietary approaches you choose, you will probably be able to stick to it most successfully if you allow yourself to eat some carbohydrate-rich foods in a controlled fashion.

Fiber

No section on diet would be complete without a few words about dietary fiber. The virtues of dietary fiber have been widely stressed, and rightly so. In experimental animals, the same number of calories, administered with fiber, causes less weight gain than if the fiber is omitted. Fiber has also been associated with a decreased rate of bowel cancer. You will find that the menus and recipes provided in "Resources" are relatively high in fiber. It occurs naturally in cereals (most notably bran), vegetables, and fruit.

Summary

In summary, there have been major advances in our thinking about dietary options to help carbohydrate addicts to keep their cravings— and their weight—in check. I have outlined three separate programs. Two of these approaches (those of the Hellers, and of Sears) emphasize that carbohydrate intake should be limited, at least for part of the day. Two of these approaches (those of Judith Wurtman and of the Hellers) recommend that favorite foods be eaten, within certain limits and guidelines. As I have mentioned before, different approaches may work for different people. Or you may find it useful to combine different elements of the various approaches to create a dietary program that works for you.

Stress Management

If you are a seasonal person, you have the advantage of being able to predict that at some times of the year your energy level will be low, and you may find it difficult to accomplish certain tasks; at other times of the year it will be high, and you may be able to tackle all sorts of things. You can use this information to regulate your stress level throughout the year. Some stresses are unpredictable and cannot be planned, but many can be anticipated. These include purchasing a new house, moving, starting a new job, beginning a major undertaking, and many other projects that we impose upon ourselves. Beware of setting spring deadlines and delivery dates on projects. Be careful not to take on too many commitments during the summer months, when you are feeling good and expansive, to prevent yourself from becoming overwhelmed during the winter. Undertake difficult projects at that time of year when you feel best. For example, if you find entertaining difficult during the winter months, and have social obligations, perhaps you would be better off tackling them in the summer. By the time winter rolls around, you will then feel free to entertain only if you really wish to do so.

Many people use the summer months for the creative aspects of their work, and the winter months to consolidate and work on more humdrum tasks. Our original seasonal patient, Herb Kern, adopted this pattern. An engineer for Bell Laboratories, he conceived his best ideas and conducted his most exciting experiments in the summer; he then wrote up his data—a more routine task—in the winter months. There is evidence that some famous composers, most notably George Frederick Handel and Gustav Mahler, were seasonal and did most of their composing in the summer months.

Anticipate those predictable burdens that come up in the winter and try to handle them in advance. These may include such chores as Christmas or Hanukkah shopping, which could be done before the seasonal low sets in. This has the added benefit of allowing you to avoid crowds of last-minute shoppers. You can even wrap gifts, buy your cards, and address the envelopes well ahead of time. If you want to write that long note to people with whom you communicate perhaps only once a year, a letter in late August might serve just as well to catch them up on the news as would one in December. Such advance planning can go a long way toward taking the burden out of the holidays, and allowing you to enjoy the social aspects of the season without feeling overwhelmed by the duties that go along with them.

Other ways of preparing for the winter may include cooking large batches of your favorite foods and freezing them in small portions, stored in containers that can go straight into the microwave. This can be done both at the beginning of the winter and on weekends during the winter, minimizing the amount of cooking you have to do during the week. If you work during the day, you may find it helpful to eat your major meal at lunchtime, thereby saving yourself from having to cook it when you get home at the end of a long day. Also, anticipate your clothing needs before winter sets in. The last thing that most people feel like doing when they are depressed is going shopping for clothes and having to look at themselves in all those mirrors.

Paying for help and services can be a wise use of money in the wintertime. You can use some of that money you are not spending on the socializing and shopping you do in the summer to pay others to help you with difficult chores. Such solutions might include taking your clothes to the laundry, hiring a cleaning service, and buying take-out dinners. Parents can have a particularly hard time meeting the demands of small children when they are feeling depressed, and paying for extra child care (or home care) can provide a great deal of relief. If you have some money to spare, think of ways in which you may be able to solve a problem by hiring someone else to do chores, such as grocery shopping and housekeeping. You may find yourself coming up with some rather creative solutions.

Sometimes feelings of guilt can be an obstacle to your getting the help you need. To help you feel comfortable paying for services you may feel you should be providing yourself, remind yourself that you are not being lazy, neglectful, and all the other derisive adjectives that depressed people are so good at using on themselves. Reduced levels of energy and motivation, and inability to cope, are key symptoms of depression. Even though you may be doing many things to reduce these symptoms, these measures may not be completely effective. It is therefore very important to reduce your stresses and commitments; if paying others to help out is financially possible, it is worth it for your mental health.

Getting help can also save money in the long run. By paying someone to take care of certain chores, you may have more time and energy to devote to your job, and thereby may manage to hold on to it. Overloading your boat with too many things may cause it to capsize. For example, it is false economy to skimp on help with chores if your job is at stake.

A major problem for depressed people is concentrating and remembering things. Many seasonal people have developed methods of coping with these difficulties. One woman I know has developed some tricks to help her remember things in the winter. For example, she keeps a very careful calendar, writing everything down, and doesn't assume that she will remember things that she would recall easily in the summertime. She cross-indexes the people she relies on for help of various kinds under a section "H" for "Help." This section includes addresses and phone numbers of plumbers, home repair people, and even her doctors, whose names she often forgets in the winter. She leaves notes for herself on the back door, where she will see them as she goes out of the house, and writes notes to herself late at night about what she needs to do the following morning. She also notes down other information, such as friends' birthdays and directions to people's homes.

For many SAD patients in their fifties and sixties, retirement offers a particular type of relief from stress. One man in this age range, who had worked for many years as an architect, told me, "I have been free of all SAD symptoms for the past three years since I retired, and I recommend it to everyone." Retirement, like relocation, is a major life decision that involves many considerations, including the loss of a meaningful job, reduced income, and having to structure the days that were previously filled up with work. The dilemma was articulated recently by a husband and wife who recently consulted me regarding how best to manage the wife's SAD symptoms. She had been a head nurse on a busy unit for many years and was finding it increasingly difficult to function effectively during the winter. Her husband, also a professional and very supportive of his wife, was concerned that she would feel even worse if she lost the daily structure that her work afforded her. When I explained that the work appeared to be generating more stress than comfort, his wife expressed great relief at the idea of either quitting her job or giving up the head nurse position and working part-time in a way that gave her more control over her hours. When he heard how she felt, her husband noted that they would have more than enough money to enable her to do that, and he supported her decision. I have little doubt that when the wife is able to sleep in, get outdoors in the middle of the day and enjoy the winter sunshine, work as much as she pleases, and have the freedom to pursue other interests (long put on hold), she will deal much more easily with her winter symptoms.

As far as stress management is concerned, the bottom line is this: *Nurture your resources and use your creativity to find shortcuts and ways to conserve your energy to help keep you going through the down season.* There must be all sorts of other strategies for minimizing stress, which I have not as yet come across. See if you can discover some new ones yourself.

Sleep Restriction

One surprising way to handle the sluggishness associated with SAD may be to sleep less. This may seem odd, since we usually think of sleep as refreshing and as providing extra energy, but it may actually increase depression. The writer Robert Burton (1577–1640), in his classic *The Anatomy of Melancholy*, noted that

> sleep . . . may do more harm than good in that phlegmatick, swinish, cold, and sluggish melancholy. . . . It dulls the spirits, if overmuch, and . . . fills the head full of gross humours, causeth distillations, rheums, great stores of excrements in the brain and in all other parts.

Some modern researchers agree with Burton's sentiments and have shown that sleep deprivation can have antidepressant effects.

Forcing yourself to wake up at 7:00 or 8:00 A.M. instead of 10:00 or 11:00 may have a salutary effect on your mood and energy level.

Support Groups

Just as patients with numerous other conditions have found support and comfort in associating with others who are similarly afflicted, so some patients with SAD have been helped by associations that deal with SAD in particular and mood disorders in general. Several of these organizations are listed in the "Resources" section of this book. Patients who have been involved with these organizations report many benefits from this association, including access to the latest information about the condition and its treatments; the support and friendship of fellow sufferers; and devices and strategies that others have found to cope with the problem. If you want to start a chapter of one of the support groups in your area, you can write to the national head offices whose addresses are provided in "Resources" for information as to how to go about doing so.

Acceptance

Sometimes, even with the best therapy, mood control is not perfect. As long as the lows are not too low or too long, a measure of acceptance can sometimes be very therapeutic. I counsel acceptance only after every reasonable means to counteract depressive symptoms has been tried. For example, I have one patient whose moods have not been successfully controlled, despite all manner of treatments. Bright light helps her, but only to a modest degree. We meet at intervals, discuss possible approaches, and evaluate new ideas for treatment as they come up. But she has reached a degree of acceptance of her condition and is not willing to try new approaches that appear to hold little advantage over those she has tried before. I support her acceptance while we both search for a better long-term solution.

Acceptance often comes slowly, bit by bit, rather than all at once. There is a great temptation each year, as spring arrives, to think that the problem is over, only to have it reappear again the following fall. I have seen many reactions to this familiar experience. For example, one woman I know has had SAD for the past fifteen years. It was first diagnosed six years ago, and she has been treated with light therapy, antidepressant medications, and psychotherapy, with considerable success. Her depressions no longer disable her as they used to, but she is still less energetic, enthusiastic, and effective in the winter than in the summer. Last winter, for the first time, she felt enraged at the limitations the condition imposes on her—the way in which her life seems to flip-flop between feeling good and feeling depressed every six months. This anger is one more phase in her slow journey toward acceptance.

It can be useful to regard some degree of fluctuation in energy, mood, and ability to function as part of the ordinary ebb and flow of life. This idea is often in opposition to our ideal for ourselves. Many of us expect to function happily and at peak levels at all times. By expecting this, we often place unreasonable demands on ourselves, which would require machine-like efficiency to carry out. A great measure of contentment can be attained by accepting the inevitable. This is perhaps more in keeping with Eastern than with Western thinking. For example, an ancient Chinese text, the Nei Ching, advises people to behave in certain specific ways during each season; it recommends, for example, that during winter people should go to bed early and get up late in the morning. The message is to yield to the physical and emotional changes that come with the changing seasons, rather than to oppose them. After you have done all you can to reverse the unpleasant and disabling symptoms of SAD, that is not bad advice. But before resigning yourself to your problems, there are certain specific types of treatment that should be tried—most notably, medications and psychotherapy. These treatments are discussed in the chapters that follow.

There are many different types of approaches you can take to help yourself cope with winter depression (or, for that matter, any type of depression). A first step requires the recognition that the difficulties associated with depression—low energy level, pessimism, lack of motivation, low self-esteem, and withdrawal, to name just a few—are symptoms of an illness, not flaws in your character. They require understanding rather than judgment and condemnation, serious attention rather than denial and minimization. The first person who needs to understand them and take them seriously is you, the depressed patient. This is helpful in itself. In addition, if you are a seasonal depressive, changing the environment may be quite beneficial. Brighten your living and work areas; travel to sunny places in the winter; or, if all else fails, relocate permanently to a better climate.

Exercise moderately and regularly in a way you find enjoyable. Find a companion to join you, and help each other stick to your routine. Diet sensibly. Don't deprive yourself of carbohydrates, and try different dietary approaches until you find one that works for you. Limit your stresses. Don't make commitments during your summer highs that you are unable to keep in the winter. Anticipate predictable chores and use your creativity to figure out solutions to them ahead of time. Keep informed. New things are being discovered all the time—and yesterday's insoluble problem may have a solution today. If you're the kind of person who derives comfort from others who are in a situation similar to yours, join a support group of fellow sufferers, or establish your own. Finally, *accept* that which you cannot change. Life has its ups and downs, and no one understands that better than the SAD patient.

Despite all our modern discoveries, it is still valuable to look back at ancient wisdom. As far as SAD is concerned, no ancient writer offered more cogent advice than the physician A. Cornelius Celsus provided to melancholics during the reign of the Roman emperor Tiberius:

> Live in rooms full of light
> Avoid heavy food
> Be moderate in the drinking of wine
> Take massage, baths, exercise, and gymnastics
> Fight insomnia with gentle rocking or the sound of running water
> Change surroundings and take long journeys
> Strictly avoid frightening ideas
> Indulge in cheerful conversation and amusements
> Listen to music

CHAPTER 8

Psychotherapy and SAD

For many people with seasonal difficulties, psychotherapy has proven to be invaluable. Indeed, most of the seasonal people I have described in this book have received psychotherapy at some time in their lives, and most have found it to be beneficial. For example, one woman in her fifties recently sought psychotherapy to cope with the aftermath of a divorce; for one young man, therapy was valuable in dealing with difficulties that arose at work. Others have found it extremely helpful in understanding and coming to terms with events that happened in their childhood, but that continue to exert a detrimental influence on their adult lives. However, not everyone with a seasonal problem needs or will benefit from psychotherapy. How do you decide when therapy is necessary?

Having made the decision to enter therapy, what sort should you seek? There are dozens of different types. Which ones will work best? And how do you find and choose a therapist—someone in whom you can put your trust? You generally tell your therapist your deepest and most private thoughts. How do you know whether you can trust him or her to treat these precious thoughts and feelings with respect? How do you know whether he or she is competent, will understand your problem, and will know the appropriate thing to say or do about it?

Once in therapy, how do you manage to integrate psychotherapy with light therapy or antidepressant medications? How do you know whether the therapy is working? All these are difficult questions, yet they are often foremost in the minds of those in search of some form of psychological help. I attempt to answer them below.

When Should You Consider Entering Therapy?

Suppose you suffer from winter depressions. We now know that these often result from light deficiency. Let us therefore assume that you seek out a therapist qualified to advise you on light therapy, undergo the treatment, and find that this takes care of many (if not all) of your symptoms. In addition, you follow all the advice outlined in Chapter 7. We can consider two opposite outcomes, though of course there are many gradations in between. In the one outcome you feel good. Finally you have an explanation for all these seasonal difficulties; moreover, you have a way of treating and controlling them. This frees you to get on with your life—to love and to work, as Sigmund Freud would say—and also to enjoy yourself. Your relationships grow stronger and more fulfilling; you are successful at work. You are justifiably proud of your accomplishments and enjoy the fruits of your labor. And you even find some free time to do whatever it is that you enjoy the most. Do you need psychotherapy? Of course not.

Now let us imagine a different scenario. Your seasonal symptoms have responded. You no longer sink to the depths of depression, familiar to you for so many years. All should be well, but it is not. Something is amiss. Perhaps you feel stuck where you are. You have been following certain routines and activities that once were fulfilling but now aren't. Some change is necessary, but nothing suggests itself to you. Persisting in the same course gets you nowhere in this mission. At this point, psychotherapy can be beneficial. It can help you define the problem and search within yourself for solutions that may be very difficult to find on your own.

I am reminded of a fly trying to escape from a room by banging against a window. He does not realize that the door behind him is open. He can see the world he longs for stretched out in front of him, but his ignorance dooms him to bang his head repeatedly against the windowpane. Fruitless, repetitive behavior of this kind is commonly found in people, too, and can be helped by psychotherapy. The example of a woman who gets into a series of relationships with men who mistreat her has become almost a cliché in recent years. However, like all clichés, this one is grounded in reality, and the pattern is all too familiar. So is the situation of the man or woman who repeatedly fails, just when success appears to be within reach. It has often been said that the neurotic does not remember, but repeats; most clinicians have seen this pattern many times.

Freud provided insights into the compulsion to repeat, tracing it back to childhood events. An image that comes to us from our age of computers is that some bug has been incorporated into the software that causes the program to make the same error again and again. To follow this analogy a little further, insight-oriented psychotherapy can be seen as an attempt to track down the problem in the software and reprogram it to succeed rather than to fail. If we return to the vignette of the fly and the windowpane, we can compare the process of psychotherapy to showing the fly that there is another way out of the room—through the open door. A wonderful, therapeutic sense of freedom accompanies a new way of seeing a problem and new strategies for dealing with it.

One type of programming error that is frequently responsible for unhappiness involves our self-esteem. In growing up, we may have incorporated incorrect or derogatory images and opinions of ourselves into the software of our brains, and these may continue to haunt us into adult life. Apart from our upbringing and early childhood experiences, there are other influences that shape our self-esteem from both the outside world and our own internal experiences. For example, suffering from repeated depressions—long stretches of inability to function properly—can have long-term detrimental effects on self-esteem and self-image. Even after these depressions are treated, self-esteem problems may persist, and may require psychotherapy in order to be properly resolved.

Many examples of people with self-esteem problems come to mind. "Melissa," an artist in her early forties, is a case in point. Intelligent, talented, attractive, and with a charming personality, she nonetheless grew up believing that she should aspire to be an empty-headed blonde. According to the voices of her upbringing, women were supposed to be pretty but vacuous, available to support the men in their lives. Signs of burgeoning talent were viewed as danger signals, which might scare off eligible men. Women were meant to conceal their talent and intelligence and to draw men out. After graduating from high school, Melissa went on to get a degree in counseling, choosing this more "appropriate" profession over the artistic areas that were her real love. Two marriages followed, which were unhappy, except that the second one resulted in a lovely daughter.

After entering the Seasonal Studies Program at the NIMH and having her winter depression treated with light therapy, Melissa entered into psychotherapy. In the course of therapy, she was able to understand how she had been programmed to believe she had to become someone at odds with the person she really wanted to be. Therefore, no matter what she did or how successful she was at it, it didn't feel right to her. She was a fine mother, a talented artist, a good friend to many, and a delightful person, but things still didn't feel right. She was not fulfilling those early programs and her parents' expectations of her. Once she understood this in therapy, she was able to change her expectations of herself and recognize that these new expectations, which were quite compatible with what she truly wanted to do, were legitimate. Psychotherapy has been a liberating experience for her. Whereas light reversed the symptoms of her winter depression (something that no amount of psychotherapy would have been able to do), psychotherapy helped her understand and come to terms with problems from her past (something that no amount of light therapy, by itself, would have been able to accomplish).

Melissa's story is one of many. I have frequently seen such successful and liberating effects of good psychotherapy. Her story also shows how well psychotherapy and other forms of therapy can work together. If there are significant problems of the sort outlined above, which persist after treatment with light therapy or medications, psychotherapy should be strongly considered.

Types of Therapy

There are many different types of therapy available, and, depending on where you live, therapists may be more or less abundant. How does the consumer choose? Some of the more commonly practiced types of therapy are summarized below. More detailed information can be found by consulting the "Further Reading" list in the "Resources" section at the back of the book. I should emphasize that most skilled therapists combine elements derived from different schools of therapy, much as a skilled chef would combine different ingredients to prepare a gourmet meal. I am generally quite suspicious of people who believe that only one narrow school of thought carries the key to curing all psychological problems. People are far too diverse and complicated for such simple solutions.

Elements common to all therapies are understanding, support, and provision of hope. These elements are critical. It is very important for a depressed person to feel understood by someone who has seen other depressed people and has helped them through their illness to recovery; to know that there is someone out there who understands how bad depression can get; who is available through the dark days. Depression is a condition where hope is lacking. The present seems bleak, the future even bleaker. These are symptoms of the illness, rather than realistic appraisals of the situation and its prospects. The therapist needs to make this clear to the patient, as well as to explain why there is good reason to be hopeful—and indeed there is. Depression is almost always reversible. Beyond these general points, there are certain specific types of therapy.

Cognitive Therapy

Cognitive therapy, developed by Dr. Aaron Beck, is quite helpful in SAD. It is based on the idea that a depressed person's thinking is distorted, and that this in turn leads to depression. During one SAD patient's depressed periods she would feel stupid, even though she had tested very well in school and had all sorts of academic laurels to her credit. When she became depressed, she believed that she was a fraud and that teachers had given her good grades because they liked her, not because she had deserved them. Depressed people often describe themselves as frauds who have managed to trick people into thinking that they are smart or talented, but who eventually will be exposed and shown up for the incompetent individuals they believe they are.

According to the principles of cognitive therapy, depressed feelings result from distorted thoughts. Pointing this distorted thinking out to the depressed individual often helps the depressed feelings go away. So the following imaginary conversation might take place between a patient and therapist in a therapy session:

PATIENT: I am a fraud; I didn't deserve all those compliments.

THERAPIST: If you are a fraud, how did you manage to trick so many people?

PATIENT: I'm just crafty. Mom always told me I used to try to get away with things.

THERAPIST: But you have tricked so many different people over so many years. Is it not possible that you were not tricking them after all—that their perceptions were accurate—and that now you are tricking yourself into believing that you do not have the talents that must have been necessary in order to achieve what you have?

PATIENT: Yes, but I feel incompetent. I can't do anything properly.

THERAPIST: Well, let's review what you've done this past week and check whether your perception is correct in this regard.

The therapist then reviews the week, and it soon becomes clear that the patient has done many things quite competently. Perhaps the patient has not met his or her own high expectations at every turn, but the outcome is quite acceptable. And anyway, how could anyone perform at peak level every single week, during all seasons? The therapist invites the patient to examine all these distortions systematically, and in so doing can help him or her change them, which may result in a lessening of the depressed feelings.

In dealing with people who have SAD, part of cognitive therapy involves pointing out that many of the difficulties they experience are symptoms of their seasonal condition; that these symptoms have an explanation; that they can be reversed; and that they do not reflect character flaws. Depressed people find all sorts of insults to hurl at themselves: incompetent, lazy, bad, immature, and deserving of punishment, to name just a few. The depressed person is generally very unfair to himself or herself, and part of the therapist's role is to point this out.

To the credit of those working in the field of cognitive therapy, they have actually studied this treatment scientifically and have demonstrated its effectiveness with certain depressed patients. Such systematic studies have not been performed for many other types of therapy.

Behavior Therapy

In behavior therapy, as its name implies, the focus is on behavior. Its theoretical origins come from work on learning. Like the dogs of the famous Russian psychologist, Pavlov, who were conditioned by the presentation of food to salivate at the sound of a bell, we have been conditioned to respond in certain ways as a result of the experiences we have had. In some cases, these learned behaviors may actually make our problems worse. For example, as a result of feeling repeatedly depressed, a person may avoid getting together with people and may become socially isolated. Such isolation will deprive him or her of the pleasures and satisfactions that may come from human interactions, which may well make the symptoms of depression worse.

In treating a patient, the therapist may focus on maladaptive behaviors, such as not calling friends or allowing bills and other chores to pile up until they feel overwhelming. It's up to the therapist to help the patient face and tackle these tasks. Behaviors regarded by both patient and therapist as constructive or positive are rewarded. For example, a patient and therapist may construct a program where the patient goes shopping for a long-desired item as a reward for taking care of the bills. There are all sorts of variations on this theme. Behavior therapy can be particularly helpful for individuals who are phobic of certain situations—for example, flying, taking elevators, or being in crowds. The patient is gradually encouraged to confront these situations in an attempt to make them less anxiety-provoking.

Behavior therapy is sometimes combined with cognitive therapy, and the patient may be given "homework" assignments, which are aimed at dealing with both behavioral problems and cognitive distortions. Such cognitive problems may inhibit actions that could make the patient feel better. For example, someone looking for work might think, "I'm not good enough for that job, so there's no point in my applying for it." A man who is interested in a woman might think, "She'll never accept my invitation; I may as well not ask her." By helping the patient to face these fears and negative thoughts, which are often not founded on fact, the therapist encourages the patient to take some risks and to do things that might make him or her feel better. A great deal can be accomplished by combining cognitive and behavior therapy.

Insight-Oriented Therapy

Insight-oriented therapy was first proposed by Freud, who pointed out the value of acquiring insight into our unconscious processes. Although this type of therapy is extremely difficult to study scientifically in a way that meets the rigorous requirements of modern clinical research, it is the experience of trained observers that insight-oriented therapy can be extremely helpful.

I have seen people benefit tremendously from psychotherapy—not just because of having someone to talk to, but as a result of acquiring specific insight into their problems. Therapists carefully share this insight with patients, who are encouraged to use it and thereby reach a new and more useful understanding of their problems.

Many of my patients with SAD have benefited greatly from insight-oriented psychotherapy. For example, one woman in her mid-forties went into psychotherapy to help resolve the guilt she felt at having been the only healthy child out of six siblings. A middle-aged man with SAD struggled for years on his Ph.D. dissertation but was unable to complete it—not because of any intellectual limitation, but because it raised anxiety in him about competing with his father, who had been much less successful than he had.

There have been many recent advances in psychotherapy, as in other forms of medicine. Traumas as apparently different as combat stress, rape and child sexual abuse have sharpened our understanding and appreciation of the long-term consequences of psychological injury. There has been substantial debate as to whether Freud and his followers did justice to the serious injuries of those abused in childhood. Although Freud was sympathetic to these early traumas, interpretations based on his theories frequently sought to resolve the symptoms resulting from these traumas by focusing too much on the notion that the symptoms arose from the drives and needs of the patient (the child's own sexual or aggressive feelings), rather than on the symptoms as predictable psychological consequences of the perpetrator's behavior. Such skewing of emphasis has often resulted in a patient's feeling personally responsible for these early traumas and missing the relief that comes with acknowledgment of the reality of the injury. Modern psychotherapists should be familiar with these new developments. In certain situations, various techniques, such as imaging and hypnosis, may be brought into the therapy to assist in the retrieval of early traumatic memories. But this should always be done in the context of a solid alliance between patient and therapist, and the primary focus should always be on the stability and well-being of the patient.

Other Types of Therapy; Cautions

Other types of therapy that may be helpful include group, family, and couple therapy. The SAD patient's problems affect—and are affected by—the people in his or her life. Often, bringing these people into the therapeutic process can accelerate improvement. No doubt there are other helpful psychotherapeutic strategies, but my goal here is not to be exhaustive. Rather, I would like to emphasize that lights and medications do not solve all the psychological problems in all cases of SAD. Some people may find psychotherapy, in conjunction with these other treatments, to be extremely useful. But psychotherapy is not necessary for everybody. If light treatment or antidepressant medications leave a person feeling happy, fulfilled, and free to live as he or she chooses, there is no need for psychotherapy.

Like all effective treatments, psychotherapy is not without hazards. Probing around in a person's past and stirring up buried secrets, although extremely helpful in some cases, is not universally so. Psychotherapy can amplify feelings of depression and anxiety, and it should only be performed by a skilled and properly trained therapist. The therapist should also be familiar with the biological treatments of depression, so that the patient is not allowed to spin his or her wheels discussing childhood conflicts while a raging depression goes untreated. This situation remains unfortunately all too common.

Choosing a Psychotherapist

It is extremely important that you choose your therapist carefully. It is surprising to think that many people who might take several days researching a car purchase—consulting consumer reports and friends, going to several dealers, and test-driving cars—might head straight for the Yellow Pages to find a therapist. A therapist is someone with whom you need to be able to share your most important personal secrets. That person's judgment, training, and suitability for *you* should be the primary basis for your choice. How do you find such a person?

I believe that recommendations from other professionals are the best guide. Find a health professional whom you respect and who has some knowledge of you as a person—a medical doctor, psychologist, or social worker. Explain to this person, briefly, the type of problem you are dealing with. Then ask his or her opinion as to who might be best suited to helping you. If possible, I would encourage you to ask more than one professional, to see whether the same name appears on more than one list. Once you have obtained one or two names, set up an appointment to interview each therapist. He or she should, of course, ask you questions about your problem. Consider whether the questions are on target. Does the therapist appear to be exploring the problem thoroughly, asking about it from different angles? Does he or she seem to understand what you are saying—not just intellectually, but also emotionally? Does he or she appear to be empathic—that is, on the same wavelength as you are? These early impressions are important, and should be taken into consideration in making your decision.

You are certainly entitled to ask the therapist questions. What is his or her background and training? Does he or she subscribe to any particular school of therapy? If these questions are asked in an ordinary, matter-of-fact manner, they should be met with ordinary, matter-of-fact replies. Any defensiveness about the replies, questions in response to the questions, such as "Why do you want to know?"; or interpretations, such as "It seems as though you suspect my competence," might reasonably raise your suspicion about insecurity on the part of the therapist.

At the end of the initial consultation, the therapist should provide a formulation of the problem—a diagnosis and some clarification of the issues—as well as specific recommendations about treatment. Some-times, however, if the situation appears to be complicated, more than one meeting may be necessary before the therapist is ready to provide a formulation and recommendations. It's important for you to consider this formulation and these recommendations as just *one* way to see the problem. There may be other ways to see it as well, and you may wish to seek other opinions before making up your mind about which therapist you want to see.

These early impressions and experiences are particularly impor-tant. Later on, when the therapy is underway, you may find yourself having all sorts of feelings toward the therapist. Many of these may be based not only on the therapist's behavior, but also on a reluctance to tackle painful and difficult psychological issues or on experiences that you have had earlier in your life. These experiences, known as "resistance" and "transference," were described first by Freud. Resistance represents the unconscious reluctance to face painful thoughts, feelings, or memories that have been covered up to protect you psychologically. Although this cover-up may be helpful for a while, ultimately it may prove harmful, and there may be some value in uncovering the psychological material. Transference is the process whereby feelings toward important people in your life are transferred to the therapist or analyst, who has actually done nothing to elicit them.

When you are dealing with resistance and transference, you may be tempted to leave therapy in order to run away from these new insights and discoveries. A skilled therapist will usually be able to help you feel safe and less threatened by the painful material being uncovered. Impulsive actions on your part while this is going on are usually best avoided until the matter is explored and understood. If these feelings persist for too long, however—and only you can tell how long to persevere—it may be that the therapy is not working well for you. At that point a consultation with another therapist is often worthwhile. In choosing a consultant, try to find someone with special expertise in your type of problem. It is probably best to obtain a referral from someone other than your current therapist, so that the second opinion is as independent as possible.

CHAPTER 9

Antidepressant medications

The administration of antidepressant medications is a subtle art. Prescribing them is not quite the same as prescribing laxatives or blood pressure pills. Antidepressants can—and should—change the way people taking them feel, the way they see their world and themselves. Proper use of them requires close communication between doctor and patient. The psychiatrist should help the patient interpret the internal changes that are taking place, and should use this information to choose the right medication or combination of medications, as well as the best dosage. It's a tricky business and should be undertaken only by someone who knows what he or she is doing.

People have all sorts of reasonable concerns about taking antidepressant medications. If you are one of these people, you may have been counseled all your life to avoid and suspect drugs that make you feel good. Now, along comes a doctor who tells you that taking such drugs may be the very thing to do. Will the drugs harm you? Will you feel too good and get hooked on them? If you feel better, is it a result of the pills rather than your own efforts? You may always have been told to take responsibility for your life, to examine the roots of your problems and solve them from the ground up. Now someone is telling you not to worry about roots and origins. Just take the pills and you'll feel better. Can it be so simple?

This chapter deals with many of these common concerns about taking antidepressant medications. For those who have already decided to take these medications or are currently being treated with them, there is also a section on the most commonly used drugs, their advantages, and their side effects.

Common Concerns About Taking Antidepressant Medications

The thought of taking a mood-altering drug often triggers associations with drug peddlers, to whom we all have been advised to "just say no." So why should anyone react differently toward a doctor who suggests antidepressant medications? There are several important differences between these two scenarios. Recreational drugs are taken in an uncontrolled way to change the mood of the moment, thus providing an immediate "high." These drugs are addictive, and withdrawal often results in serious symptoms, including crashing depressions. Antidepressant drugs do not generally cause an immediate "high," nor can they be regarded as addictive. With recreational drugs, one often needs increasing amounts to get the same mood-altering effect; this is not so with antidepressants. Since their introduction over thirty years ago, they have been shown to be highly effective in providing long-term relief for the symptoms of depression.

Some people may feel that taking an antidepressant is the easy way out, evading the responsibility for finding the root of the problem and solving it. This idea stems from their assumption that somehow the depression is their fault, a result of something they have done. This concern is especially common because one of the symptoms of depression is for people to feel excessively responsible for their situation. It is therefore logical for them to think that they should be able to fix it themselves. However, most experts now agree that clinical depression is caused by a biochemical abnormality with a genetic basis.

If depression is genetic and biochemical, how can it be the patients' fault? And why shouldn't they treat the problem as they would any other medical illness? Would people with diabetes, for example, consider giving themselves daily insulin injections to be comparable to shooting up regularly with heroin? Or, for that matter, would they think that they were responsible for their problem with producing insulin and that they should figure out a way to fix it themselves?

Many patients are afraid that when they take antidepressant medications, they will lose control of themselves or their thinking. They are concerned that after taking these medications they will become different and lose their identity. In addressing this concern, it is important to realize that a person feels different about himself or herself when depressed, as compared with when he or she feels well. Which of these two sets of perceptions is the real person—the sad and weary soul who feels that he or she has never done anything worthwhile and doesn't deserve anything, or the fundamentally healthy and intact individual who happens to be suffering a temporary setback? One of the most painful things about depression is that it changes a person's self-image. In my experience, when a patient has been effectively treated with antidepressants, the result is much closer to the "self" that the person would prefer to be, than to the depressed individual he or she was before.

One reason why it is difficult for patients to accept the medical model of depression is that there is no good laboratory test for it. This is where a comparison to diabetes or high blood pressure falls short. In diabetes, high levels of glucose are present in the urine and the blood. This can be detected simply by dipping a stick into urine and watching the chemicals on the tip change color. In a case of high blood pressure, the abnormal numbers can simply be read off the blood pressure machine. But in a case of depression, laboratory tests generally come back negative. In the past few decades there has been considerable excitement about hormonal tests for depression, but after an initial wave of enthusiasm, these proved undependable. So for now, all that remains to the diagnostician is the patient's account of his or her story; accounts by the patient's relatives; a track record of the damage caused by the illness, such as failing grades, poor job performance, and unsuccessful relationships; and how the patient actually looks. At first glance, this may seem like slim evidence on which to make the diagnosis of a psychiatric disorder, and an insufficient basis for prescribing antidepressant medications. However, the trained clinician is generally able to diagnose depression easily and reliably. Sometimes just a glance across the waiting room, the angle of a person's gait, or a few sentences articulated over the telephone are enough to give the clinician a good idea of how a depressed person is doing.

The brain is an elusive organ to study. Its processes have not as yet yielded their secrets to modern technology in the same way as those of the pancreas, heart, kidney, and liver have done. This is bound to change as technology advances. But despite its elusiveness, researchers who attempt to study the brain are at an advantage over students of these other organs, in that a person can directly report on events going on within the mind. Feelings, thoughts, sensations, and impulses all reflect underlying brain processes. These experiences can be communicated to a clinician and monitored over time. In my experience, these clues provide sufficient evidence for the diagnosis and treatment of most cases of depression.

Many people are concerned about how long they will have to remain on medications. This is easier to predict for patients with SAD than for those with other forms of depression, because SAD is usually a self-limiting condition. When summer comes, symptoms generally resolve. In some cases, however, medications may be helpful even in the summertime. Another concern that I have heard from time to time is a fear that antidepressant medications will cause some permanent physical change or damage. Fortunately, chronic side effects are rare and there is no evidence whatsoever that any long-term damage to the brain occurs.

Side Effects of Medications

Concerns about side effects are common and valid. People vary greatly in their propensity to develop side effects. On one end of the spectrum is the individual who develops none at all; on the other end is the person who develops them toward a host of different antidepressants, at dosages so low that no beneficial effects are possible. Because of this wide variability, a psychiatrist often chooses to start with a low dosage of the medication of choice and to increase the amount after seeing how well the patient tolerates the low dosage.

The specific side effects of antidepressant medications differ from drug to drug and are discussed below at greater length under each specific heading. In general, however, common side effects include sedation, weight gain, dizziness, and a cluster of symptoms known as "anticholinergic side effects." This last group reflects the tendency of many antidepressants to block the effects of a certain part of the nervous system called the "cholinergic system." This system is responsible for keeping the surfaces of membranes moist; causing the muscular walls of tubular organs, such as the bowels, to contract smoothly, and opening up sphincter muscles, which serve as valves—for example, in releasing urine. When these functions are blocked, the resulting side effects include dry mouth, blurred vision, constipation, and difficulty in passing urine.

The Pros and Cons of Using Antidepressant Medications

In deciding how we wish to lead our lives, we are continually doing cost–benefit analyses, which is another way of saying that we weigh the pros and cons and make our choices accordingly. Most of these analyses are so routine that we are barely aware that they are taking place. Is the risk of having a car accident worth the potential benefits of going to the supermarket to do the shopping? Is the risk of a plane crash worth the benefits of a Caribbean vacation? And so on. Sometimes, when the decision is of unusual magnitude, we become more aware of the cost–benefit analysis that is taking place.

A cost–benefit analysis should certainly be undertaken every time medications are used. What good is this medication likely to do? What harm might result? In the case of antidepressant medications, this analysis should be a shared process between patient and therapist, perhaps to an even greater degree than for other forms of medicine. The reason for this is that many of the symptoms of depression, such as sadness, guilt, and low self-worth are hidden, and known only to the patient. The same applies for side effects. The psychiatrist largely depends on the patient's evaluation of how bad both symptoms and side effects are. In addition, since the patient has to live with both the symptoms of the illness and the side effects of the medicine, it seems only fair that he or she should have the major say in whether the medications should be used or not.

So where does the psychiatrist fit into the picture? He or she is the expert on both the illness and the medications, having seen other cases before, and having noted how they have responded to different types of antidepressants. However, the psychiatrist cannot know for sure how a drug will work in any particular case. It is necessary to educate the patient about the nature of the illness, the available treatment options, and their potential benefits and possible risks. The psychiatrist should summarize his or her experience with both the drug and the illness, and show how it pertains to the patient's particular situation. The patient, in turn, should share his or her hopes, fears, and previous experiences with medications. Together, they should balance the pros and cons. Through such a dialogue, the best decision is likely to be made.

Although most medications can cause a wide array of side effects, many of these are extremely unusual. In my own practice, I tend to discuss the commonest side effects of a particular medication and to note that other side effects may occur. I also recommend that my patients ask their pharmacist for the medication package insert, which they may or may not choose to read, but which is useful to have available to refer to if any questions arise. If while on medications you should develop any physical or psychological changes that have not been fully discussed, or about which you feel concerned, you should not hesitate to contact your psychiatrist by phone, rather than wait for the next session.

Before making a decision, some people want to know the worst-case scenario. What is the worst thing that can happen if they do or do not take a medication? The answer is the same in either case: In a rare, worst-case scenario, the course of action can be fatal. In exceptionally rare instances, for example, a person may have an allergic or exaggerated reaction to a medication, which could prove fatal. (This is possible, incidentally, with any medication, including over-the-counter preparations.) It is much more likely, however, for depression to prove fatal, and I'm not referring only to suicide. There are studies showing that both the incidence of sickness and the death rate are higher in depressed patients than in the rest of the population. A depressed person may be distracted or uninterested in the world, and may be more likely to walk across a street carelessly or to use an electrical appliance without taking all the necessary safeguards. A depressed person may also neglect his or her health; for example, a woman may not get regular gynecological check-ups or may ignore a breast lump that she finds. So depression is really not a trivial, innocuous illness.

However, since these worst-case scenarios are rather rare, they should generally be given rather limited weight in the cost–benefit analysis, just as the risk of a fatal accident is not generally regarded as an important reason for not going to the supermarket. Those outcomes that are far commoner should be given greater weight.

In general, it has been my experience that the cost–benefit analysis greatly favors the use of antidepressant medications, especially when depression is moderate to severe, when the individual is relatively healthy, and when nonmedical alternatives (such as light therapy) seem unlikely to do the job by themselves. In addition, people with seasonal depressions seem to respond well to medications, and I cannot think of a single patient of mine who could not be helped to *some* degree by a combination of light therapy and antidepressant medication. On the other hand, if depressions can be treated successfully without medications, this course is generally preferable.

Medications Commonly Used in SAD

I want to emphasize that antidepressants should be administered only by qualified professionals. The patient's efforts would be well spent in locating and consulting such a professional. Once the doctor has been chosen, the patient should generally defer to his or her judgment about which medicine is best for a particular clinical situation. However, the patient is entitled to an explanation of why that particular drug has been selected and to a discussion of its advantages and disadvantages compared with other possibilities. The discussion in this section is intended to provide information about some of the most useful medications available for the treatment of SAD in particular, and depression in general. However, the decision to administer antidepressants and the choice of medication should only be made by a licensed professional who has had a chance to interview and examine the patient in question.

There are many different types of medications available for treating depression. The choice of which drug to use first is an educated guess, based on the clinical picture of the patient and on the therapeutic and side effect profile of the medication. Because there is no scientific method at this time for reliably predicting the best antidepressants for particular patients, administering them often proceeds by trial and error. If the first choice doesn't work, the next should be tried. I have seen some patients who have tried many different drugs without success and then finally hit on the right one. It's a bit like having a large bunch of keys and trying each in turn until you find the one that turns a lock. But once the lock turns, the door opens, and new vistas appear. So it is for the depressed patient who finally feels better and is able to enjoy life once again. It may be helpful to bear this image in mind if the first or second antidepressant fails to deliver its promised effect; otherwise, it is easy to become discouraged and give up prematurely when the next key on the bunch may be the right one.

All antidepressants take time to work. At least two weeks should be allowed after the medication has been administered in *sufficient dosage* before a judgment about its effectiveness can be made. Because of the wide variation in susceptibility to side effects, psychiatrists often choose to start a medication at a low dose and increase the dose gradually, as noted above. This precaution obviously increases the time before the medicine can have its full effect. Therefore, in severely depressed people, it may be desirable to start at a higher dose and increase more rapidly. One minor problem with starting at a low dosage is that the final dosage may appear to be huge compared to the initial one, whereas in fact the initial one was very small.

Although antidepressant medications may be used instead of light therapy in some patients with SAD, they are usually used to supplement it. Light therapy may be only partially effective in eradicating the symptoms of SAD, and this partial effect may be enhanced by medications. In addition, if light therapy is used in conjunction with antidepressants, it is often possible to get by with smaller doses and correspondingly fewer side effects. It is often necessary to adjust the dosage with the changing seasons-increasing it as the days become shorter and darker, and decreasing it as the days become longer and brighter.

The Selective Serotonin Reuptake Inhibitors

In the brief space of a few years the selective serotonin reuptake inhibitors (SSRIs) have moved up the list to the drugs of choice in treating the winter depressive symptoms of SAD. As their name implies, these drugs are believed to be more specific than older antidepressants in their therapeutic function, which is believed to reside in their capacity to block the reuptake of the neurotransmitter serotonin into nerve terminals. This allows serotonin to transmit its message to the next neuron for a longer duration. Since the depressive symptoms of SAD are believed to be due to deficient transmission of signals from one serotonin neuron to another, increasing these signals is thought to be helpful in reversing these symptoms. Although some older antidepressants had the same biochemical effect, they had many other biochemical effects as well, which resulted in side effects and made the older drugs unpopular with many patients. That is not to say that the newer drugs are without side effects, which I discuss below. But in general these side effects are less marked and more acceptable; as a result, the discomfort associated with being on antidepressant medications has been greatly decreased. A real advantage of these newer drugs is that they are low in anticholinergic side effects—for example, dry mouth, blurred vision, and constipation—which are often quite unpleasant.

In addition to having fewer side effects, the SSRIs are very effective in reversing the symptoms of SAD. Although this has been apparent to the many patients and clinicians who have used these drugs over the past several winters, the observation was supported more recently by a controlled study by Dr. Siegfried Kasper in Germany, who compared light therapy with fluoxetine (trade name: Prozac) and found them to be equally effective after a five-week trial. As with all antidepressants, one should expect that it will take several weeks before these drugs begin to work, although some people report benefits sooner. The effectiveness of these drugs for SAD is one of the reasons that makes researchers suspect that SAD may result from an abnormality in brain serotonin systems. Other SSRIs available on the U.S. market include sertraline (trade name: Zoloft) and paroxetine (trade name: Paxil).

Although some people feel almost no side effects on these drugs, others are less fortunate. Side effects that have been most widely reported with the SSRIs include nausea, upset stomach, irritability, anxiety, and sedation. Side effects that have been underreported, in my opinion, include sexual difficulties and weight gain. Early reports suggested that sexual difficulties were quite rare with these medications. This does not appear to be the case, and several of my patients on these medications have complained of decreased interest in sex, decreased sexual arousal, and difficulties in reaching orgasm. One report by Dr. Frederick Jacobsen suggested that the drug yohimbine (trade name: Yocon) was capable of overriding the sexual difficulties associated with fluoxetine. In the few cases where I have prescribed this solution, however, patients have found it to be unsatisfactory.

There have been reports of weight *loss* associated with fluoxetine, which has even been advocated as a medical treatment for obesity. Although weight loss is fairly common in the first weeks after patients start using the drug, in my experience this weight is regained later. In fact, patients often end up weighing more than they did before starting the medication, despite all attempts to diet.

Although fluoxetine can be activating, it can also result in periods of intense somnolence that can sweep over a patient in waves. These bouts of sleepiness may occur at predictable times—for example, in the middle of the afternoon. In other cases, patients may find it very difficult to wake up at their customary time and may need to sleep in longer in the mornings. Others have reported intense yawning and falling rapidly asleep at night instead of drifting off gradually. As can be seen from these different effects, altering brain serotonin functioning can have opposite effects in different people.

I have also seen fluoxetine have opposite effects in the same people at different times of the year. In winter the drug may be quite activating, reversing the lethargy and fatigue that afflict so many SAD sufferers. In spring, however, the drug may have an opposite effect, making a patient sluggish and lethargic. If this possibility is not recognized, it would be easy for the psychiatrist to believe that the patient needs *more* rather than *less* medication, which would tend to compound the lethargy and fatigue. These seasonal differences in response to antidepressants that work on the serotonin system may be based on seasonal variations that have been documented to occur in serotonin concentrations in the hypothalamus. Given these variations, one would expect that the dosage of medications may need to be varied over the course of the year in people with seasonal mood changes.

There are other side effects of the SSRIs, which, although infrequent, can be distressing to those who suffer them. These include headaches; tooth grinding and jaw pain; and itching skin or pins-and-needles sensations. One of the most controversial side effects alleged to occur with fluoxetine is the propensity for it to cause suicidal or violent actions. There has been considerable debate on this topic, with special-interest groups lining up on both sides of the fence.

Although some people on these drugs have in fact committed such acts, the question remains unanswered as to whether the drugs were in any way responsible for them. It has been long known to psychiatrists that when patients are emerging from the lowest depths of their depressions, but are not yet feeling completely better, they are at greater risk for suicide. They may still feel awful, but may be more activated and more inclined to do something impulsive about it. Whether the risk is greater on the SSRIs than on any other type of antidepressant is debatable. But even the existence of such a possibility underscores the importance of having antidepressants closely monitored by someone who is experienced in their use.

The SSRIs can alter sensations in different ways. Whereas one of my patients complained that his senses were dulled and that his experience of life appeared to lose its luster and sparkle to some degree, others have reported enhancement of certain sensations—for example, sensitivity to light. One patient, for example, who had previously had no difficulty falling asleep when his wife's bedside lamp was on, found that the brightness of the light transmitted through his eyelids made it quite impossible for him to fall asleep after he began to take Prozac. Another reported that his sensations were vividly enhanced in ways that brought back to him intense memories of his childhood. For example, when he was on the medication he would walk into a house, smell food, and become overwhelmed by memories of his grandmother's delicious cooking of many years before. On another occasion, he was tramping over some fallen leaves and was powerfully reminded of an enjoyable camping trip he had undertaken as a boy.

It is possible that fluctuations in this man's brain serotonin system, induced by the Prozac, sensitized him to recall these vivid and enjoyable childhood memories when presented with a cue from the present, such as cooking food or fallen leaves. Perhaps we should call this type of response the "madeleine effect," named after the French pastry, a madeleine, that Marcel Proust describes in *Remembrance of Things Past*. When, as an adult, the hero of the novel bites into a madeleine soaked with tea, the memories of his childhood come flooding back to him. Our modern counterpart to Proust's hero did well on Prozac, which prevented his SAD symptoms from developing. We know that the seasons are associated both with powerful memories of things past and with changes in brain serotonin systems. Shifts and fluctuations in serotonin systems may also account for the symptoms of SAD, the antidepressant effects of light (and Prozac), and the "madeleine effect."

One question that always arises when someone develops a side effect on one of the SSRIs is whether there is any possible advantage to switching to another member of the same drug family. Despite our limited experience with the newer SSRIs, the answer to this question appears to be "yes." Sometimes these differences are predictable. For example, Prozac tends to be a more activating drug than Zoloft, and may therefore have advantages for those whose depressions are characterized by sluggishness and lethargy. Zoloft, on the other hand, tends to be more sedating and may have advantages in patients with mixed anxiety and depression, who may feel pleasantly calmed down by the drug. These are generalizations, however, and there is no telling for sure how a person is going to respond to any given antidepressant. In some situations, one SSRI may have advantages over another for reasons that could not have been predicted. Practically speaking, what this means is that if one SSRI doesn't work well or results in unacceptable side effects, it is worth trying another.

One noteworthy difference between the different SSRIs is the time needed to excrete them from the system. This tends to be far longer for Prozac than for Zoloft or Paxil. Whereas the latter two drugs are generally excreted from the system within a few days, levels of Prozac and its active breakdown products can be detected in the blood for weeks after the medication is discontinued. In certain situations, this delay in excretion can be a problem. For example, it may take longer for a troublesome side effect to subside, and a patient certainly needs to wait longer before starting another medication that may interact adversely with Prozac—most notably one of the monoamine oxidase inhibitors (MAOIs), which are discussed below. But in many situations, this difference in excretory profiles is of no practical importance. Another difference between drugs is that Prozac tends to push up the levels of other drugs in the bloodstream more than Zoloft. As long as a psychiatrist is aware of this effect and monitors the situation adequately, this property should not generally be a problem.

Although the list of side effects outlined above may seem imposing, the SSRIs are generally well tolerated and a significant advance over the older antidepressants. Millions of people have benefited from them, and many who are on these medications are hardly aware that they are taking any drug at all.

Bupropion (Wellbutrin)

Bupropion (trade name: Wellbutrin), also relatively recently introduced into the U.S. market, shares with the SSRIs the advantage of having a relatively low level of anticholinergic side effects as compared with the older antidepressants. In other words, constipation, dry mouth, and blurred vision are not generally problems with this drug. It tends to be activating and energizing and is therefore good for depressed patients who feel sluggish and lethargic, as opposed to those who are anxious and agitated. Although there have not as yet been any controlled studies of this drug in SAD patients, clinical and uncontrolled study results are encouraging.

Although one of the known effects of Wellbutrin is to help delay the reuptake of the neurotransmitter dopamine, no one really knows whether that action is instrumental in its antidepressant effects, the basis for which is not well understood at this time.

Wellbutrin has certain advantages over the SSRIs; most notably, it is less likely to cause sexual side effects and is, in my experience, less frequently associated with long-term weight gain. Its disadvantages are that it may not be as effective as the SSRIs for certain people; it is more likely to cause anxiety and irritability; and in some cases it may elevate the heart rate. The most serious side effect of Wellbutrin, which is quite rare, is that it may induce seizures. In this regard it is not completely dissimilar to most of the other antidepressants, which may also induce seizures, although slightly less frequently than Wellbutrin. For all the reasons I have just outlined, I usually save Wellbutrin for my second choice, reserving it for when the SSRIs are not fully satisfactory.

Desipramine and Imipramine: Old Faithfuls

I call desipramine (trade names: Norpramin and Pertofrane) and imipramine (trade name: Tofranil) "Old Faithfuls" because they have been around for a long time and they continue to be useful weapons in our arsenal against depression. They are generally well tolerated and quite effective. I know of several patients with SAD who have responded well to them. Side effects are generally quite tolerable with desipramine. It may make some people feel energized or "wired," and others a little sedated. Anticholinergic side effects (dry mouth, constipation, blurred vision) are relatively mild, though they may be real problems for some people. Pulse rate and sweating may increase, and dizziness may be experienced upon standing. Although these side effects are inconvenient, they are rarely dangerous. Imipramine tends to be a little more sedating than desipramine and produces more anticholinergic side effects.

These two drugs are members of a larger family known as the "tricyclic antidepressants." Other members of the tricyclic family are also often prescribed for depression. Amitriptyline (trade names: Elavil and Endep), which is commonly prescribed, is very sedating and very anticholinergic, and often causes more side effects than the other tricyclics. Because of these side effects, I rarely use it as a first-line drug in treating depression. Doxepin (trade names: Sinequan and Adapin) is another tricyclic that I don't use as a first-line drug, because it too is sedating and has prominent anticholinergic effects. Sometimes these sedative properties can be used to advantage in people with insomnia. Most SAD patients, however, have just the opposite problem—they sleep too much. The last thing they generally need is something that is going to make them even sleepier.

Trazodone (Desyrel)

Trazodone (trade name: Desyrel) is structurally different from the tricyclic antidepressants, but shares some of their properties. It seems particularly attractive for the treatment of SAD patients because, like the SSRIs, it works on the serotonin system. For this reason I have prescribed trazodone for a number of patients when light therapy alone has not been sufficient, and have been pleased at the favorable outcome. Although it tends to be very sedating (a property that can be exploited in those with insomnia), several SAD patients I have treated with trazodone have tolerated the drug well and benefited from it. In my experience, trazodone is not generally sufficiently antidepressant if used by itself, but is often quite effective when given in conjunction with other antidepressants. In addition to sedation, side effects of trazodone include feelings of heaviness and weight gain.

The Monoamine Oxidase Inhibitors

Specific monoamine oxidase inhibitors (MAOIs) include phenelzine (trade name: Nardil), tranylcypromine (trade name: Parnate),and isocarboxazid (trade name: Marphan). The MAOIs have a long and checkered history in the United States. They were the first drugs found to be effective in treating depression, and they were discovered serendipitously. Patients with tuberculosis (TB), who happened to be depressed, became less so when given an anti-TB drug related to the MAOIs. This observation led to the development of other, more effective MAOIs. In my experience it is unusual to have to prescribe the MAOIs in patients with SAD, who generally respond well to the drugs noted above, which are safer and cause fewer side effects.

The MAOIs inhibit the enzyme monoamine oxidase (MAO), which is found in both the brain and the bowels. It is thought that this action may be responsible for their antidepressant effects. MAO (pronounced M-A-O, not like the name of the late Chinese leader) breaks down substances called "biogenic amines," of which norepinephrine and serotonin are two examples. By inhibiting the enzyme, the MAOIs promote the build-up of monoamines in the brain. It has been suggested that depression may result from a functional deficiency of these biogenic amines, and that the MAOIs may exert their antidepressant action by causing these amines to accumulate in the brain.

The MAO enzyme is also produced in the bowel, where it has the important function of breaking down certain substances in food that, if absorbed, can be harmful. These substances are present in yellow cheeses, red wines, liver, and all broken-down proteins (such as marinated meats, pickled fish, and any food that is partly spoiled). *All these foods should be strictly avoided by patients on MAOIs.* There are also certain drugs, most notably over-the-counter cold preparations and diet pills, that should not be taken in combination with MAOIs. If a patient who is taking MAOIs should happen to take some of these over-the-counter medications, or should eat one of the forbidden foods noted above, a serious and rapid rise in blood pressure may result. Before a patient starts taking one of these drugs, this particular hazard, known as a "hypertensive crisis," should be thoroughly discussed with the psychiatrist, who should provide both oral and written instructions about the precautions necessary to avoid it, and the steps to be taken if it should arise.

Unfortunately, the hypertensive crisis mentioned above is not the only difficulty one can encounter when using the MAOIs. Other bothersome side effects include insomnia, daytime drowsiness, weight gain, and decreased sexual pleasure. In addition, care needs to be taken when combining MAOIs with other drugs, including antidepressants.

So why use these drugs at all? Because they can be extraordinarily effective in some people, who may experience virtually no side effects while taking them. Many people have been greatly helped by them, and for this reason they have once again emerged as useful tools in the treatment of depression. In deciding to use the MAOIs, both psychiatrist and patient should make a careful cost–benefit analysis; this should take into account the availability of alternative, safer medications, as well as all the necessary information about the patient's medical background.

Lithium Carbonate

Originally used as an agent for treating mania, lithium carbonate has been recognized as a versatile mood-regulating medication. It can be used as a general mood leveler, to inhibit the development of both manic and depressive episodes, as well as an antidepressant. It can be used either alone or in combination with any of the antidepressants mentioned above.

The idea of taking lithium is very scary to many people. Perhaps they associate it with extremely disturbed people whose behavior is out of control, or regard it as dangerous. But, in fact, lithium is frequently a very helpful and well-tolerated drug in the treatment of depression in general. In my experience, however, it is not especially valuable in the treatment of the typical winter depressions of SAD. It does not usually appear to exert a powerful antidepressant effect by itself. In addition, the medications mentioned above generally work quite well in SAD without lithium.

Lithium can be very useful, however, in controlling the hypomanic symptoms that affect some SAD patients in spring and summer. Although there is no reason to treat such patients simply because they may feel exuberant or be more active and energetic than others, these behavioral changes may accelerate to such a degree that they cause problems for the patients or those who have to deal with them. Hypomanic people tend to get into arguments easily, act impulsively in ways that they may later regret, and have disturbances in their perceptions of reality that can be problematic. For example, hypomanic people may overestimate their financial holdings and spend more money than they can afford. Clearly, such behavioral changes cause problems, which can be minimized by early recognition and by prompt and appropriate treatment. Restricting light exposure— for example, by keeping bedroom window shades down or wearing very dark wrap-around glasses—may be helpful for hypomanic patients. However, it is often difficult for them to go along with these recommendations, and medications tend to be the most effective solution. In such situations, lithium can save the day.

Common side effects of lithium include increased thirst, increased urine volume, and hand tremors. Some nausea and abdominal discomfort may be experienced, but these are often transient and may be minimized by taking the medication with meals. Other side effects include weight gain, memory difficulties, and skin rashes. It is usual to have lithium blood levels checked at intervals, because if they are too high, symptoms of toxicity may result. These include nausea and diarrhea, vomiting, markedly increased tremor, and coordination difficulties. These should be rare, however, if the drug is properly monitored. If toxicity occurs, the patient should drink plenty of fluid and contact his or her psychiatrist immediately or go to an emergency room. Long-term side effects, in the form of kidney or thyroid problems, may occur. Fortunately, kidney damage is rare. Interference with thyroid function is somewhat more common, but it can easily be treated with oral replacement of thyroid hormone.

Combining Antidepressants with Light Therapy

Over the past decade, antidepressant medications have frequently been combined with light therapy. Studies of light therapy have shown that it works just as well in patients who are also on antidepressant medications as in those who are not. In clinical practice, using these two types of treatments together has its advantages. First, the combination is often more effective than either of the treatments administered alone. Second, it is often possible to take lower dosages of medications (and therefore to have fewer side effects) if light therapy is used as well. Finally, it may be possible to spend less time in front of the lights if medications are used as well.

A possible disadvantage of this combined strategy is that the treatments may accentuate each other's side effects. For example, patients may be more likely to experience hypomanic symptoms if they are on a combination of light therapy and medications than if they are on either treatment alone. Another area where a potential for problematic interactions between treatments has been suggested is the possibility of damage to the eyes. Although there are theoretical reasons for raising such concerns, there have been no reports to date of any damage to the eyes resulting from a patient's being on a combination of light and antidepressant therapy. If you are on such a combination, however, it is prudent to be aware of the theoretical problem and to alert your ophthalmologist to all the details of your clinical situation when you get your eyes checked.

Combining Antidepressants with Each Other and with Other Forms of Therapy.

In practice, it is frequently necessary to combine different antidepressant medications with each other. The next chapter, which deals with combining therapies, describes one patient in whom such a combination was useful. A full discussion of how to combine different medications requires considerable expertise on the part of the psychiatrist and goes beyond the scope of this book. It is important, though, for you to be aware that such options exist in case you don't respond to any of the individual medications that you try. Combining antidepressants with other forms of therapy makes good sense, as these treatments tend to enhance one another's effects.

Conclusion

To summarize, many people have concerns about being on antidepressant medications, and these concerns should be fully discussed with the psychiatrist. Once they are carefully explored, and answers to some of the more common questions are provided, the medications become more acceptable and less scary to most patients. In all cases of depression, the psychiatrist and patient should measure the benefits of taking the antidepressant and balance these against the potential side effects. There are many different types of medications. The choice of a specific drug is an educated guess, and several may need to be prescribed before the best one, or best combination, is found. These drugs should be prescribed by a skilled and qualified psychiatrist who has a specific knowledge of the patient. The outlines provided above are just descriptions of the effects these drugs may have and of my own experience with them; they are not intended as recommendations. It's important to remember that antidepressants frequently work well in conjunction with light therapy in SAD patients, allowing smaller doses of medications to be used.

CHAPTER 10

Combining different types of treatment

Although, for ease of organization, I have dealt separately with all the different types of treatment that may be helpful for patients with SAD, in practice they are often best used in combination. In this brief chapter, I describe how I personally handle my own winter difficulties and those of one of my patients, who needed a combination of many different treatment interventions.

My Own Personal Winter Routine

When people ask me whether I suffer from SAD myself, I am honestly unable to answer them with any degree of certainty. For many years now, I have taken a series of measures to prevent myself from finding out the answer to that question. I suspect, though, that without all these measures I might not do too well, especially since my work as a SAD researcher means that winter is my busiest and most stressful season.

My typical winter day begins at 4:00 A.M., when my dawn simulator is set to turn on my bedside lamp. Although I am still asleep at that time, I can imagine the lampshade gradually becoming brighter as the light enters the pupils of my eyes through my closed eyelids. At 5:15 A.M. my first alarm clock begins to ring, and the process of turning it off ensures that my head comes out from under the covers and my eyelids open wide enough to let in a fair amount of light. By 5:30 my bedside lamp has reached its maximum intensity. At that time, a light box (set on a timer three or four feet from my head) goes on, and my eyes are exposed to about 2500 lux of light. Believe it or not, I have usually fallen back to sleep by that time, though I am probably stirring

179

and aware that the end of the night is rapidly approaching. It takes the second alarm clock, set for 6:00 A.M., to bring that message finally home to me, and I am able to get out of bed fairly easily. This stands in sharp contrast to those days when for some reason the lights do not come on, and I feel that I have to drag myself out of a coma in order to get up. Luckily my wife is also somewhat seasonal, so she does not object too vigorously to this early morning sound-and-light show.

I try to get to the gym or take a long walk outdoors three or four times a week before work. At one point I hired a personal trainer to help motivate me, but now I work out with a friend who luckily does not suffer from SAD and is willing to put up with my morning bearishness. I find that unless I make a commitment to meet someone at a set time, the temptation to play hooky is very great. Somehow, at 6:00 A.M. on a winter's day, the argument that regular exercise helps give me the energy I need to get through the day is not persuasive enough to propel me into the dark world. But after exercising I always feel good, and the sauna at the end of the work-out is an added incentive. On days when I don't work out, I may sleep in an extra hour and have breakfast with the newspaper in front of a 10,000-lux light box. I also have a light box at work, and I read, write, or answer phone calls while sitting in front of it.

By now, I rarely have to calculate how much light exposure I have had on a given day and how much more I need. It has become quite instinctive, and I can tell that when I am feeling sluggish and lethargic, I need more light. On the other hand, when I have had too much light, I feel as if I have drunk too much coffee—a sort of edginess, a feeling of being "wired." It is important to develop this ability, because light requirements vary over the course of the winter, and no single regimen will work all the time. For this reason, I would encourage you to focus your attention inward to evaluate whether you have had the right amount of light, and to adjust your light exposure schedule accordingly.

My wife and I have bright lights in different parts of the house. We have actually had some light boxes bracketed to the ceiling and walls of our bedroom, to which we can retreat on a winter's evening and imagine that we are on some Caribbean island. We have also had a Sunlight Pipe (see Chapter 7) installed in our upper hallway, which used to be quite dark, but is now often well illuminated with natural light.

Luckily for me, these steps have been sufficient to keep me on an even keel through the winter. I still don't feel as good in the winter as I do in the summer. I often have to let nonurgent chores pile up during the winter and tackle them in the spring, when I have more energy and motivation to do so. One thing I plan to do differently in future years is to take my vacation in the winter and head south, rather than taking the summer vacations that psychiatrists more traditionally enjoy.

I last had my eyes checked about two years ago, at which time I had been using light therapy for eleven years, and I was pleased that the ophthalmologist found no problems. I guess I'm due for another check-up sometime soon.

The way in which I have structured my winter days works for me, and I offer it as a detailed example of how one person has succeeded in preventing the symptoms of SAD. But remember, everyone is different; strategies that work for me may not work for you. It has taken me some time to learn all the tricks I've just described—ways to make life easier for myself during the difficult winter months. In a similar way, you too can be creative in finding those strategies that work best for you or someone you care about.

The Lesson from Sara's Story: Throw the Kitchen Sink at It

Every now and then, I encounter a patient with SAD whose symptoms are either so severe or so resistant to simple remedies that every measure has to be taken to overcome them. I have to throw the kitchen sink at the problem. "Sara" was such a person.

Sara was a sales representative in her late thirties, married and without children, who lived and worked in rural Massachusetts. She had suffered from problems with the winter since she was seventeen years old, and had received help for them in the form of psychotherapy and medications (amitriptyline [Elavil], imipramine [Tofranil], monoamine oxidase inhibitors [MAOIs], and lithium), which helped to a small degree. Because of her winter depressions, she realized that she needed to gear down in the winter, get more sleep, and get out of a destructive relationship, which made her feel bad about herself. Life became much more difficult for Sara in the two years before she consulted me, starting with a serious depression that occurred, quite uncharacteristically, during the summer shortly after she changed jobs—from one in which she traveled around in her car to one in a windowless office. Sara remained depressed through the summer and into the next fall and winter; she was still depressed when I saw her at the end of the second summer.

What followed was an extensive series of interventions to help free Sara of her depressions. She kept a careful log of her moods, so that we could accurately evaluate the effects of these interventions. Light therapy (10,000 lux for up to one and a half hours per day), plus regular aerobic exercise initiated in early October, didn't help much. After a month, I prescribed one 20-mg capsule of fluoxetine (Prozac) per day, and a few days later she went to Florida on vacation for a week. For the first time in months, her mood moved into the normal range. On her return we increased her light treatment to two hours per day, one hour in the morning and one hour in the evening. She remained in reasonably good spirits until December, when her depression once again became a problem.

I raised her Prozac to two capsules per day and reminded her to keep exercising. Within a few weeks she was feeling somewhat better again, but that didn't last for long. In December she went down to Mexico on vacation and her depression lifted, only to relapse shortly after she returned home. She hooked a bright bedside lamp up to a timer, which she set to go on an hour before she was due to wake up in the morning. In addition, she worked at increasing the brightness of her indoor lighting both at work and at home. Although she managed to keep working, she suffered from fatigue and depressed mood, and winter felt like one long chore. Finally, in March of the next year, for the first time in over two years, she switched out of her depression in a solid way; we were able to discontinue all forms of treatment, including medications.

Given the serious difficulties that Sara had suffered despite multiple treatment interventions, she and I began to discuss strategies to minimize her SAD symptoms the next winter. I recommended that she purchase a dawn simulator and a portable light box, which would give her more flexibility and control over her environmental light the following winter. We brought her husband—an extremely supportive and understanding man—into our therapy sessions so that he could be involved in all discussions about plans that might affect him, and could also provide suggestions of his own. Sara decided to plan several brief trips to Florida as a "safety net" for the forthcoming winter, to use when the depression became too bad. Not only did this idea prove extremely valuable, but just knowing that the plan was in place was a great comfort to Sara. We also used the summer to work in psychotherapy on some traumatic experiences that Sara had suffered in early adulthood. Free of depression, she was able to obtain some relief from the burden of these painful experiences.

Sara began to feel depressed again in early August, and I started to treat her with a combination of light therapy (one to two hours per day) and Prozac, at first one capsule every other day. As she entered the winter, it became necessary to increase the dosage of Prozac. She exercised regularly and began to use a dawn simulator in an attempt to hold the time of dawn (albeit an artificial dawn) constant as the days became shorter. By mid-December her depression deepened once again and was severe enough to warrant the addition of bupropion

(Wellbutrin) to the Prozac. On a combination of light therapy (two hours per day), daily aerobic exercise, Prozac (40 mg per day), and Wellbutrin (300 mg per day), she felt reasonably well and was able to continue to work and to deal with issues in her psychotherapy. One of these issues was her need to learn to take good care of herself, especially given the stress of her serious SAD symptoms.

She did use her planned time away to good effect, and her three one-week vacations, scheduled for December, January, and February, all significantly lifted her spirits. She was able to tell her husband just how bad she felt at times during the winter, and he began to appreciate their need to make major lifestyle changes to accommodate her problem. Together they chose a community in Florida to which they are planning to relocate, and when spring came they bought a house there. I have little doubt that in Florida the winters will be easier for Sara. She plans to find a job that allows her to spend time outdoors during the day. She is aware that her SAD symptoms will probably not disappear completely, but that she will have to continue to work on them, though presumably far less intensively than she has done while living in the north.

I have deliberately included a story of someone who has found neither a quick nor an easy path to recovery. The last two winters have, however, been significantly better than the preceding two—and there is every reason to hope for better winters ahead. Sara has felt happy and productive for at least some of the time during the winter months, and her feelings of depression have been more limited and contained. At no time in the last few years has she felt the loss of hope that characterized her earlier depressions. Her bond with her husband is good, and they have been able to have fun together in winter as well as in summer. She has also been able to come to terms with—and dispatch—some of the psychological demons from her past, and feels better and stronger for it.

I include Sara's story as a message to those of you out there whose path to recovery has also been difficult. Don't despair. There are all kinds of things that can help, either individually or in combination, and I recommend that you try different approaches at the advice and under the supervision of a qualified professional. Keep well informed and up to date on the latest research developments. Even if you don't completely overcome your SAD symptoms this winter, who knows what new discoveries next winter will bring?

CHAPTER 11

"How can I help?": Advice for family and friends

It is good to know that other people—friends and family—can be a terrific source of comfort and support to someone with SAD. This chapter is addressed to you, the family members and friends of seasonal patients, in an attempt to help you be a comfort to the patient.

Things to Do

1. *Understand the problem.* Recognize that the seasonal mood problem is a real affliction. This may be hard to appreciate. After all, the seasonal person looks okay. There are no obvious wounds or abnormalities. All the tests have come back normal. So what is the fuss about? It is especially difficult for people who have never themselves been depressed to understand what it feels like. Even people who experience mild seasonal changes, which are at worst a nuisance, have a hard time understanding how bad people with SAD can actually feel. More mildly afflicted friends and relatives sometimes feel that they also have to contend with the same sort of difficulties. Yet they pick themselves up and get on with their lives, so why can't the SAD person do the same? It is important to realize that severity makes a big difference. Depressed people have major difficulties in functioning. I would encourage you to read some of the stories in the earlier part of the book, to gain insight into how disabling the problem can be.

It can be helpful to think of SAD as similar, in certain critical ways, to a physical illness. The example of diabetes often comes to mind. It is a condition in which the pancreas does not make enough insulin, which results in an abnormality of glucose metabolism. We do not know what the underlying abnormality is in SAD, but I would wager that it resides somewhere in the brain, where some chemical process does not function normally, resulting in all the symptoms of the condition. Somehow, light that enters via the eyes plays an important role in this key chemical process. During the short, dark days of winter, when there is not enough light in the environment, the brain chemical abnormality becomes manifest in the form of SAD symptoms. Bright light reverses the symptoms, presumably by correcting the underlying abnormality. If your friend or relative had diabetes, you would understand that insulin shots and a special diet were necessary to help control the condition. Similarly, your friend or relative with SAD needs extra light and can benefit tremendously from your support. You can help, for example, by keeping your friend or relative company while he or she is sitting in front of the lights.

Once you understand the mood and energy problems of SAD, you will be able to handle them better. For example, if your spouse falls behind in paying the bills or carrying out various chores when winter arrives, it will be much easier for you to put up with the resulting inconvenience if you recognize that you are probably dealing with SAD symptoms rather than laziness. If you want to find out more about the condition and its treatments, you may find parts of this book helpful. Another way to learn about SAD is by joining a recently formed nationwide support group, open to patients and other interested people, called the National Organization for Seasonal Affective Disorder (NOSAD). Further information about this organization can be obtained by writing to: NOSAD, P.O. Box 40133, Washington, D.C. 20016.

2. *Just be there.* Don't feel you have to do anything specific. Your undemanding presence and company will be experienced as soothing and helpful. Even though the seasonal person may appear withdrawn and unfriendly, he or she will often appreciate having company. As one patient I know puts it, "I want my friends to tolerate me sitting solemnly in a corner reading a magazine. I like people to be around but not asking very much of me, because I don't have very much to give." Another patient echoes this need for understanding, noting that when a seasonal person is depressed, "you get into a place where it's hard for another person to relate to you unless he really cares about you, has known you for a while, and understands your seasonality." She recognizes that "people don't like their friends to change. It's hard for the people you live with," but she requests of her friends that they do not expect her to be "bubbly and full of myself like I am in the summer . . . just accept me the way I am."

3. *Encourage the seasonal person.* Remind the person that this is a passing phase—that he or she has not always felt this way, and can and

will feel better again. A person who is lethargic and uninspired during the depths of the winter may be kind, friendly, charming, or witty at other times of the year. Remind him or her about the good times; when the person is depressed, it's easy for him or her to forget that they ever happened.

It's important for you to bear in mind that when someone is depressed, everything that he or she has been told about depression—for example, that it is a legitimate and transient illness—is easily forgotten. At such a time, because you understand what is happening, you can help tremendously simply by saying, "Hey, you're forgetting, this is your winter problem. It will pass."

4. *Help with simple things.* Sometimes even shopping or laundry can feel like a huge chore to the depressed person. Offers on your part to help out with these will generally be greatly appreciated. One of the earliest members of our seasonal program worked out such an arrange-ment with her family. They had a system of rotating household chores, so that each family member would do a certain one for a given week. Some of them, such as tidying up the house, were easier, whereas others, such as cleaning the bathrooms, were more difficult. During the winter, the children understood that their mother was not able to tackle the more difficult chores, and all agreed that she should be exempt from bathroom duty during those months.

The best way to find out what help is needed is to ask. Examples include going to the grocery store for a friend; fixing breakfast for your spouse or getting the kids off to school while he or she sits in front of the lights; sitting and talking to a friend or loved one while he or she does the laundry or pays the bills; or helping him or her wake up in the morning (which is so difficult for a person with SAD). All these things will be remembered and rewarded by a deepening and strengthening of your relationship.

These are some of the things that you, as friends and relatives, can do. They don't take a lot of effort, but they do make a big difference.

5. *Try to understand the seasonal person when he or she is in the other (hypomanic) phase.* Sometimes it's difficult to understand the high side of SAD as well. Someone who has been hibernating all winter and suddenly springs into action with more energy than anyone else may be hard to take. As one patient puts it, "I think it's easier to love someone who's down and depressed and hurting in some way. But please remember to love her when she's happy and successful as well." It may also be helpful to point out *tactfully* that the seasonal person is going a bit fast for you and most other people, and that it may be useful to get some help to slow down a bit. Wearing dark glasses during daylight hours may help people slow down at such times if they are too "wired."

When people are a bit high, they can become argumentative. If you are a friend or relative exposed to such querulousness, you would do well to choose carefully what issues are discussed. The husband of one of my seasonal patients, who has learned the value of this strategy over the years, avoids confronting his wife on minor issues. He observes, "If we have a conflict, it's going to be over something worthwhile."

A patient who is showing poor judgment or impulsiveness, or who doesn't sleep, should be encouraged (or taken) to see his or her psychiatrist.

Things to Avoid

1. *Don't judge and criticize.* The seasonal person is already feeling bad about not functioning up to his or her normal standards, and about letting you and other friends and family members down. Very often the person is his or her own harshest critic, measuring his or her own actions and finding them wanting. To have these criticisms confirmed by someone the person loves and respects can be extremely painful, may further undermine his or her self-esteem, and could enhance feelings of depression and worthlessness. A tendency to judge and criticize the seasonal person is very understandable, but it stems from a fundamental misinterpretation of his or her behavior. It is based on the misconception that the seasonal person is willfully declining to do certain things (such as meet social obligations or follow through on commitments), or, at the very least, that he is being self-indulgent, weak-willed, and giving in to things.

You may well be tempted to think back on some difficult or unpleasant thing that you had to do in the past, and to feel a little self-righteous about it. Resist that temptation. Everyone is different. You may be able to overcome feelings of lassitude, fatigue, and lack of motivation, but this may not be possible for your seasonal friend or family member. It may be helpful for you to think back to some time when you were feeling weak, tired, or out of sorts, perhaps because of a physical condition, such as an infection or operation. Imagine how you would have felt to be criticized at such a time for not meeting your obligations with sufficient energy or enthusiasm.

One young man who has been in and out of seasonal depressions for the past several years still finds it difficult to convince his friends that he has been suffering from an illness. They continue to regard his months of withdrawal and impaired functioning as a character disturbance or failure of will. As a result of this, he is beginning to re-evaluate these friendships; he wonders whether he might not be better off to choose friends with a greater capacity to understand and tolerate differences in behavior, as well as an ability to care about him even when he is not functioning at peak level.

2. *Don't take the seasonal person's withdrawal personally.* You should not assume that the person is mad at you or uninterested in being friends with you. One patient thinks back on friends who have called her during her down times and said, "Well, I've called you the last three times. Do you really want to be friends any more?" She observes,

> That kind of situation seems to pop up all the time in the winter. I understand that other people need certain things from a friendship, but it comes at a time when even getting up to answer the phone is a major effort—"Who is it going to be? What do I have to talk about now?" The best kind of friend is someone who is willing to keep calling you and to keep saying, "Do you feel like doing anything?" I'm not saying that friends should baby you, nor do they have to sit there and hold your hand. It's very simple: Just accept someone who is in a different place.

The same person recalls hurtful conversations with friends who have not understood her difficulty. "They say, 'Oh, yeah, here you go again,' and it's sort of mocking. They just don't understand."

If you, the friend or family member, do not understand the nature of the problem, you are likely to feel rejected when the seasonal person doesn't return your telephone call or doesn't call you for a few months. You may assume that the person doesn't like you or doesn't value you. If you make these assumptions, it is understandable that you would feel hurt and angry. It is a mistake, however, to assume that the seasonal person doesn't care about the friendship; moreover, it is likely to cause you to become more demanding, insistent, or rejecting. By reacting in these ways, you put pressure on the seasonal person to do the very thing he or she finds most difficult during a depressed period—namely, to initiate and maintain social interactions. Confronting the seasonal person about this inability to do so adds to his or her feelings of failure. Once again, understanding the nature of the problem will cushion you against taking the seasonal person's behavior too personally and will pour balm rather than salt on the injured relationship.

3. *Don't assume that it is your responsibility to make the seasonal person feel fine.* It's not likely to work, and you will probably end up feeling frustrated and irritated at your failure. When you feel responsible for bringing a person out of a depression and have failed to do so, you are likely to feel guilty and angry. You have sunk so much energy into trying to reverse the situation that you may be inclined to

see the depressed person as having caused you to fail. You will then be more likely to blame him or her for making you feel that way. You may attribute your "failure" to a willful attempt on his or her part to resist all help, and, in your anger, may feel inclined to say that if the person is not willing to accept your helping hand, he or she deserves to remain in a slump. As I have noted already, anger tends to get turned on the depressed person just when he or she feels least capable of coping with even the most ordinary things in life, let alone problems with a dear friend or relative. The key to not getting angry is understanding the problem and not feeling responsible for fixing it. But do remember that simple things, such as being there for your friend or family member, can make an enormous difference, even if the person is not able to show it right away. Your mere undemanding presence can be a comfort; your encouragement and nondepressed perspective can provide crucial support; and help with the simple chores of everyday life will be greatly appreciated.

CHAPTER 12

Research on SAD and light therapy

Since the description of SAD as a condition and the first controlled study of light therapy were published in 1984, research in this area has burgeoned. Elements of this research are present throughout this book. In this chapter I try to bring you up to date on some of the major developments not dealt with elsewhere.

SAD as a Disorder

The validity of SAD as a distinct psychiatric disorder was given the blessing of the American Psychiatric Association in the 1987 edition of its diagnostic manual, the DSM-III-R, which included a version of the seasonal syndrome among the traditionally accepted psychiatric conditions. The condition is also slated for inclusion in the newest version of this manual, the DSM-IV.

This acceptance was based on findings that patients with SAD have certain features that make them different from other depressed patients. These include the predictable seasonality of their moods, their sensitivity to environmental light, and their favorable response to bright light therapy, none of which has been nearly so well documented in nonseasonally depressed patients. There are, however, still many unanswered questions about how SAD patients differ from other depressed people, and these remain the subject of ongoing research.

Controlled Studies of Light Treatment

In a "controlled study," researchers compare treatments that differ from each other, usually in only one important way—the way that is thought to be of key significance in the effect. There are, of course, special problems associated with designing well-controlled studies of light treatment. One problem is the "placebo effect," the bane of the clinical researcher. If a person expects that a treatment will be helpful, then the treatment may help for psychological reasons, rather than because it contains some special active ingredient. Researchers have wondered to what extent the placebo effect explains the efficacy of bright light in SAD. Although dozens of controlled studies have been performed to date, and many researchers are by now convinced that the effect of light is more than a placebo, skeptics persist and studies continue to address this question.

As one of the researchers involved in light therapy studies notes, the placebo effect is real. There is much about it that we still don't understand, and it offers important clues into the mind's ability to heal itself. I would thoroughly agree. Light therapy, like all therapies, exerts a placebo effect as one aspect of its efficacy. But as those who have used light therapy successfully for many years will testify—after many attempts to stop light treatments during the winter have led to relapse, and restarting treatment has been accompanied by merciful remissions—there is far more than a placebo effect involved in this powerful treatment modality.

Besides the placebo effect, another factor that we had to consider in interpreting our early results was sleep deprivation. In and of itself, sleep deprivation can have antidepressant effects, and we wondered whether this might be the explanation for our early success with morning light treatment. Subsequent studies showed that although sleep deprivation might itself have antidepressant effects in SAD, the light treatment worked well even when there was no sleep deprivation at all. In one study, Dr. Thomas Wehr and I turned the question around. Could it be, we wondered, that exposure to more light during the night in people who are being sleep-deprived is the reason for why sleep deprivation is an antidepressant? To answer this question, we sleep-deprived a group of depressed people in bright light and in pitch dark. We found that sleep deprivation worked under both conditions, and concluded that both light therapy and sleep deprivation are effective treatments, and they they probably work in different ways and are not responsible for each other's efficacy.

The various elements of light therapy that are important for its effects have been well studied, in part to establish that light's antidepressant effect is specific and not merely a placebo, but also to guide clinical practice. As I have mentioned, our early controlled studies of light therapy for SAD at the NIMH involved comparisons between bright and dim environmental light. The dimension being tested in those studies was the intensity of the light. We predicted that the bright light would be effective and the dim light ineffective in treating SAD, and this prediction was borne out by the results of three separate studies with the light box. The same prediction was not borne out, however, in our studies with the Light Visor, the results of which are therefore ambiguous (see Chapter 6).

Other parameters of light treatment that have been controlled are the part of the body to which the light is exposed, the color of the light, and the timing of treatments. In several of these studies, researchers have been able to demonstrate differences between those conditions that they predicted would be active and those they predicted would be inactive controls. Studies dealing with which elements of light therapy are important for its antidepressant effects are discussed more fully in Chapter 6. In one ingenious controlled study of light therapy, performed by Dr. Ybe Meesters and colleagues in The Netherlands, researchers compared bright light with "imaginary light," which they asked their patients to contemplate as part of daily meditation sessions. They found that the real light treatments worked better.

As conviction grows that light is an effective treatment for SAD, fewer studies are being undertaken to address the question of the efficacy of light. More research is presently being directed toward finding out what other conditions might benefit from light therapy, what the underlying biological abnormalities in SAD are, and how light therapy exerts its often dramatic effects. I deal with each of these topics in turn.

The Anatomy of Light

If we consider that the portal of entry of the antidepressant effect of light is the eyes, then what are the anatomical pathways within the nervous system along which this effect might be transmitted? Light waves that strike the retina are converted into nerve impulses that pass toward the brain along tracts of nerve fibers. One tract directly connects the retina to a part of the brain known as the suprachiasmatic nuclei (SCN) of the hypothalamus. The SCN are thought to constitute the body's clock.

Much has been written about the body's internal clock, and it would be worth our while taking a moment to consider it—especially since light (and darkness, for that matter) is known to be able to influence the timing of this clock, and some believe that this influence is the basis for the antidepressant effects of light in SAD. A "clock" implies a device that keeps time regardless of what is going on around it—whether it is night or day, whether you are on land or at sea, or whether you are on earth or in outer space. And indeed, this applies to the human body's clock. It has been shown, for example, that people who are kept in isolation from all external time cues maintain their daily rhythms. In fact, their rhythms are not exactly "daily" (twenty-four hours in cycle length), but "almost daily" (or "circadian," as they are more appropriately termed). In fact, human rhythms in isolation run at a cycle length of approximately twenty-five hours. In our regular lives, of course, we are not isolated from time cues, and it is these time cues that reset our body clock to a twenty-four hour rhythm on a daily basis.

Most important among the time cues responsible for the daily resetting of our body clock is the rhythm of light and dark. This rhythm has been known for decades to be very important in the regulation of the biological clock in other species. It is only relatively recently, however, that its importance in regulating the human clock has been appreciated. To some extent, our delay in recognizing the importance of light and dark in regulating our rhythms resulted from researchers' using light that was not bright enough to have a powerful impact on the clock. But that is not the full explanation, because it turns out now that even lower intensities of light, such as those resulting from ordinary indoor lighting, can have profound effects on our circadian rhythms.

All species studied so far, from the smallest single-celled organism right on up the evolutionary tree, have been observed to have a biological clock. If something—such as this internal clock—has been so faithfully conserved through million of years of evolution, we can assume that it has a rather important biological function. All evidence suggests that it does—that the biological clock influences most of our physical functions (when we are drowsy or alert, sleep or wake, and eat or go hungry), as well as the timing of our hormonal secretions and other biological processes. These behaviors are mediated by a rich array of neural connections spreading from the SCN to the different parts of the brain that govern these functions. One of these connections is to the pineal gland, which secretes the hormone melatonin at night, in a rhythm generated by the SCN.

The biological clock receives inputs from the external world; one of the most important of these inputs is the daily rhythm of light and dark, information about which is conveyed through the nerve tracts from the retina. The influence of light and dark on biological rhythms in humans has been extensively studied in recent years. One of the most studied of these rhythms is the pattern of melatonin secretion. It was, after all, the suppression of human melatonin secretion by bright light that ushered in our studies of the effects of light in humans, and it is a theme to which I return later.

Besides having direct effects on the SCN, nerve projections from the retina pass to other regions of the hypothalamus as well, and these areas may also be influenced by patterns of light and dark. The hypothalamus as a whole is a central processing unit, responsible for keeping us in balance with the outside world. It also regulates many vital functions, including sleeping, eating, temperature, sex drive, and mood—in other words, the very functions that are disturbed in depressed patients. It seems highly likely that depressed patients have some biochemical abnormality in the hypothalamus. In the case of seasonal depression, this abnormality is manifested when there is not enough environmental light. Conversely, bright environmental light is capable of reversing this abnormality. It would seem plausible to suggest that the nerve impulses traveling from the retina to the hypothalamus in response to bright light correct a biochemical abnormality of the hypothalamus in patients with SAD.

Additional Applications of Light Therapy

Following the success of light therapy for SAD, researchers and clinicians have looked for other potential applications of this novel form of treatment. These applications fall into three categories: (1) attempts to influence circadian (approximately daily) rhythms and the body clock; (2) the treatment of other disorders that show seasonal variation, with winter worsening; and (3) nonseasonal psychiatric disorders. I discuss each of these applications in turn.

Light Therapy as a Way of Influencing the Body's Clock

There are several circumstances in which the body's clock is out of sync with the outside world and its rhythm of day and night. For some people this state of being "out of sync" is temporary—for example, when they fly across many time zones and develop jet lag, or when they work changing shifts. For others, though, being out of sync is not a temporary state resulting from special circumstances, but a permanent state resulting from some internal abnormality of the body clock. People with such abnormalities include those who are extreme "night owls"—who cannot fall asleep until very late at night and cannot wake up easily at conventional hours. This condition is known as "delayed sleep phase syndrome" (DSPS). On the other end of the sleep–wake spectrum are those with "advanced sleep phase syndrome" (ASPS), who tend to fall asleep early in the evening and wake up early in the morning. Many elderly people fall into this category. All of the circadian rhythm disturbances mentioned above have two things in common. First, they all result in discomfort and difficulties if the individuals concerned are expected to adhere to a schedule that is at odds with their biological clocks and are not free to sleep and wake when they choose. Second, they can all be helped by appropriate modifications in exposure to light and dark.

Understanding how exposure to light and dark can affect the timing of the body's clock requires some appreciation of what is known as the "phase response curve." All creatures studied to date, from single-celled organisms to human beings, have been found to exhibit a phase response curve to light. This curve describes the relationship between the time of an animal's twenty-four-hour day when it is exposed to light and the resulting effect on the animal's circadian rhythm on subsequent days. For example, in the case of human beings, light exposure late at night tends to push circadian rhythms later on subsequent days. On the other hand, light exposure in the early hours of the morning—say, at 6:00 A.M.—tends to push circadian rhythms earlier on subsequent days. So you can see how researchers can calculate a person's phase response curve by exposing that person to light at different times of his or her twenty-four-hour day and measuring the effects of that exposure on the person's circadian rhythms on subsequent days. I should point out that keeping people away from light (in other words, in the dark) has an effect on their circadian rhythms that is approximately opposite to the effect of exposing the persons to bright light at that same time of day.

Delayed and Advanced Sleep Phase Syndromes

From what I have told you about the human phase response curve, you can figure out for yourself how you might be able to treat someone who is an extreme "night owl" with bright light and dark. You should expose such a person to bright light in the morning and keep him or her away from bright light in the evening, both of which treatments would tend to shift his or her circadian rhythms earlier. In fact, my colleagues and I at the NIMH conducted just such a study. We asked patients with DSPS to sit in front of a 2500-lux light box for two hours each morning for two weeks. During those same two weeks, we asked them to wear dark, wrap-around goggles from 4:00 P.M. until sunset, and to stay in dimly lit rooms in the evening hours. Sure enough, these people fell asleep more easily at night, woke up more easily in the morning, and were less drowsy during the day.

Some people become indignant at the idea that an unusual sleep pattern should be classified as a disorder. Why, they ask, should someone be declared ill simply because he or she is out of phase with the rest of the world? I would agree completely that having an unusual type of sleep pattern does not in itself mean that someone is suffering from a disorder. In fact, for people with late night jobs, such as actors or bartenders, a delayed sleep pattern may fit in well with their lifestyle. Clearly, one way to adapt to having a circadian rhythm pattern that is out of the ordinary is to adapt one's lifestyle to fit one's rhythms. Unfortunately, this is not possible for everyone. When extreme "night owls" choose—or are required—to live on a 9:00 A.M. to 5:00 P.M. schedule, they are likely to encounter problems. For example, I have seen stockbrokers and accountants who are unable to succeed at their jobs because they can't get to work on time, and therefore miss out on the crucial early morning hours. The problem is not uncommon among adolescents and young adults, who may struggle—at times unsuccessfully—to get to their early morning classes and have school difficulties as a consequence. Many of these people find that even when they can get their bodies to class, their minds really want to stay in bed, and they find it impossible to concentrate.

The distress and difficulty that many "night owls" suffer as a result of the discrepancy between their biological clocks and the schedule they are required to maintain may be quite sufficient to justify considering the condition a disorder. But it is certainly treatable. Many subjects from the NIMH study on DSPS continued to use light therapy in the morning long after the official study was over. In some cases the treatment substantially improved the quality of their lives, enabling them to go to sleep earlier at night, wake up earlier in the morning, and (most importantly) to concentrate and focus on their work in the morning hours.

ASPS, a condition found most frequently among the elderly, responds to a pattern of light exposure opposite to that required for treating DSPS. Bright light exposure should be administered in the evening hours, and subjects should be kept in darkness in the early morning hours.

Jet Lag

Jet lag is a condition in which the rhythms of the body clock are temporarily out of sync with those of the external world as a result of traveling across several time zones. The condition can persist for up to ten days, depending on the number of time zones crossed and the individual's capacity to shift his or her circadian rhythms into sync with the outside world. In its milder forms, jet lag can be a nuisance, causing people to wake up when they want to sleep and doze off when they should be awake. Imagine how annoying it would be to travel thousands of miles to see some legendary tourist attraction, only to find yourself standing in front of it, unable to keep your eyes open. But jet lag can be more than an annoyance, because the resulting disorientation can cause errors of performance or judgment. Consider, for example, the difficulties a businesswoman would encounter trying to negotiate a deal at a time that would be 4:00 A.M. in her home town. Even though it may be midafternoon at her destination, for her it feels like 4:00 A.M. and her body is telling her it's time to sleep, just when she is supposed to be at her sharpest.

An understanding of the phase response curve can allow a person to treat his or her own jet lag. Appropriately timed exposures to bright light and darkness can greatly diminish the length of time necessary to shift a person's rhythms into sync with local time. For example, instead of a week of jet lag following a transatlantic trip, proper treatment with light and dark may shorten the adjustment time to one or two days. Understanding exactly when to administer bright light and dark to overcome jet lag is more complicated than treating DSPS or ASPS. In the latter two conditions, we know that light exposure in the early morning hours will shift circadian rhythms earlier and that light exposure in the evening hours will shift rhythms later. We know this because we have a good idea where the phase response curve is in relation to the hour of the day.

When people travel across time zones, however, their internal body rhythms (including their phase response curves) remain in the same position as they were at the point of departure for several days after they arrive at their destination, until they have shifted into the new time zone. This makes it much more complicated to calculate when someone should be exposed to light or to dark in order to shift his or her circadian rhythms in the right direction to speed up adjustment. Such timing is crucial, since exposing someone to light or dark at the *wrong* time on the phase response curve may actually shift rhythms in the *wrong* direction, *delay* adjustment to the new time zone, and *increase* the duration of jet lag. Exactly how to calculate when someone should be exposed to light or dark after traveling across several time zones is a topic beyond the scope of this book. For those who wish to learn more about it, I would recommend a book written by my colleagues Drs. Dan Oren, Walter Reich, and Thomas Wehr and myself, called *How to Beat Jet Lag: A Practical Guide for Travellers* (Holt, 1993).

Shift Work

Just as those suffering from jet lag experience distress as a result of being fatigued when they are supposed to be alert, and suffer from sleep difficulties, so do shift workers, who can be considered to be recurrently "jet-lagged" as a result of their shifting work schedules and the resulting disruption of their sleep times. Not only can the circadian problems of shift workers result in discomfort (or even physical illness) in the workers themselves; sleepiness on the job and errors in judgment can result in serious industrial accidents. It has been pointed out, for example, that the nuclear accidents at Chernobyl and Three Mile Island both occurred in the early hours of the morning, and researchers have speculated about the degree to which worker error resulting from fatigue and circadian disruption might have been responsible.

Just as properly timed exposure to bright light and dark can be used to help those suffering from jet lag, it can also be used to help shift workers adjust to the demands of changing shifts. One well-publicized successful use of this strategy is in the training of astronauts. The astronauts on the space shuttle, for example, may need to take off at night, when they would normally be going to sleep. Proper adjustment of their circadian rhythms in the days leading up to the take-off can result in their being wide awake and ready to go at midnight. Once up in space, astronauts generally work in shifts that require being asleep and awake at times different from their usual sleep–wake schedules. Once again, judiciously timed light and dark exposures in the days before take-off can enable them to do so comfortably and effectively.

Not all shift workers are as fortunate as the astronauts in the ease with which a carefully designed program of exposure to light and dark can be implemented to help them adjust to changing shifts. The astronauts are an especially committed group of workers, willing to undergo all sorts of rigors in order to accomplish their job optimally. More importantly, though, the management at NASA is highly responsive to the needs of the crew members, and willing to allow modifications in their training program that will help them perform to the best of their abilities. This is by no means the case with all shift workers and those responsible for their work schedules. Rotating workers rapidly among day, evening, and night shifts may make it impossible for them to adjust to one shift before being changed to another, even with the best-planned light or dark interventions.

As with jet lag, it is complicated to work out exactly when shift workers should be exposed to light and dark in order to speed up their adjustment. There is no easy formula that can readily be applied, and, to date, there is no good manual for shift workers to consult. One of the leading researchers in this particular area, Dr. Charmane Eastman, warns against simple remedies such as "Try thirty minutes of bright light each morning." She points out that light, if administered at the wrong time, can sometimes delay adjustment to the new shift. Environmental influences, such as sleeping and waking at certain times, can help the shift workers adjust to a new schedule. Unless light and dark signals work in the same direction as these social time cues, the resulting competition between influences may delay adjustment.

Eastman points out that, just as in the case of jet lag, people are more or less flexible in their ability to shift their circadian rhythms to meet the changing schedule demands of their jobs. For some reason, people who are "morning types"—that is, those who are at their best in the morning hours—seem, in Eastman's experience, to have a harder time adjusting to shifting work schedules than evening types. Also, older people seem to have more trouble adjusting to shift work than younger ones. Eastman's advice to shift workers is to try to sleep routinely at the same time of day—a piece of advice that may be impossible for those on rotating shifts. For those on the night shift, the biggest problem tends to be the temptation to sleep at night when they are off duty, which disrupts their circadian adjustment when they get back to work again.

Insomnia

Patterns of light and dark are capable of influencing circadian rhythms with respect not only to their timing, but also to their amplitude (or strength). If you think of circadian rhythms (for example, of alertness or body temperature) as waves—with the peak of the wave being the highest temperature or level of alertness, and the trough being the lowest level—then the strength or amplitude of the rhythm is the difference between these two extremes. There is evidence that when people have circadian rhythms of low amplitude, they may have difficulty falling or staying asleep. This happens, for example, in far northern countries during the weeks of continuous winter darkness. The artificial indoor lighting may be inadequate to provide sufficient contrast between daytime and nighttime light levels. The result is midwinter insomnia—a condition of disrupted sleep that afflicts many people living at very high latitudes during the winter.

There is some evidence that even for those insomniacs who do not live in the far north, light therapy may have some value in improving the quality of their sleep. This may apply not only to those with difficulty falling asleep (such as the DSPS patients discussed above) or those who wake early (such as the ASPS patients discussed above), but also for those who have difficulty staying asleep.

Dr. Scott Campbell and colleagues at New York Hospital–Cornell University Medical Center in White Plains, New York, successfully treated a group of elderly patients who had difficulty staying asleep. The patients received bright light exposure for two hours in the evening. Following the treatments, patients woke up less during the night and showed an overall increase in sleep, even though they did not spend more time in bed. In other words, their sleep efficiency increased. This type of treatment can be as effective as sleeping medications, without the side effects. Light treatment for insomnia is certainly worth further research, to evaluate its scope and limitations in the management of this common and distressing condition.

Light Therapy for Other Seasonal Psychiatric Disorders

Just as seasonal variation in its symptoms was a clue that SAD might respond to changes environmental light, so researchers have wondered whether any other seasonally varying conditions might prove similarly responsive. Our group and others have found that subgroups of patients with eating disorders (both bulimia and anorexia nervosa), obsessive compulsive disorder, panic disorder, and schizoaffective disorder show a degree of seasonal variation, with symptoms worsening during the winter. All of these patients would be good candidates for trials of light therapy, though it is too early to say in what percentage of patients such therapy would be useful. Dr. Raymond Lam and colleagues in Vancouver have treated a small number of bulimic patients with light therapy, and preliminary results are encouraging. More work is needed, however, before we get too excited about the prospects of light therapy for these patients. Dr. Hakan Yoney and I treated a small number of obsessive compulsive disorder patients with bright light, but observed no improvement in their symptoms. Dr. Siegfried Kasper and colleagues in Germany have had more success in this regard, and they feel that the potential value of light for this condition is worth exploring further.

Light Therapy for Nonseasonal Disorders

Two nonseasonal conditions that have been intensively studied deserve special attention: nonseasonal depression and premenstrual syndrome (PMS).

Nonseasonal Depression

Dr. Daniel Kripke of the University at California in San Diego has been a pioneer in the area of light therapy for nonseasonal depression. He has undertaken several studies in which he has compared bright white light with dim red light in the treatment of this condition. In the largest of these studies, he compared three hours of each type of light in the evening for one week, and found bright white light treatment to be superior. In a separate study, Mary Moffit and Dr. Sonia Ancoli-Israel, working in the same department as Kripke, treated a small number of elderly depressed patients with two hours of light in the late morning for ten days, and observed in their patients a small but significant antidepressant effect.

More recently, Kasper has taken a different approach. He has investigated whether light therapy can enhance the improvement in patients who have not fully responded to an antidepressants. Specifically, he administered two hours of bright light in the morning for five weeks to a group of patients who had already been treated with—but had not responded to—the antidepressant fluoxetine (Prozac). Although he observed very little improvement within the first week of light therapy (which was the entire duration of the studies by Kripke), he observed far greater improvement over subsequent weeks. By the fifth week, patients who had been treated with bright light (in addition to fluoxetine) were substantially better than those patients on fluoxetine plus a control treatment.

In summary, although the response to bright light in nonseasonal depressives is less dramatic than in SAD, the results are encouraging thus far. They suggest that light therapy might best be used in combination with antidepressants and should be tried for several weeks before being regarded as unhelpful.

Premenstrual Syndrome

PMS, more recently termed "premenstrual dysphoric disorder," is a condition that affects women of menstruating age in the week or two before their period. Common symptoms of this condition include mood changes, such as depression, anxiety, or irritability; these may be accompanied by physical discomfort, such as feelings of being bloated, breast swelling, and joint pains.

When Dr. Barbara Parry worked in the Seasonality Clinic at the NIMH, she observed that female patients with SAD frequently also suffer from PMS, which tends to get worse in the winter and tends to improve along with the symptoms of SAD when patients are treated with light therapy. She went on to wonder whether PMS, even in the absence of SAD, might not also respond to light therapy. Parry has subsequently conducted controlled studies of light therapy for PMS. In the most recent and well-controlled of these, she observed no difference in antidepressant effect among three different treatments: bright white light in the morning; bright white light in the evening; and dim red light. Although this result does not allow us to conclude with confidence that light therapy is of value in PMS, Parry's opinion, after treating women with PMS for some time, is that bright white light—whether administered in the morning or the evening—appears to have ongoing value in preventing the symptoms of this condition.

Light therapy of an unusual kind has long been reported to be beneficial in women with irregular menstrual cycles. As early as 1967, Edmund Dewan reported that such irregular cycles could be stabilized by the light of a 100-watt bulb of a bedside lamp, left on overnight. Kripke and his colleagues replicated this finding by treating women with irregular periods by means of a similar lamp, left on overnight between the tenth and fourteenth days or the thirteenth and seventeenth days of their menstrual cycle (the first day of bleeding was counted as the first day of the cycle). Although the medical implications of this observation—now rather solidly established—are unclear, it does suggest that light, operating via the eyes, can influence reproductive functioning in women.

Dr. Erick Turner at the NIMH has studied a woman who was in the process of entering the menopause, and in whom the typical menopausal symptoms of "hot flashes" occurred only during the winter. Bright light treatment in the morning abolished these hot flashes, which recurred when treatment was stopped.

Although the research of Dewan goes back at least twenty-five years, it is only in the past few years that researchers, stimulated by the success of light therapy in SAD and other conditions, have again addressed the potential value of light in regulating reproductive function. Further interesting findings in this area can confidently be expected in the years to come.

Possible Causes of SAD and Mechanisms of Light Therapy's Effects

"What are the biological abnormalities in SAD?" and "How does Light therapy work?" are among the questions most frequently asked by my patients and colleagues alike. We do not as yet have any certain answers to them, but a great deal of research has been done in this area, and some interesting results (both positive and negative) have emerged.

You don't need to read this section in order to understand how to recognize and treat SAD. It is presented particularly for those curious individuals who feel the need to have the most up-to-date research information, regardless of whether it benefits them directly or not.

Several theories about the underlying causes of SAD and the mechanisms of action of light therapy have been advanced. Some are mostly of historical interest, while others represent directions of continuing research. Even though there are connections between the different theories and they are not mutually exclusive, I discuss each of them separately for the sake of simplicity. I have been selective in choosing those theories that have been most thoroughly explored and those I regard as most promising.

Melatonin

One of the earliest hypotheses proposed by our group was that the symptoms of SAD were caused by an abnormality in melatonin secretion or an abnormal response to melatonin. After all, it was the suppression of melatonin by bright light that had stimulated our interest in light therapy in the first place. Was it not possible that light therapy was working by acting on the pattern of nocturnal melatonin secretion? Certainly there is a wealth of evidence in other animals pointing to the pivotal importance of melatonin secretion in regulating all sorts of seasonal rhythms, from the behavior of single-celled algae to the reproductive cycles of sheep and cattle. Might the symptoms of SAD not be one more example of a melatonin-mediated seasonal rhythm?

We investigated the hypothesis in several studies and came up with mixed results. First we treated SAD patients with a drug called atenolol, which suppresses the secretion of melatonin (just as light does), to see whether patients would respond to that drug as they do to light therapy. Overall, the drug was no better than a placebo, though there seemed to be a few convincing atenolol responders. In a second study, we treated patients with light therapy; then, after their symptoms responded, we gave them melatonin to see whether their symptoms would return again, which would suggest that melatonin secretion might have been responsible for the symptoms in the first place. Once again, the results were mixed. Although some symptoms got worse after melatonin was given, patients did not seem to relapse to the same degree as when light therapy was discontinued. Finally, we administered light therapy at times of day when melatonin is secreted and when its secretion would therefore be suppressed by light (early in the morning and late at night), and compared this with light treatment given at times of day when no melatonin is secreted (late morning and early afternoon). Both types of treatment proved equally effective, suggesting that suppressing melatonin secretion is not a critical aspect of the antidepressant effects of light.

Given the results of our melatonin studies, which at the time looked discouraging, we went on to explore other research questions. In retrospect, perhaps we expected too much of the hypothesis, were too greatly discouraged by the negative findings, and did not sufficiently pursue the partly positive ones. Since our early studies were conducted, there have been some new suggestions by other groups that melatonin secretion may indeed be involved in SAD and the antidepressant effects of light.

Dr. David Schlager at the State University of New York at Stony Brook has used another melatonin blocker called propranolol (which is in the same family as atenolol, the drug we had used) to test the melatonin hypothesis. He treated SAD patients with propranolol in the morning, and selected those patients who appeared to respond to this drug for a controlled study of propranolol versus a placebo. He found a greater relapse rate in those patients who were switched to the placebo than in those left on propranolol. The results of this study suggest, first, that propranolol given in the morning may have some value in the treatment of SAD patients; and second, that suppression of melatonin may after all be relevant in the treatment of SAD.

Cara Hoffman, a medical student working with Dr. Susan Swedo at the NIMH, examined the urines of children with SAD and nonseasonal controls, looking for a breakdown product of melatonin. She found exaggerated levels of the breakdown product in the urines of SAD children, suggesting that they might secrete too much melatonin. Adults with SAD have not, however, been shown to secrete exaggerated amounts of melatonin.

In summary, the findings from investigations of the role of melatonin in SAD are mixed. Although we cannot say that melatonin secretion is important in causing the symptoms of SAD, there is still sufficient interest in the area to warrant further exploration. Some people have questioned what role melatonin normally plays in our bodies and whether its suppression by light therapy might be harmful in any way. We have little understanding of the normal role of melatonin in humans, though we believe that it may help keep circadian rhythms in sync with the light–dark cycle. Melatonin is suppressed by light therapy only when light is administered late at night or early in the morning. We have no reason to believe that suppression of melatonin by light therapy should cause any physical problems.

Circadian Rhythms

Several theories have attempted to relate SAD to abnormalities in circadian rhythms and the beneficial effects of light to the restoration of these rhythms to their normal pattern. Most important of these theories is that advanced by Dr. Alfred Lewy and colleagues, who suggested that most patients with SAD have abnormally delayed circadian rhythms, like patients with DSPS. According to this theory—the "phase shift hypothesis"—light treatment in the morning improves the depressive symptoms of SAD patients by shifting their rhythms earlier, to a normal position in time. Light treatment in the evening, on the other hand, should make their SAD symptoms worse. Although some studies showed superiority of morning versus evening light treatment (though no worsening after evening treatment), many studies showed no difference in outcome when patients were treated at different times of day. In addition, though some studies showed evidence of delayed circadian rhythms in SAD patients, other studies did not. Taken together, these contradictory findings do not convincingly support this particular form of circadian rhythm hypothesis. Other circadian rhythm theories have also been suggested and are being tested, but there is currently too little evidence in support of these theories to warrant discussing them further here.

The Eye

Several researchers have wondered whether the key to understanding SAD—and the antidepressant effects of light—might reside in the eye. Dr. Dan Oren and colleagues at the NIMH have studied this problem most extensively, and have concluded that the eyes of SAD patients function very similarly to the eyes of non-seasonal individuals. Dr. Raymond Lam and colleagues, on the other hand, have found certain subtle abnormalities in the electrical patterns generated by the eyes of SAD patients. One of their findings has been replicated by Dr. Nori Ozaki and colleagues at the NIMH. Because there is an overlap in the values obtained from SAD patients and from nonseasonal controls, these subtle abnormalities are of no value as diagnostic tests for SAD. Nevertheless, they do suggest that SAD patients may be less sensitive than normal to light perception—and they may be clues to why SAD patients develop symptoms when environmental light levels are too low and why they need more light than other people during the winter.

The Stress Response Axis

As Bridget, one of our earliest SAD patients (see Chapter 1), observed, "I should have been a bear. Bears are allowed to hibernate; humans are not." She was referring to an observation that many SAD patients have made—that if they are left alone to rest, they do not feel depressed. It is only when they are stressed or challenged, when demands are made of them, that they are unable to rally themselves, and they feel depressed as a consequence. This observation—together with the general sluggishness that SAD patients experience—led Drs. Jean Joseph-Vanderpool, Phillip Gold, and me to hypothesize that SAD patients may have a physiological abnormality in their capacity to respond to stress.

One way to test this hypothesis is to inject a hormone called corticotrophin-releasing hormone (CRH), which is normally secreted by the hypothalamus. CRH, as its name implies, stimulates the pituitary gland to release corticotrophin, an important hormonal mediator of our response to stress. Corticotrophin levels in the plasma can be measured and provide an indication of the degree to which the pituitary has responded to CRH. We performed this study in SAD patients and controls, and found that SAD patients responded with abnormally low corticotrophin levels following CRH injection. Light therapy restored this response to a level that more closely resembled a normal response. This study suggests that an abnormal response to stress may be part of what is wrong in SAD patients; correcting it may be part of the way in which light therapy works. Even if this theory is correct, it is only a very partial explanation and needs to be connected to other theories.

Serotonin

I have left for last the theory that currently holds the greatest interest for me personally and that is a focus of my ongoing research. Serotonin is one of several neurotransmitters (nerve chemical messengers) responsible for passing electrical signals from one nerve cell in the brain to the next. Nerve cells containing serotonin are widely distributed throughout the brain, connecting with, among numerous other groups of cells, those of the SCN (the body's clock; see "The Anatomy of Light," above) and those responsible for secreting corticotrophin. So any theory that hypothesizes some abnormality in serotonin secretion in SAD could also explain abnormalities in circadian rhythms—since these rhythms are regulated by the body's clock—and in the hormonal response to stress.

There are many reasons for hypothesizing that abnormalities in brain serotonin systems may be at the basis of SAD. First, seasonal rhythms in serotonin concentrations in the hypothalamus have been described, with lowest levels being registered during the winter months. Second, there is evidence that dietary carbohydrates increase the production of brain serotonin. As noted elsewhere in this book, SAD patients crave carbohydrates and feel energized when they consume them. Although they do not know that by eating carbohydrate-rich foods they are increasing their brain serotonin levels, they may sense at some level that they are correcting a deficiency. Third, the antidepressant medications called selective serotonin reuptake inhibitors (see Chapter 9), such as fluoxetine (Prozac), sertraline (Zoloft), and paroxetine (Paxil)—which increase the amount of serotonin available for nerve signal transmission—all appear to reverse the symptoms of SAD. Dr. Siegfried Kasper compared Prozac to light therapy in the treatment of a group of SAD patients and found the two treatments to be equally effective. Dr. Dermott O'Rourke and colleagues at MIT studied another drug that promotes serotonin transmission, d-fenfluramine (which is not currently available in the United States), and found that it too was helpful in treating patients with SAD. Fourth, light exposure has been shown to stimulate serotonin-containing nerve cells in the brain and to increase concentrations of serotonin in the hypothalamus in rats.

To test the hypothesis that the symptoms of SAD might result from too little brain serotonin, several colleagues (Drs. Frederick Jacobsen, Jean Joseph-Vanderpool, Diego Garcia-Borreguero, Dennis Murphy) and I evaluated the response of SAD patients and controls to a drug that stimulates the same sites (receptors) on which serotonin acts. We injected the drug, called m-CPP, into patients and controls in winter and summer and in light-treated and untreated conditions. We found that injections of m-CPP induced short-lived feelings of activation and increased energy in untreated patients with SAD—feelings that were not experienced to the same degree after patients had been treated with light or during the summertime. Besides these exaggerated behavioral responses, untreated patients also showed exaggerated secretion of the hormone prolactin—a response that was also reduced to normal levels following successful light treatment. Interestingly, even though behavioral and prolactin responses were *exaggerated* in untreated patients and *decreased* by light therapy, corticotrophin secretory responses were *blunted* in untreated patients and *increased* by light therapy.

We interpreted our findings as follows: When SAD patients are exposed to too little environmental light, such as during the winter, they produce too little serotonin, which is responsible for the symptoms of SAD. This deficiency of brain serotonin leads to increased sensitivity in the sites (receptors) upon which serotonin normally acts. When these receptors are then stimulated by the drug m-CPP, exaggerated responses (in behavior and secretion of the hormone prolactin) are observed. When SAD patients are treated with light or during the summer, more serotonin is produced in their brains, and the symptoms of SAD improve. This increase in serotonin production reduces the sensitivity of serotonin receptors to their normal levels. When these receptors are stimulated by injections of the drug m-CPP, they lead to behavioral and hormonal responses that resemble those of non-seasonal people. The response of corticotrophin to m-CPP runs counter to this pattern. We believe that this is because the stress response axis is abnormal in SAD, possibly as a result of chronic serotonin deficiency.

Conclusion

We really do not know exactly why some people get SAD while others do not, or how light therapy works. Researchers continue to struggle with their theories and hotly debate one another over the relative merits of these different explanations. The discussion above must surely reflect my own bias toward those theories that I regard as most promising. Another researcher's list of theories and the amount of space he or she would choose to allocate to explaining each of them would no doubt look very different. Those who want to read articles with emphases other than my own will find them well represented in the scientific literature. I share with many of my readers a sense of the frustration at a mystery as yet unsolved, and look forward to the years to come, in which accumulating clues will no doubt reveal in full detail the secrets of SAD and the mechanisms of action of light therapy.

PART 3

Celebrating the Seasons

CHAPTER 13

A brief history of seasonal time

So far, I have discussed the seasons in terms of the discomfort and disability they can cause, and have considered light largely as a medication. These aspects, however, are only a few of the ways in which light and the seasons affect the mind. The seasons provided an impetus for the development of our solar calendar, and have helped us come to terms both intellectually and emotionally with the passing of time. The fluctuations in mood, energy, and vitality that may be experienced with the changing seasons have infused many people with a creative drive that has been the source of many of their finest achievements. These internal changes, coinciding as they do with those in the natural world, have inspired artists and writers to express, in paint or in words, the shifting beauty of their landscape. It is these other aspects of light and the seasons that are the subjects of this section.

Although the solar calendar may seem commonplace to us, since we use it on a daily basis, its discovery was not intuitively obvious to ancient humans. Rather, it was the more obvious monthly cycle of the moon that formed the basis for our earliest measure of time. The calendar helped ancient civilizations predict the changing seasons and decide when to plant their crops. A major problem with the lunar year, which consisted of twelve months, was that it fell short of the 365-day solar year by several days. As a result, the lunar year shifted gradually out of phase with the seasons. In an attempt to correct these shifts, certain societies inserted extra months at intervals into their lunar calendar to keep it in line with the solar one.

The Egyptians have been given credit for developing the solar calendar. They used their ability to predict where the sun would fall on a given day to illuminate their obelisks and add drama to their religious festivals. Many societies have since used the similar principle of knowing where a slab of light or shadow would fall on a particular day—for example, the winter or summer solstice—to enhance their sense of awe at a mysterious yet predictable universe. The solar calendar (as measured, for example, by the sundial) worked well, and still does, in predicting the changing seasons.

The problem of anticipating seasonal changes in the world around us has not been exclusively a human one. For many animals, especially those that live at some distance from the equator, it is crucial to be able to anticipate when it will be cold or hot; when food will be scarce or plentiful; and when to mate, migrate, or hibernate. The sheep needs to anticipate when to give birth, so that there is food enough to enable the newborn lamb to survive. The weasel must anticipate when to transform its dirty brown coat into one that is sleek and white for camouflage against the snow. The buck needs to time the growth of his antlers so that they will be at their full splendid size by the end of the summer, to enable him to fight his competitors for the doe of his choice. In order to time such events correctly, all of these animals have evolved complex physiological programs that depend for their accurate timing on information from the physical world. The environmental time cue of greatest importance across a multitude of species is the length of the day, which is a function of the solar year.

We know now that seasonal changes are not confined to animals, but occur in humans too. Many normal individuals surveyed in the northern United States report that their energy and activity levels are highest in the summer and lowest in the winter; in winter they eat more, gain weight, sleep more, and prefer sweet and starchy foods. These behavioral changes—similar in nature to those seen in SAD patients, though milder in severity—could be viewed as adaptive to the energy demands of winter, since they appear to have an energy-conserving function. These seasonal changes are probably triggered by certain environmental factors such as daylength or temperature, which vary seasonally. Thus our solar calendar and the calendar of our biological responses both follow the annual course of the sun across the sky. The discovery of the solar calendar by the Egyptians (a product of human intellect), and the seasonal patterns of human biology (shaped over thousands of years by the forces of evolution), have thus both used the sun and the seasons as the most dependable and meaningful markers for charting time over long periods.

Quite apart from the practical need to measure time, we have also had to deal with the emotional impact of time's passing. Over the course of time we receive the gifts of life, health, youth, children, and the rewards of our labors; yet, in time, we lose them all. We are subject to aging, disease, the destructive forces of our fellow human beings, and finally death. How do we come to terms with all these losses, as well as with the burden of the errors we have made?

These are age-old problems, and ancient civilization found a novel solution to them: Simply abolish time. Wipe it out and start all over again. Thus, in ancient times, people engaged in cleansing rituals at the end of each year, purifying themselves of the dirt and sin they had accumulated over the previous year. They could then enter the new year fresh and clean. All sorts of complex rituals were developed. For example, sins would be transferred to a goat, and the animal would be driven out of the area—the proverbial scapegoat. Not only were one's sins abolished, but the slate of time was itself wiped clean. Ancient humans lacked a sense that one year led to the next—a concept of time that has been termed "linear" or "historical." Instead, they believed in cyclical time, "the myth of the eternal return," which happens to be the title of a fascinating book on the subject by Mircea Eliade.

Around the time of the winter solstice, it was traditional to extinguish and rekindle fire. Even in modern times, the festivals that take place around the time of the winter solstice are celebrated with lights: the colored ones on Christmas trees and the candles on a Hanukkah menorah. In some cultures the winter solstice coincides with the new year, and the extinguishing and rekindling of fire can also be regarded as symbolizing the obliteration of time past and the start of new time. Alternatively, such activities may be viewed as a celebration of (or prayer for) the return of the sun's light following the winter solstice. The use of light in these rituals may also serve to lift our spirits during the darkest days of the year.

Cyclical time was common in many ancient societies. The Greeks conceived of history as cyclical and developed the idea of a "Great Year" many thousands of solar years in length. The Great Year, which they believed corresponded to the rotation of the heavens, had a Great Summer, when planetary forces would combine to destroy the earth by fire, and a Great Winter, when the world would be overwhelmed by water. The Indians had a similar concept of a cosmic cycle, called a Mahayuga, which was thought to last four million years.

It seems likely that the obvious seasonal changes in the world around us, and our internal changes in mood and behavior—together, perhaps, with the wish to abolish the past—all contributed to the development of a cyclical sense of time. In the past few centuries, however, a linear or historical sense has prevailed. This sense of time is familiar to every schoolchild who has had to construct a dateline showing how certain events occurred over the years. An integral part of this concept is that these events took place in a certain sequence, and that in certain critical ways, the clock or calendar cannot be turned back. Thus, for example, World War II took place in part because of unresolved issues from World War I. Dropping the atom bombs on Japan put an end to World War II—an event that could not have happened four years earlier, since the atom bomb had not yet been invented. The dropping of the bomb ushered in an age in which nuclear warfare is an ever-present possibility. This has changed the nature of war and the whole way in which we view our world. Thus, nowadays even schoolchildren become thoroughly familiar with the concept of linear or historical time that moves in one direction only.

The Jews have been credited with the development of the sense of linear time. Calamities that beset the children of Israel were interpreted by the prophets as the result of the wrath of God—proof that the people needed to reform their ways. The prophets thus forced the people to turn away from a purely cyclical and ever-renewing sense of time and face the consequences of their actions. This concept was continued in Christianity, which sees time as a straight line that traces the course of humanity from its creation through redemption to the present. The Chinese, in their descriptions of successive dynasties, have been credited with independently coming up with a linear sense of time, and such a sense was surely present in the mind of one thirteenth-century Japanese sage, Dogen, who observed, "Time flies more swiftly than an arrow and life is more transient than the dew. We cannot call back a single day that has passed."

According to Eliade, the conflict between the two different perceptions of time—cyclical and linear—continued into the seventeenth century, after which the latter view gained ascendance. This was in keeping with the development of science, the theory of evolution, and the idea of human progress, all of which were believed to proceed in a linear way. Despite this linear trend, both Jews and Christians have continued to celebrate cyclical time in the form of seasonal rituals and festivals. There has been a renewal of interest in cyclical time in the twentieth century. Historians such as Oswald Spengler and Arnold Toynbee have considered the problems of periodicity in history. The works of two important modern writers, T. S. Eliot and James Joyce, are, in Eliade's view, "saturated with nostalgia for the myth of eternal repetition and . . . the abolition of time."

One of the reasons it took modern psychiatrists so long to rediscover SAD might have been the ascendance of linear over cyclical time. According to a linear way of thinking, a psychiatrist might consider, for example, a female patient with three episodes of winter depression as follows: Three years ago, in October, she broke up with her boyfriend and became depressed for several months. By April she recovered, moved, and found a new job. She was not able to function for a prolonged period in this position, however; she became depressed, and lost the job in December. The next March she entered into a new relationship, which seemed to lift her spirits. She was well until about a month ago (October), when her relationship difficulties resurfaced, and she has since become markedly lethargic, withdrawn, and depressed.

In the past few decades, however, psychiatrists have once again become interested in cyclicity in the form of biological rhythms. It was this developing interest that served as a major precursor to the rediscovery of SAD.

CHAPTER 14

Polar tales

I have frequently been asked, "Haven't they studied SAD in Scandinavia? Don't they get a lot of it over there?" In recent years, since our work from the NIMH first appeared, several Scandinavian research groups have begun work on the subject. Before then, however, there was little or nothing about it in Scandinavian medical literature. Given the degree of light deprivation so far north, one wonders about this gap. Does it mean that the condition—or indeed, any seasonal change in mood or behavior—is very rare in those people, or is there some other reason why they have not studied it? One Swedish psychiatrist provided a witty answer to my question about the prevalence of SAD in Scandinavia. "Either everyone there has it," he replied, "or no one does."

It certainly appears as though some Scandinavians have the problem. Dr. Tront Bratlid in Norway has come across many patients with the symptoms of SAD, and Dr. Andrés Magnússon in Iceland notes that "Everyone seems to have some relative who takes to bed for the whole winter." Cases that sound like SAD can also be found, according to him, in Icelandic myths. Seasonal changes in behavior are reportedly rife in the general population in Scandinavia. According to some observers, these seasonal rhythms seem to be so widespread that most people just take them for granted. This may be the reason why they did not gain the attention of the medical community until reports started appearing from other parts of the world.

In fact, some of the best descriptions of the behavioral effects of circumpolar winters come from outsiders. One early outsider, Dr. Frederick Cook, who went on a nineteenth-century expedition to Antarctica as ship's doctor to the *Belgica*, described how the ship was trapped in the ice during the Antarctic winter and how the crew suffered from isolation and the harsh weather conditions. Of all of these, the darkness appeared to affect the men most. According to Cook, they "gradually . . . became affected, body and soul, with languor." He described other psychiatric problems among the crew, and concluded that "The root cause of these disasters was the lack of the sun." He treated his men with direct exposure to an open fire and found that this seemed to help them, perhaps more because of the heat than the light. For sixty-eight days the sun was not seen until, once again, it appeared above the horizon "like a small, withered orange."

Dr. Cook also provided us with a description of seasonal rhythms of sexual drive among the Eskimos:

> The passions of these people are periodical, and their courtship is usually carried on soon after the return of the sun; in fact, at this time, they almost tremble from the intensity of their passions and for several weeks most of their time is taken up in gratifying them.

Such shifts in sex drive, with a surge of interest in the spring continuing into the summer, almost certainly affect people living at lower latitudes, though to a lesser degree. Many societies have created spring rituals that incorporate elements of sexuality or fertility, which coincide with the burgeoning of nature outside and rising sexual passions within.

An excellent description of the psychological effects of the dark days on the people of Tromsø in northern Norway was provided by Joseph Wechsberg, who wrote an article in *The New Yorker* called "*Mørketiden*," which means "murky times." Tromsø, which lies 215 miles north of the Arctic Circle, has forty-nine sunless days during the winter. Wechsberg observed that "the people talked a lot about *mørketiden*, and at the same time protested that they were not affected by it." He reported that people felt tired; had difficulty getting up in the morning and accomplishing their work; and suffered from disturbed sleep, low energy level, and actual depression. In other words, many of these people complained of the symptoms of SAD. One man he interviewed even observed that the depression seemed to be a particular problem among women.

Wechsberg described an opposite pattern of behavior in the summer. People rarely seemed to feel tired and often did not feel like going to bed. They were active at all hours of the night. There was widespread celebration as people headed for the country to "fish, hunt, have fun." As a result, it was difficult to get any work done. I have experienced similar effects of the long Arctic summer days myself while visiting Alaska in May, when the days were over twenty hours long. My family and I were extremely energetic and didn't get the feeling of winding down that ordinarily comes at the end of the day. We had to remind ourselves to go to sleep at two o'clock in the morning, or else we would have stayed up all night.

Wechsberg observed that in winter, the people of Tromsø kept their indoor lights on constantly during the day. One woman reported missing the sun so much that she gravitated toward the window. The return of the sun after forty-nine dark days was celebrated as *Soldag*, or "Sun Day." Children were sent home early from school that day and all work stopped by noon. The first rays were greeted with tears, prayers, and special wishes. Some people, unwilling to wait for this day, flew to southern Norway to see the sun.

Apparently, the physicians of Tromsø agreed that a study of the effects of *mørketiden* was long overdue. This was in 1972. Since then, some work has been done in Norway on midwinter insomnia, but it was only after SAD was described and treated with light in the United States that studies began in Tromsø. Why did it take so long? It is possible that the investigators' own seasonal rhythms interfered with their ability to study the problem. In the winter, it is conceivable that their low energy level did not provide them with the creativity or enthusiasm to undertake such a study, whereas in the summer, they might have been too busy enjoying the long, sunny days. It is also possible that the stoicism of the northern people caused them to understate the difficulties associated with *mørketiden* and to deny the extent of the problem. Finally, it might have required an outsider such as Joseph Wechsberg, who did not take *mørketiden* for granted, to describe the full extent of the problem. This may account for why the Scandinavians were not the first to describe SAD. I believe that my own upbringing, in a climate where the seasons were mild, enabled me to recognize the dramatic nature of the seasonal changes in North America. As in Edgar Allan Poe's story "The Purloined Letter," sometimes that which is right under one's nose is most difficult to observe.

CHAPTER 15

SAD through the ages

The relationship between depression and the seasons was first observed over two thousand years ago by Hippocrates, who noted, "It is chiefly the changes of the seasons which produces diseases." Aretaeus, in the second century A.D., recommended that "Lethargics are to be laid in the light and exposed to the rays of the sun, for the disease is gloom." Yet it is only in the late twentieth century that seasonal depression has entered the diagnostic manual of psychiatric diseases, and light therapy has been seriously considered as a treatment for winter depression. How can we account for this long hiatus? Why did it take medical science so long to rediscover the wisdom of the ancients? This rediscovery is not the result of some technological breakthrough, examples of which are to be found in so many other areas of medicine, for the elements needed to make this discovery—our powers of observation, the charting of mood changes over time, and bright light—have been available for ages. Rather, this rediscovery was a result of advances in our understanding of psychiatric diseases and our changing concepts of time.

The following are three historic cases of SAD, described some three centuries apart. Clinically, they have certain distinct resemblances to one another and to modern-day descriptions of SAD. What I find fascinating about these cases is how they illustrate the different ways in which the physicians of the time conceptualized SAD, and what they can teach us about the changing concepts of time and mental illness over the centuries. During the era when the first case was described (the seventeenth century), medical science was still under the powerful influence of the humoral theories of disease that had held sway since the times of ancient Greece. The second case was described in the nineteenth century, at a time when the impact of the physical environment on mental illness was considered of great importance to those suffering from mood disorders. The final case was described in the middle of the twentieth century, when psychoanalytic theories had the greatest influence on our approach toward mental illness.

Anne Grenville

She was the daughter of the Bishop of Durham and the wife of a minister, but it was not for these reasons that Anne Grenville, who lived in England in the late 1600s, is remembered in history. Rather, it is because of her extraordinarily well-documented psychiatric problems and the prominence of the physicians whom she consulted. We owe this thorough documentation to an ongoing battle between her father and her husband. Her father claimed that she had always been healthy, and, according to her sister, she had been driven to madness by her husband. Her husband's annoyance at Mrs. Grenville's psychiatric problems was compounded by financial difficulties, which were further aggravated by his father-in-law's reluctance to pay the expected dowry.

Mrs. Grenville appears to have suffered from a cyclical mood disorder. According to one physician she consulted, "There are twin symptoms, which are her constant companions, Mania and Melancholy, and they succeed each other in a double and alternate act; or take each other's place like the smoke and flame of a fire." Her problem would probably not have received so much medical attention—at least nine prominent physicians saw her—had it not been for the troublesome nature of her manic episodes. One physician, a prominent Frenchman, described these episodes as follows:

> The first oncoming of this recurrent disease shows itself by mild insomnia, unusual talkativeness, propensity to laughter, practically continuously. . . . But as the illness increases, her periods of wakefulness become more extended, or if she does fall asleep, her condition is worsened as a result of the sleep; silence succeeds talkativeness, morosity, laughter . . . and finally, she sometimes rages against her attendants and attacks anyone she meets in a petulant manner.

It is not uncommon for mania to begin as an euphoric condition and progress to a state of irritability and anger. As the following description by two English physicians of the alternate phase of Mrs. Grenville's condition indicates, she also suffered from recurrent depressions: "From time to time the symptoms of melancholia proper also put in an appearance; she carries on her ordinary tasks and duties in a gentler manner, sometimes taciturn, timid, and sorrowful, without a trace of savageness."

The seasonality of her symptoms—particularly her tendency to become manic in the summer—was well documented. For this reason, one of her doctors suggested special treatments "at the approach of the dog days." The dog days are the six hottest weeks of the year, named after the dog star, Sirius, the brightest star in the firmament. Once a year the dog star rises in direct alignment with the sun, and the ancients believed that during this time, its effects combined with those of the sun to produce the intense heat of July and August.

Mrs. Grenville's case is not exactly typical of most SAD patients I have seen, whose manic symptoms are generally less prominent. In addition, although her manias clearly occurred in the summer, and we are told that these alternated with her depressive episodes, we are not told specifically that the depressions occurred in the winter, though it seems likely that they did. Her depressions were probably less well documented than her manias, because depression is often regarded as less of a problem by a patient's relatives. The patient frequently takes the opposite point of view, seeking help when depressed, but not when manic.

Many theories were advanced to explain Mrs. Grenville's condition, and on the basis of these, several treatments were suggested—all, unfortunately, to little avail. The explanations of her illness showed the continuing influence of the humoral theories of the ancient Greeks, according to which a person was composed of four humors: blood, yellow bile (choler), black bile (melanchos), and phlegm. These humors were thought to be associated with the four seasons: spring, summer, autumn, and winter, respectively. Different types of climates—cold or hot, moist or dry—were thought to act upon the different humors, altering their relative influence on a person. So were different constellations and planets. The result of these influences on an individual's innate disposition was thought to result in one of four temperaments: sanguine, choleric, melancholic, or phlegmatic.

Melancholia, as its name implies, was considered to result from an excess of black bile. The planet Saturn was thought to exert an influence on this condition. In one artistic portrayal of the four humors, the melancholic describes his nature as follows:

> God has given me unduly
> In my nature melancholy.
> Like the earth both cold and dry,
> Black of skin with gait awry,
> Hostile, mean, ambitious, sly,
> Sullen, crafty, false, and shy.
> No love for fame or woman have I;
> In Saturn and autumn the fault doth lie.

The idea that black bile was responsible for melancholia was extended by Aristotle to account for mania as well. According to him, black bile, which he regarded as being naturally cold, "produces apoplexy or torpor or despondency or fear." However, if the black bile became overheated, "it produces cheerfulness, accompanied by song and frenzy." In keeping with this thinking, several of Mrs. Grenville's doctors attributed her condition to "atrabilious ferment"—in other words, black bile. According to one of the doctors,

> The whole aim of our treatment must be at least to blunt that ferment, if we cannot entirely destroy it. This was the purpose behind the treatments proposed by the learned Doctor Bellay of Cleves: namely, cooling medicines, aperients, gentle evacuants, and occasionally hypnotics. The hope is, by these remedies to be able to suppress the force and energy of that atrabilious humour; for which purpose, especially as a preventive measure, you must see that every year at the beginning of spring you use the well-established remedies to provoke a flow of the haemorrhoids by the application of leeches.

The twin legacies of the ancient Greeks to the treatment of Anne Grenville were the humoral theory of disease, which tied melancholia to the seasons, and a cyclical view of time. The Greeks saw history as cyclical, with the rotation of the stars in the heavens resembling the rotation of the seasons, but on a much larger scale. With these theoretical views of the world, it was quite natural for them to emphasize the influences of the seasons on the lives of human beings.

The Case of M

Approximately 150 years after Anne Grenville was treated for her problems, a patient whom we know only as "M" consulted a famous French psychiatrist, Esquirol, who described his case as follows:

> M, a native of Belgium, forty-two years of age, of a strong constitution and transacting a very large business, consults me at the close of the winter of 1825. Observe the account which is given me by him. "I have always enjoyed good health, am happy in my family, having an affectionate wife and charming children. My affairs are also in excellent condition. Three years since, I experienced a trifling vexation. It was at the beginning of autumn, and I became sad, gloomy, and susceptible. By degrees I neglected my business, and deserted my house to avoid my uneasiness. I felt feeble, and drank beer and liquors. Soon I became irritable. Everything opposed my wishes, disturbed me, and rendered me

insupportable, and even dangerous to my family. My affairs suffered from this state. I suffered also from insomnia and inappetence. Neither the advice nor tender counsels of my wife, nor that of my family, had any more influence over me. At length, I fell into a profound apathy, incapable of everything except drinking and grieving. At the approach of spring I felt my affections revive. I recovered all my intellectual activity, and all my ardor for business. I was very well all the ensuing summer, but from the commencement of the damp and cold weather of autumn, there was a return of sadness, uneasiness, and a desire to drink, to dissipate my sadness. There was also a return of irascibility and transports of passion. During the last autumn and the present winter, I have experienced for the third time the same phenomena, which have been more grievous than formerly. My fortune has suffered, and my wife has not been free from danger. I have now come to submit myself to you, sir, and to obey your directions in every thing."

After many questions, I offered the following advice. "A hospital will not benefit, but on the contrary, injure you. . . . In the month of September, you should go to Languedoc [in the south of France] and must be in Italy before the close of October, from whence you must not return until the month of May." This counsel was closely followed. At the close of December he was at Rome. He felt the impression of the cold, and the beginnings of a desire to drink were manifest, but shortly disappeared. He escaped a fourth attack by withdrawing himself from the coldness and moisture of autumn. He returns to Paris in the month of May, in the enjoyment of excellent health.

This beautiful early description of SAD, and the inspired treatment that was so successful in the case of M, are impressive to a modern psychiatrist. It appears that Esquirol's treatment of M with climate modification was not an isolated event, for he observed that it was the practice of English physicians to send their melancholic patients into the southern provinces of France and Italy, "thus protecting them against the moist and oppressive air of England."

Esquirol acquired his enlightened approach from his mentor, Phillipe Pinel, the French psychiatrist renowned for removing the chains from patients in a Paris mental hospital. Pinel had strong reservations about "the usual routine of baths, bloodletting, and coercion," the standard treatment for mood disorders at the time; he suggested instead a "moral treatment" that relied more on empathy, understanding, and encouragement.

Pinel also drew attention to the importance of the physical environment in modulating mood. For melancholics, he pointed out "the urgent necessity of forcibly agitating the system, of interrupting the chain of their gloomy ideas, and of engaging their interest by powerful and continuous impressions on their external senses."

With such a renowned mentor behind him, Esquirol went on to make his own original contributions to psychiatry. He noted that depression could result from many different causes and ought to be treated in different ways, "not . . . limited to the administration of certain medicines." In his view, "Moral medicine, which seeks in the heart for the cause of the evil, which sympathizes and weeps, which consoles, and divides with the unfortunate their sufferings, and which revives hope in their breast, is often preferable to all other." However, he also stressed the importance of the physical environment, recommending "a clear sky, a pleasant temperature, an agreeable situation with varied scenery."

The late nineteenth and early twentieth centuries saw the development of bright artificial light as a therapeutic modality. In fact, Niels Finsen of Sweden was awarded one of the first Nobel Prizes for medicine for his work on the effects of artificial light on the tuberculosis bacillus. Bright light was used for many conditions, including depression. A leading British psychiatrist, Dr. J. G. Porter Phillips of the Bethlehem Hospital in London observed in 1923:

> Since the energising influence of sunlight on all living matter is so well known, it is surprising that therapists have not made greater use of this natural curative agent.
> In the province of psychological medicine it is generally accepted that no institution, from a structural point of view, is complete without its solarium. . . . In addition . . . several mental institutions have already installed apparatus for the production of artificial sunlight.
> Even to the lay mind, it is obvious what a stimulating and beneficial influence artificial sunlight can exert on those whose fund of energy is seriously depleted by nervous or mental disorder, especially during the dull, sunless, and depressing months of our British winter.

The Unmarried Clerk

The next published case of SAD was reported a century after Esquirol's description of patient M, and on the other side of the Atlantic. In the United States in 1946, Dr. George Frumkes published in the *Psychoanalytic Quarterly* the case of a thirty-year-old clerk. Frumkes described the patient's history as follows:

> [He] was recovering from a depression of a type he had had each year for the past ten years. Although he knew he would be better in the spring and summer, he wanted to be treated so that the depressions would not recur. They began in August or September and continued about six

months. During the spring and summer he was overactive and too confident, without excitement or unseemly behavior. After the recurrence of the first few cycles, he was never free from the fear of the autumnal depression. This constant threat interfered with his freedom of action in his business and in his relationship with women.

The depressions were heralded by the observation that he was sweating excessively; then he felt vague anxiety, followed by the fear that he would not be able to do his work. Later came feelings of unworthiness and inefficiency. He was convinced his work suffered because he was slow, because he had to check his work four times, and [because] he dreaded anything new and avoided making decisions. He tried to evade as much work as possible without attracting attention, and he avoided contact with superiors and fellow workers. Despite the great effort it cost him, he never missed a day's work. He felt he had no right to indulge himself. He was certain that his deficiencies were apparent to everyone. If he could have afforded to do so he would have remained in hiding in the South for six months. If criticized, he would suffer keenly and be incapable of defending himself. Praise or affection caused him suffering because he felt he was an impostor not deserving such consideration.

He was especially uncomfortable in cold weather, but there was not a constant relationship between the depth of the depression and the drop in temperature. Certain signs foretold his recovery: he would take out his camera, make strokes as if he were playing tennis, and become interested in girls. In his overactive phase he was with as many as four girls a week; he was restless, prided himself on doing the work of three men, and devised new office systems.

Frumkes followed up this excellent description, which will sound familiar to all SAD sufferers, with an extensive history of the patient's background: His parentage, family relationships, childhood, and employment background were all reviewed. His sex life was a particular focus of attention: Descriptions of his sexual development, the sleeping arrangements in the family, masturbatory practices, dating patterns, and dreams and fantasies about sex take up well over half the article.

In attempting to explain the patient's depressions, Dr. Frumkes departed from the simple and straightforward prose used to describe the patient's symptoms and launched into a convoluted psychoanalytic interpretation. According to his formulation, the patient's depressions

began about the time he learned that masturbation was not a unique sin of his; when there was a decrease in the intense, conscious feeling of guilt. The depressions represented a redistribution of the punishment in the psychic economy. . . . Masturbation for him was an unconscious infantile sexual striving for his mother, and the associated hostile impulses connected with this drive.

Frumkes also suggested that the depressions might have represented "memorial observances of the births of his brothers and sisters." Such explanations for the development of manic and depressive episodes were frequently offered by U.S. psychiatrists in the 1950s and 1960s. I have read through many medical records of manic–depressives treated at the New York State Psychiatric Institute during these years, and have been impressed by some of the ingenious formulations, which purported to explain both depressions and manias in terms of childhood experiences.

Frumkes treated his patient with psychoanalysis. Although he did not specify the frequency of sessions and length of treatment in his paper, I would assume that he met with the patient four or five times a week over several years, as is customary in traditional psychoanalysis. Frumkes reported that "as the treatment progressed, the depressions diminished in regularity and intensity. The patient undertook work of a nature he had formerly dreaded. A year following treatment he wrote that he had had no disturbances of mood, that he was married and felt well."

It is difficult to know quite what to make of this reported outcome. It seems as though the patient did indeed have sexual conflicts, and it is quite conceivable that the analytic therapy was helpful for them. However, my experience with SAD makes me question the likelihood that the treatment made a significant impact on his annual depressions, though he might have worried less about them.

It is interesting to consider that in the same year in which Frumkes published his case, a German physician, Dr. Helmut Marx, reported using bright artificial light to treat four men who had become depressed in the dark days of an Arctic winter. Marx's work was impressive, in that he recognized the recurrent nature of winter depressions and even described the overeating that often accompanies the condition. Not only did he identify light deficiency as a trigger for this condition—and bright light as an effective treatment—but he also correctly suggested that light acted via the eyes to influence the hypothalamus. All these insights are in agreement with our views of SAD and light therapy some fifty years later. Marx's report, however, was unknown to modern psychiatrists until very recently, and had little influence on patterns of psychiatric treatment or research.

How, in the course of the century between the cases reported by Esquirol and Frumkes, did the importance of the physical environment get lost? In my view, the main reason for this was the powerful influence of Sigmund Freud. Although the discovery of psychoanalysis contributed enormously to our understanding of the human mind, it also obscured our consideration of alternative hypotheses—for example, the simple possibility that depressions could be related to regular changes in climatic variables.

Freud also made his mark on our view of time. He had two opinions on the subject. First, he asserted that the information that was repressed into the unconscious mind remained unaltered by the passage of time. His was a linear, historical view—of time as an arrow. Like the Dead Sea Scrolls, resting in their earthen jars in a cave until they were discovered, unaltered by time, so the repressed memories of childhood were buried in the unconscious, to be discovered later by the analyst. Freud's second opinion on time perception in the mind was that "In the id there is nothing corresponding to the idea of time." He summarized these two views as follows: "The processes of the system Ucs. (the unconscious) are timeless; i.e., they are not ordered temporally, are not altered by the passage of time, in fact bear no relationship to time at all." Although his colleague, Wilhelm Fleiss, believed in the importance of cyclical processes in the mind, there is little evidence that Freud regarded such a cyclical sense of time as being of any major importance. So it was in the United States, as the second half of the twentieth century unfolded, that psychiatry, heavily influenced by the writings of Freud, lost its grip on time as an important consideration in evaluating psychiatric conditions; this applied both to cyclical time and to the longitudinal evaluation of individuals over time. Rather, the psychological associations of the moment were what mattered. Like a hologram in which a fragment contains an image of the whole picture, everything was contained in the present, in the cross-section of the mind that appeared there and then to the analyst.

As for the biological developments in psychiatry in the second half of the twentieth century, the big news was the development of psychotropic drugs, which could reverse psychosis, depression, and mania. These were the single most important factor in emptying out our state mental hospitals and "deinstitutionalizing" their patients. The consequences of such deinstitutionalization—for example, homelessness and street people—have caused new problems, but there is little question that the discovery of effective psychotropic drugs was a major breakthrough for psychiatry.

However, these drugs were regarded as suitable only for more disturbed patients, whereas those who were able to function in the outside world, like Frumkes's patient, were more likely to receive only psychotherapy. To some degree, a two-class system of psychiatric patients resulted. Since most patients with SAD do not require hospitalization, most would have been grouped in the healthier class and given insight-oriented psychotherapy.

Two trends in modern psychiatry were responsible for paving the way for the rediscovery of SAD and light therapy. First, standard methods of identifying discrete psychiatric conditions were developed; and second, the concept of cyclical time was once again appreciated. The development of criteria for identifying psychiatric syndromes came from a group of psychiatric diagnosticians at Washington University in St. Louis. This group emphasized the importance of examining the longitudinal course of an illness, rather than relying primarily on the mental state of the patient as presented to the psychiatrist at any given moment. As for cyclicity and behavior, the great strides made in the past few decades in understanding biological rhythms in animals were applied to people. Pioneering human studies in Germany and the United States showed that humans have an endogenous circadian system resembling that of other animals. The medical importance of cyclical time was thus rediscovered.

The NIMH group, led by Dr. Thomas A. Wehr, expanded on earlier observations by other circadian rhythm experts to develop the idea that disturbances of biological rhythms may underlie cyclical mood disorders. The cycle of day and night, light and dark, is crucially important in modulating daily rhythms in animals. It was logical, therefore, that light should recapture the interest of psychiatric clinicians and researchers, who had abandoned it some fifty years before. Into this environment came Herb Kern, scientist and patient, with fifteen years of documented seasonal cycles of depression and hypomania, to usher in the modern era of SAD and light therapy.

CHAPTER 16

Creating with the seasons

Great Wits are sure to Madness near ally'd,
And thin Partitions do their Bounds divide.
—JOHN DRYDEN

The association between genius and insanity is ingrained in our culture. We are told about the "thin line" that exists between the brilliant artist and the mad person. Is there any truth to this assertion? Have great artists of the past indeed suffered from psychiatric disturbances, and, if so, what forms have these disturbances taken? Where do seasonal responses fit into this picture, if at all? Does sensitivity to light—a cardinal feature of patients with SAD—seem to go along with sensitivity to our exterior and interior worlds?

The Link among Mood Disorders, Creativity, and the Seasons

The concept that genius and madness are somehow connected goes back at least to the time of Aristotle, who observed that "No great genius was without a mixture of insanity." He added, "Those who have become eminent in philosophy, politics, poetry, and the arts have all had tendencies toward melancholia." The Roman playwright Seneca echoed this view, noting that "The mind cannot attain anything lofty so long as it is sane." For centuries this belief persisted, and melancholia was somehow endowed with cultural value. Genius was regarded as a "hereditary taint" transmitted in families, along with mental illness.

It is only in our century, however, that the subject has been a matter of serious study. Dr. Nancy Andreasen was the first researcher to study the relationship between creativity and mental illness, using modern psychiatric diagnoses. She interviewed thirty creative writers

229

at the prestigious Iowa Writers' Workshop about their own backgrounds and those of their close relatives, and compared their responses with those of thirty control subjects. She found a substantially higher rate of mental illness among the writers and their family members. She had approached the study with the belief that there would be an association between schizophrenia and creativity. To her surprise, it was not schizophrenia but disorders of mood regulation—especially those involving a tendency to mania or hypomania, in addition to depression—that distinguished the writers from the control group. She concluded that the traits of creativity and mood disturbance appeared to run together in families and could be genetically mediated.

More recently, Dr. Kay Redfield Jamison studied a group of eminent British writers and artists for evidence of psychiatric illness, seasonal variations in mood and productivity, and the perceived role of intense moods in their creative processes. She selected these artists and writers on the basis of objective acclaim, in the form of prestigious prizes and other types of acknowledgment. She interviewed them extensively and found very high rates of mood disorders in the group. Over a third had been treated for mood problems, the great majority with medications or hospitalization. Poets were most likely to have required medication for depression and were the only group to have required treatment for mania. Playwrights had the highest total rate of treatment for mood disorders, but a high percentage of this group had been treated with psychotherapy alone. Exceptional among the writers in regard to their mood stability were biographers, who reported no history of mood swings or elated states. Although these writers were as outstanding as the others in terms of their objective achievements, they were perhaps a less creative group, in the sense that writing a biography may not be as purely "creative" an act as writing a poem or a play.

Almost all subjects (with the exception of the biographers) reported having had intense, highly productive, and creative periods. Most of these lasted between one and four weeks. These episodes were marked by "increased enthusiasm, energy, self-confidence, speed of mental association, fluency of thoughts, elevated mood, and a strong sense of well-being." They sound very much like "hypomanic" episodes, without the behavioral disturbance that this term implies. It is extremely interesting that 90 percent of Jamison's group reported that very intense moods and feelings were either integral to, or necessary for, the development and execution of their work.

Investigating the association among seasons, mood, and productivity, Jamison found a strong seasonal pattern of mood changes among artists and writers, with highest mood scores in the summer and lowest in the winter. Peak periods of productivity, while also seasonal, occurred in the spring and the fall. It seemed that as mood increased from spring to summer, so productivity declined to some extent, picking up again in the fall. Those who had been treated for mood disorders had a sharper decline of productivity in the summer than the other subjects.

How can one explain this drop-off in creativity in the summer, as the subjects' mood continued to improve? A few possible explanations come to mind. When people are too euphoric, they are often not able to produce to the best of their ability. Their thoughts may race too quickly and their focus may be scattered. There is a tendency to start many tasks but not to follow through; distractibility is a problem. Those subjects in Jamison's study who had been treated for mood disorders might have experienced more marked highs during the summer, with greater associated difficulties in focusing and carrying out tasks. Another possibility is that an artist or writer may not wish to be creative during the summer. One writer with SAD whom I know said that she has so much fun in the summer that she doesn't want to spend her golden, sunny days bashing away at a word processor.

A new way of measuring creativity has been developed by Drs. Ruth Richards and Dennis Kinney, researchers at Harvard University. The advantage of this new Lifetime Creativity Scale is that it can be used to measure creativity in anyone, not just in those of exceptional talent. By means of this scale, these researchers were able to show a higher rate of creativity among manic–depressive (bipolar) patients than expected. But even greater creativity scores were found among the relatives of bipolar patients—those with milder mood swings or no clear-cut mood swings at all. It is quite possible that this heightened level of creativity found in relatives of bipolar patients may explain why the illness has been so successfully transmitted from generation to generation. People who carry bipolar genes may be at an advantage to survive and reproduce, by virtue of their creative abilities. People with bipolar tendencies, and their relatives, seem more likely to take risks (such as emigrating), which may be highly adaptive in crisis situations.

All these studies suggest that Aristotle was correct in linking mood disturbance and creativity. It seems as though the most creative people are those with milder forms of mood disturbance, which is in keeping with my clinical experience. Severe depressions or wild manias are not conducive to productivity. The opposite is true for mild depressions alternating with hypomanias. During hypomanic periods, thoughts and associations flow rapidly, energy and confidence levels are high, the need for sleep is reduced, and ideas are more readily generated and pursued. During mild depressions, these ideas can be critically evaluated. Ideas that are too grandiose or unlikely to succeed can be discarded, and those that look more promising in the sober light of depression can be retained and developed. Mild depressions may be conducive to the drudgery that is required for any creative venture—the daily plodding necessary for the execution of any grand scheme.

The seasonal person will easily recognize this pattern of mood swings and its relationship to creativity. The depressions of SAD are often relatively mild in severity, and the hypomanias are often relatively restrained and productive. As we now know, the mood changes in SAD patients are often driven by the amount of daylight present. Many creative artists have recognized the connection between changes in environmental light and their mood and productivity. The following section deals with famous creative people who suffered from mood disorders—especially those who showed evidence of strong seasonality or light sensitivity.

Moody and Famous: Sensitive to Seasons and Light

The list of famous people with mood disturbances is impressive. Although there was no psychiatrist with a modern diagnostic handbook around to record the mental status of most of the people mentioned in this section, abundant evidence for mood disorders exists in most cases. It is not my purpose here to be comprehensive, but only to select some illustrative examples of famous creative people with mood disorders. Among artists we have Michelangelo, Albrecht Dürer, and Vincent van Gogh; composers include George Frederick Handel, Gustav Mahler, and Robert Schumann; writers include John Milton, Edgar Allan Poe, Ernest Hemingway, and Virginia Woolf; politicians include Abraham Lincoln and Winston Churchill, who referred to his depressions as his "black dog." Sir Isaac Newton was perhaps the most eminent scientist to have suffered from manic depression.

How many of these prominent people were strongly seasonal in their mood swings or sensitive to changes in environmental light? This is hard to say with any clinical certainty, especially since SAD as a distinct entity was described long after most of these people had died. Statistically, it is highly likely that many of these people were seasonal. Figures for the rate of SAD among persons with recurrent depressions range from one in six to one in three. For reasons noted above, highly creative people with mood disorders are more likely to have SAD than other forms of mood disorder, most of which are more disruptive to productivity. Beyond such general statistical information, however, we do have specific clues about seasonality and light sensitivity in several cases.

Among writers, Emily Dickinson is a likely candidate for a diagnosis of SAD (see Chapter 17). T. S. Eliot might be another patient for this distinguished clinic. His poetry sparkles with references to light. We learn that Eliot was instructed by his doctors to go south each winter. Could this have been to treat his SAD? We can only speculate. Milton is reputed to have suffered from summer SAD; according to one biographer, he was able to work on *Paradise Lost* during only half the year, between autumn and spring.

Still another writer with a mood disorder was the French short-story writer Guy de Maupassant. Toward the end of his life he attempted suicide and went on to die in an asylum. The following extract is from a story by de Maupassant entitled "Who Knows?", in which the narrator, who ends up in an asylum, recalls how he went to Italy, where the sunlight made him feel good. After that,

> I returned to France via Marseilles, and in spite of the gaiety of Provence, the diminished intensity of sunlight depressed me. On my return to the Continent, I had the odd feeling of a patient who thinks he is cured but who is warned by a dull pain that the source of illness has not been eradicated.

Was de Maupassant seasonal? It seems like a fair bet.

Among musicians, Handel and Mahler were most clearly seasonal. Both, we are told, did most of their creative work during the summer months. One of the most prodigiously rapid feats of composition was Handel's *Messiah*, which he completed in twenty-three days, between late August and mid-September. Mahler, who called himself the "summer composer," was fortunately an avid letter writer. His seasonal mood changes are clearly reflected in his letters. First, consider the following letter written to Joseph Steiner, June 19, 1879:

> Dear Steiner,
>   Now for the third day I return to you, and today I do so in order to take leave of you in merry mood. It is the story of my life that is recorded in these pages. What a strange destiny, sweeping me along on the waves of my yearning, now hurling me this way and that in the gale, now wafting me along merrily in smiling sunshine. What I fear is that in such a gale I shall someday be shattered against a reef—such as my keel has often grazed!

It is six o'clock in the morning! I have been out on the heath, sitting with Fárkas the shepherd, listening to the sound of his shawm. Ah, how mournful it sounded, and yet how full of rapturous delight—that folk-tune he played! Ah, Steiner! You are still asleep in your bed, and I have already seen the dew on the grasses. I am now so serenely gay and the tranquil happiness all around me is tiptoeing into my heart, too, as the sun of early spring lights up the wintry fields. Is spring awakening now in my own breast?! And while this mood prevails, let me take leave of you, my faithful friend!

Contrast that with a winter postcard sent to Friedrich Löhr, January 20, 1883:

Dear Fritz,
Simply cannot find time to write to you properly. Sending the stuff soon. My address is: . . . Am extremely depressed.
Very best wishes to you and your family,

Yours,
Gustav

But two years later, in spring, Mahler wrote to the same friend:

My dear Fritz,
My windows are open and the sunny, fragrant spring is gazing in upon me, everywhere endless peace and repose. In this fair hour that is granted me I will be together with you. . . .
With the coming of spring all has grown mild in me again. From my window I have a view across the city to the mountains and woods, and the kindly Fulda wends its amiable way between; whenever the sun casts its colored lights within, as now, well, you know how everything in one relaxes. That is the mood I am in today, sitting at my desk by the window, from time to time casting a peaceful glance out upon this scene of carefree calm.

There are many other letters that suggest that Mahler suffered from SAD.

Painters and sculptors are more difficult to diagnose in retrospect than writers, but Jamison's work would suggest that they are just as susceptible to mood disturbances. Artists, perhaps more than any other group, have struggled to portray light. In fact, the works of some can be instantly recognized by the distinctive quality of the light they portray: Turner's swirls of light; Rembrandt's splashes of *chiaroscuro*, illuminating the pensive faces of his models; and, of course, the dazzling colors of van Gogh.

Of these three painters, the only one with a clear history of a mood disorder is van Gogh. It seems very likely that he suffered from manic depression, although his clinical picture was complicated by intoxication with absinthe, the French liquor that at that time had a toxic ingredient in it. van Gogh's intimate understanding of depression is apparent in two famous sketches, *Sorrow* and *The Old Man in Sorrow*. In contrast to these sad figures is *The Reaper*, a young man striding boldly across a field with a huge, luminous sun shining in the background. van Gogh's wonderful use of light and color might make one suspect that he was extremely sensitive to light; indeed, his letters to his beloved brother, Theo, appear to bear this out. They are filled with descriptions of his feelings of sadness and joy, as well as of his sensitivity to the weather, and to light and darkness in particular. Here are a few selections:

[Autumn in Drenthe, 1883]
When I look around me, everything seems too miserable, too insufficient, too dilapidated. We are having gloomy days of rain now, and when I come to the corner of the garret where I have settled down, it is curiously melancholy there; through one single glass pane the light falls on an empty colour box, on a bundle of brushes the hair of which is quite worn down. It is so strangely melancholy that it has, luckily, almost a comical aspect—enough not to make one cry over it.

As long as the weather was fine I did not mind my troubles, because I saw so many beautiful things; but with this rainy weather, which we must expect to continue for months, I see more clearly how I have got stuck here, and how handicapped I am. . . .

[Winter in Nuenen, 1883]
Hardly ever have I begun a year of gloomier aspect, or in a gloomier mood. It is dreary outside; the fields are a mass of lumps of black earth and some snow, with days mostly of mist and mire. . . . This is what I see in passing, and it is quite in harmony with the interiors, very gloomy these dark winter days.

[Spring in The Hague, 1892]
Spring is coming fast here. We have had a few real spring days; last Monday, for instance, which I enjoyed very much. I think the poor people and the painters have in common this feeling for the weather and the change of the seasons.

In February 1888 van Gogh left Paris for Arles, in the south of France, at least in part to escape the north and seek out the brilliant and dazzling light of Provence. In van Gogh's own words,

I came to the south for a thousand reasons. I wanted to see a different light, I believed that by looking at nature under a bright sky one might gain a truer idea of the Japanese way of feeling and drawing. Finally, I wanted to see this stronger sun . . . because I felt that the colors of the spectrum are misted over in the north.

Here is a description to his brother, Theo, written from Arles in the summer of 1888:

> The loneliness has not worried me, because I have found the brighter sun and its effect on nature so absorbing. . . .
> Yesterday at sunset I was in a stony heath where some very small and twisted oaks grow, in the background a ruin on the hill and corn in the valley. It was romantic, like a Monticelli; the sun was pouring bright yellow rays upon the bushes and the ground, a perfect shower of gold, and all the lines were lovely. . . .

Here is another description of the sun by van Gogh:

> Now there is a glorious fierce heat, a sun, a light which for want of a better word I can only call yellow, pale sulphur yellow, pale lemon gold. How beautiful yellow is.
> Life is almost an enchantment. Those who do not believe in the sun here are without faith!

To sum up, creativity appears to be more common among patients with mood disorders, especially those whose condition is relatively mild, as well as among the relatives of such patients. It is quite conceivable that the genes for creativity and mood disorders are transmitted together. It is important for psychiatrists treating such individuals to understand this. Eradicating all mood swings may diminish creativity in some people, though it is likely to improve matters greatly for those whose mood swings are severe. Nowadays, when an understanding of the human genetic makeup is close at hand, and the possibility of preventing certain undesirable genes in the new generation is scientifically conceivable, we would do well to consider the beneficial aspects of certain types of emotional disturbance, while never forgetting the pain they can cause. Had the birth of all depressives in history been successfully prevented, the world we live in would be a far different place today, and not necessarily a better one.

Prominent seasonal changes in mood and behavior seem particularly conducive to creativity, and there is evidence that many creative individuals, both past and present, have experienced them.

CHAPTER 17

Words for all seasons

For centuries the seasons have inspired poets and songwriters, who have left us a glorious legacy describing the changes that occur—both in the world around us and in ourselves—as, year after year, the earth tilts and rotates around the sun. What is it that has so inspired writers over the ages? I believe it is, first, the intense feelings with which the changing seasons imbue us; second, the capacity of seasonal images to evoke memories in us; and third, the appeal of the cycle of the seasons as a metaphor for a person's life.

The seasonal changes in energy, feelings, and drives that we now recognize as common parts of the human experience are accompanied by prominent changes in the world around us: varied colors, fragrances, temperatures, and sounds. By reminding us of these specific sensations, a poet can evoke in us the feelings that often accompany them. Beyond the recreation of these feelings, and the nostalgia that comes with them, the seasons remind us of cyclical time, loss, and recovery—birth, death, and renewal.

In poetry, spring has usually been portrayed as representing reawakening, rebirth, sexuality, and joy, and for some people this is true. Yet others find spring to be a difficult and painful season. Summer is generally seen as a time of happiness and generative capability, though we know it can make some people feel depressed and others aggressive. Autumn engenders mixed feelings: Nature is intensely beautiful and summer's harvest abounds, but there are also hints of the approach of winter, and melancholy often accompanies them. Then winter comes, and with it the death of vegetation; cold, inhospitable temperatures; food shortages; the disappearance of birds and animals; and, of course, the waning of the sun's light.

The cycle of the seasons has often been compared by writers and artists to a person's life. This is a strange metaphor. One might think that a person's life would be better conceptualized as linear, extending

237

in a straight line from birth to death. But perhaps it is more difficult for us to think of our lives in such a linear way—as a segment snipped out of a long string, with a finite beginning and end. Instead, we once again embrace the concept of cyclical time—"ashes to ashes, dust to dust"— to create the more comforting image of life as a ring, round and complete.

In connecting the seasons with the cycles of human life, poets have linked spring with youth, summer with the prime of life, autumn with declining powers, and winter with old age.

Seasons and Passion

In spring, as the saying goes, a young man's fancy lightly turns to thoughts of love, and this applies to women too. So it has been since Biblical times, when Solomon, poet and lover, sang to his beloved:

> For lo, the winter is past,
> the rain is over and gone.
> The flowers appear on the earth,
> the time of singing has come
> and the voice of the turtledove
> is heard in our land.

The passions of spring have continued unabated for thousands of years. As Shakespeare observed:

> Between the acres of the rye
> With a hey, and a ho, and a hey nonny no,
> These pretty country folks would lie,
> In the spring time, the only pretty ring time,
> When birds do sing, hey ding a ding, ding:
> Sweet lovers love the spring.

Yet the spring has not always been associated with unmixed joy. With spring comes the revival of desire, which has lain dormant through the winter. There may be an inertia to overcome before the energy of spring can be fully enjoyed. Emily Dickinson, one of our most seasonal poets, described this sensation:

> I cannot meet the Spring unmoved—
> I feel the old desire—
> A Hurry with a lingering, mixed,
> A Warrant to be fair.

T.S. Eliot, in his famous lines, expressed a more painful form of spring fever:

April is the cruelest month, breeding
Lilacs out of the dead land, mixing
Memory and desire, stirring
Dull roots with spring rain.

More recently, blues singer Betty Carter observed, in the words of composer Tommy Wolf:

Old man winter was a gracious host,
But spring can really hang you up the most.

Summer has been regarded by some as a season of heady delight. Emily Dickinson wrote:

Inebriate of Air—am I—
And Debauchee of Dew—
Reeling—thro' endless summer days—
From inns of Molten Blue—

She compared herself to a bee, drunk on the light of the sun, an influence more intoxicating than any liquor brewed.

Although autumn has been regarded by some poets, like John Keats, as a "season of mists and mellow fruitfulness," a time of beauty and fulfillment, others have seen it as a sad time—a time of waning light, and a harbinger of the coming winter. Matthew Arnold, for example, wrote:

Coldly, sadly descends
The autumn evening. The field
Strewn with its dank yellow drifts
Of wither'd leaves, and the elms,
Fade into dimness apace,
Silent.

Although poets have had their differences in their views of autumn, winter has been almost universally treated as a season of despondency and unremitting gloom. According to Shakespeare, "a sad tale's best for winter." James Thomson, in his poem "Winter," of 1726, encapsulated the common view of this season:

See! Winter comes, to rule the varied Year,
Sullen, and sad.

Seasons and Memories

The poet can depend on the reader to have powerful memories and emotions associated with the seasons. The distinctive colors, smells, and characteristics that each brings serve as cues to memories of poignant events that have occurred in that season. Conversely, the memory of a significant event is often colored and modified by the season in which it happened. We can recall perhaps the quality of the sky, the weather, and the specific smells of the season. Associations such as these were emphasized by Freud in his models of how the mind works. The importance of such associations continues to be recognized by both writers and mental health professionals. They are in no way incompatible with our more recent understanding of the biological changes in mood and behavior associated with the seasons.

Such memories, reawakened by a particular time of year, have been described, for example, by Edgar Allan Poe in his poem "Ulalume":

> The skies they were ashen and sober;
> The leaves they were crisped and sere—
> The leaves they were withering and sere;
> It was night in the lonesome October
> Of my most immemorial year. . .

As the poem continues, it emerges that the speaker, driven by some compulsion that he does not understand, seeks out a path to the tomb of his beloved, whom he buried on that same October day the year before. He has repressed this memory until he comes across the tomb with the name of his beloved, Ulalume, upon it. At this sight, the sad memory of her loss penetrates him and he recalls now why the autumn, with its crisped and sere leaves, sent such a chill through his heart. Poe has thus provided us with a powerful example of how we associate important events in our lives with the seasons in which they happen.

Another such example is Percy Bysshe Shelley's poem "Adonais," where he lamented the death of Keats, which occurred in late winter. He wrote:

> Ah, woe is me! Winter is come and gone,
> But grief returns with the revolving year.

The Seasons of a Person's Life

The metaphor of the seasons as the stages of a person's life was succinctly expressed by Keats:

He has his lusty Spring, when fancy clear
Takes in all beauty with an easy span:
He has his Summer, when luxuriously
Spring's honey'd cud of youthful thought he loves . . .
His soul has in its Autumn, when his wings
He furleth close; . . .
He has his Winter too of pale misfeature,
Or else he would forgo his mortal nature.

Shakespeare also compared the final stages of a human life to winter and found both barren and dreary:

That time of year thou may'st in me behold
When yellow leaves, or none, or few, do hang
Upon those boughs which shake against the cold,
Bare ruin'd choirs, where late the sweet birds sang.

Seasonal imagery has also been used to evoke feelings about an era, as Charles Dickens did in A *Tale of Two Cities* when he labeled the period of the French Revolution as "the spring of hope . . . the winter of despair." Likewise, Thomas Hardy, looking out over the landscape at the end of the nineteenth century, saw in its dreary, wintry features a metaphor for the dead century and a confirmation of his sense of hopelessness for the future:

I leaned upon a coppice gate
When Frost was spectre-grey
And Winter's dregs made desolate
The weakening eye of day. . . .
The land's sharp features seemed to be
The Century's corpse outleant;
His crypt the cloudy canopy,
The wind his death lament.
The ancient pulse of germ and birth
Was shrunken hard and dry,
And every spirit upon earth
Seemed fervourless as I.

The Loveliness of the Light

Just think of the illimitable abundance and the marvelous loveliness of light, or of the beauty of the sun and moon and stars.
—St. Augustine, *City of God*

Light has many meanings for us, and poets and authors have used images of it to illustrate them. Besides revealing our world to us, light can, by itself, influence the way we feel. In addition to the effects of light shining from the world outside, much has been written about the "inner light."

The capacity of light to induce in us a sense of wonder and joy may be new to scientists, but writers have recognized it for centuries. In the second verse of Genesis, we are told: "And God said, 'Let there be light'; and there was light. And God saw that the light was good." Later in the Bible, in Ecclesiastes, we are advised: "Truly the light is sweet, and a pleasant thing it is for the eyes to behold the sun."

Just as light has been associated with joy, so has darkness been associated with sorrow. Perhaps no poet could understand darkness so well as the blind Milton, who wrote:

> Seasons return, but not to me returns
> Day, or the sweet approach of ev'n or morn,
> Or sight of vernal bloom, or summer's rose,
> Or flocks, or herds, or human face divine;
> But cloud instead, and ever-during dark
> Surrounds me, from the cheerful ways of men.

But even to the sighted, the dim light of winter can prove depressing. If the reader is not by now convinced that Emily Dickinson suffered from SAD, the following verse should settle the question:

> There's a certain Slant of light,
> Winter Afternoons—
> That oppresses, like the Heft
> Of Cathedral Tunes—
> Heavenly Hurt, it gives us—
> We can find no scar,
> But internal difference,
> Where the Meanings, are.

Dickinson's intuitiveness is astonishing. She not only connected her heavy mood with the quality of the light (specifically, its low angle), but she recognized that one can be hurt without any external manifestations—that inside the mind there are places where the meanings of things are recorded, where joy and suffering are experienced.

Although Dickinson pointed out that the weak and fading light can be oppressive, she also observed:

We grow accustomed to the Dark—
When Light is put away—
As when the Neighbor holds the Lamp
To witness her Good-bye— . . .
Either the Darkness alters—
Or something in the sight
Adjusts itself to Midnight—
And Life steps almost straight.

Again, this brilliant poet observed something within herself corresponding to the physiological changes that occur in the eye—and
perhaps the brain—when a person is surrounded by darkness. The eye
adapts to the dark: The pupil enlarges, and the rods, the most
light-sensitive receptors in the retina, take over from the cones, which
are responsible for ordinary vision. It is quite conceivable that a
corresponding adaptation to the dark occurs in the brain.

Flooding the dark-adapted eye (and perhaps brain) with light may
have a powerful effect on mood. Such an effect, as is produced by bright
snow on a dark winter's day, was described by T. S. Eliot in "Little
Gidding":

Midwinter spring is its own season . . .
When the short day is brightest, with frost and fire,
The brief sun flames the ice, on pond and ditches. . . .
A glare that is blindness in the early afternoon—
And glow more intense than blaze of branch, or brazier,
Stirs the dumb spirit: . . .
In the dark time of the year . . .
The soul's sap quivers.

The capacity of light to affect mood was recognized by William
James, prominent psychologist and brother of the novelist Henry
James, in his book *The Varieties of Religious Experience*. He cited an
example from the autobiography of J. Trevor, in which Trevor
described how, one Sunday morning he felt unable to accompany his
wife and sons to church, "as though to leave the sunshine on the hills,
and go down there to the chapel, would be for the time an act of
spiritual suicide. And I felt such need for new inspiration and
expansion in my life." So reluctantly he bade his wife and sons
farewell, and headed for the hills with his stick and his dog.

In the loveliness of the morning, and the beauty of the hills and valleys,
I soon lost my sense of sadness and regret. . . . On the way back, suddenly,
without warning, I felt that I was in Heaven—an inward state of peace and

joy and assurance indescribably intense, accompanied with a sense of being bathed in a warm glow of light, as though the external condition had brought about the internal effect—a feeling of having passed beyond the body. . .by reason of the illumination in the midst of which I seemed to be placed. This deep emotion lasted, though with decreasing strength, until I reached home, and for some time after, only gradually passing away.

Architects have recognized the important influence of the interior lighting of a building on the way its inhabitants feel. For example, in a recent restoration of a small London church designed by Christopher Wren, the architects went to great lengths to create the effect of daylight in the church's dome. One lighting consultant noted that he was seeking "that magical moment when you feel light becomes a material rather than something only to be in." Had similar pains been taken with the lighting in the church attended by Trevor, who is quoted above, he might not have chosen to spend his morning in the sunlight of the hills.

Trevor's response to the sunlit hills is reminiscent of the reactions of the people of Tromsø on *Soldag*, or, for that matter, of the reports by many patients with SAD following treatment with bright light therapy. Just as the darkness oppressed Emily Dickinson by acting on the place "where the meanings are," so perhaps the light exerts its uplifting effects by acting on the same part of the brain to reverse the oppressive effects of darkness. It seems reasonable to postulate, as Dickinson did, the existence of a part of the brain capable of being stimulated by light entering the eyes, and thereby registering feelings of wonder and joy. That same part of the brain, if deprived of light, might lead to sadness and despair. I would speculate that this part of the brain, so sensitive to the presence or absence of light, is located in the hypothalamus at the base of the brain.

Besides the many descriptions of the way in which light from the world outside affects our mood, there are also many reports of internally perceived light, often associated with powerful emotions and, at times, with religious conversions or other major life changes. Mircea Eliade, who called this experience "the mystic light," described many reports of such experiences by holy men of all religions, as well as by apparently ordinary people. A famous example of a mystic light experience appears in the New Testament, where Saul of Tarsus, on the road to Damascus, experienced blinding light, which resulted in his conversion to Christianity. Another can be found in the *Bhagavad Gita*, where Krishna appeared to Arjuna "with the effulgence of a thousand suns." The poet Henry Vaughan (1622–1695) described such an experience as follows:

I saw Eternity the other night
Like a great *Ring* of pure and endless light,
All calm as it was bright.

How can we understand mystical visions of light if we do not ascribe these experiences to divine intervention? I believe that the clue may lie in their resemblance to the euphoriant effects of bright light therapy in SAD patients, or to the effects on those in the far north or south when the sun returns after many weeks of darkness. During light therapy, light enters via the eyes and acts on a part of the brain "where the meanings are," inducing feelings of energy, reawakening, tranquility, harmony, and joy. Under certain circumstances, the same part of the brain may perhaps be activated either spontaneously or by some stimulus other than light.

Whatever the mechanism of such mystical light experiences, and whatever their influence on the individual may be, there seems to be little question that they occur. Their profound emotional effects are compatible with the idea that light can powerfully modify mood and behavior—a lesson I have learned from my experiences with the treatment of SAD patients.

CHAPTER 18

Seasonal artists of our time

I have enjoyed working with SAD patients for several reasons: The condition is eminently treatable, and the idea that light affects mood and behavior has always fascinated me. But beyond these considerations have been the people themselves. I have seldom met a more sensitive, artistic, and creative group. I have learned a great deal from them, starting with the very first seasonal patient, Herb Kern, a creative scientist, who discerned the patterns of his moods and wondered about their relationship to changes in light. I have learned to look at light in a new way: to discriminate between different shades of fluorescent lamps, as well as to observe the angle of the sun, the degree of cloud cover, and the quality of fog.

Among the strongly seasonal people I have known are artists of all types. Some of them have incorporated their sensitivity toward light and the changing seasons into their art, and this chapter deals with two such people. One collects wildflowers in the summer and shapes them into wreaths and garlands, to which the memories of long, sun-filled summer days adhere. The other tells stories, in which changes in light are intimately associated with changes in mood, as they are in his own life. Their stories follow, and illustrate how SAD as a condition and seasonality as a creative gift can be opposite sides of the same coin.

"Jessica": A Flower Artist

"Jessica" is a woman in her mid-forties with blond hair flowing around her face in curls, blue eyes, and a broad smile. She has suffered from SAD for years and has benefited from light treatment. But Jessica, like all seasonal people, defines herself in a much larger context than "having SAD." She is a professional, a mother, a devoted friend, and a support to many in her community—an eminently likable woman. In this chapter I do not discuss Jessica as a patient, but as an artist.

She has always felt the urge to create, but resisted it for years because it was not regarded as an acceptable way of life in her family, where her father was a doctor and her mother a nurse. Life had to be devoted to service, and art, insofar as it was acceptable, had to be a hobby. She struggled to become a counselor, but the artist in her prevailed.

I spoke with Jessica on her porch at the height of summer. She served iced, fruit-flavored tea, garnished with mint. Bees were buzzing all around us, attracted to the flowers hanging from baskets and craning toward us in splashes of color from all sides. Jessica creates her artwork from these flowers. The artist was in her studio.

Jessica did not always work with flowers; she was a photographer first. But in her creative work she has always felt in harmony with light and the seasons. Her whole body, she feels, resonates with the seasons. As she describes it,

My body is part of the day and the night. In a dry spell, when the earth is dry, I feel dry. When it is wet, I feel clogged and wet and soaked. When it's dark, I feel dark; and when it's light, I feel light. I love nature because somehow I am biologically tied to it. When the days get shorter, I almost feel a silent buzzing in my ears. It's just a presence that gets heavier and heavier as my body gets heavier and heavier. In the spring I am aware of a lightness, a peeling off, the way we peel off our clothes. As the days get lighter, I get lighter. By March I am like a plant. I can't wait to get outside and get my hands into the earth. As I water a plant and see it growing in the sunshine, I think to myself, "I am that plant. That plant is me."

Even though she suffers with the changing seasons, Jessica would hate to lose them. Even the sad, drab winter holds for her its magical images—the sun shining off snow; a fire crackling at night; the architecture of the trees, stripped of their leaves—and she would miss them if she were to move to a seasonless climate. She was once diagnosed as manic–depressive and was offered lithium to level out her moods, but she was reluctant to relinquish the buoyancy of the summer and the creative impetus provided by her alternating mood states.

Jessica is fascinated by portraying the dark, as well as the light gleaming out of that darkness. As a photographer, she loved working with lighting and had a powerful desire to master taking pictures in the dark. She thought of photographing the winter landscape at sunset, when there was snow on the ground and little lights would come on in all the houses. How could she make a picture where there was no light except these? She became obsessed with the desire to capture the darkness on a photograph. Now that she is no longer doing photography, her urge to capture the light within the darkness has been transformed into a wish to create a Christmas decoration of a miniature papier-mache house built under the roots of a huge tree. Inside there will be little caverns and rooms, covered with soft moss and furnished; these will be inhabited by little animals—mice and moles—and illuminated by tiny lights. The object is to portray the peaceful hibernation of the winter—the comfort of not having to do anything when you don't want to, but instead of being warm and snug, and resting inside some dark cavern in the earth.

These concepts were and are very different from the photographic images that Jessica wanted to convey in the summer: pictures with too much light in them. She enjoyed letting the sunspots show—"those little dappled, octagonal things you get when your lens is too close to the sun." She wished to create an effect in the viewer that would cause him or her to exclaim, "Look at all this sun! How it shone! Incredible!"

After the photographic phase of her life, Jessica worked in her husband's flower shop and developed a new way of creating with the seasons. She began to resonate with the progression of the year, as reflected in the changing flowers available at the market:

Every week something new has arrived and something else has died off. In May you have to get flowers from California: statice and caspian. But in June the yarrow starts—white yarrow and green dock. Those are the first things you watch for by the road, and suddenly, now that June is beginning, there they are. That's the beginning of the picking season. By July the dock has turned from green to brown, and then it's time to pick that. Then there's goldenrod. In late July and early August many things arrive. I go north, picking tansy from the Catskills and pearly everlastings from the Berkshires. There are about fifty varieties of goldenrod, which I pick along the way. There are grasses to pick all summer long. Then in September comes hydrangea. You have to wait until it's dry on the vine. In October there's rabbit tobacco from around Williamsburg, and pussytoes, an everlasting from the Cape Cod area. There are things to pick all summer long. I've even taken the family out on picking trips at Thanksgiving.

Flowers are Jessica's medium. She dries them and twists them into wreaths, and makes arrangements and decorations for Christmas. She also creates little animals of papier-mache. She has used her mood changes and swings of productivity, which resonate with those in the world around her, to create from nature's own bounty. She marks the changing seasons with the flowers, and they provide her with her art and her livelihood.

Robert Wilhelm: Tales of Darkness and Light

Robert Wilhelm described himself as a storyteller when he called to apply for the NIMH Seasonal Studies Program. Even on the phone I could imagine him spinning out his tales in his deep, sonorous voice, and his storytelling was on my mind when I went to interview him in his apartment. There is nothing about his appearance, or his apartment, that would suggest that he is an artist. He is in his mid-forties, with a ruddy complexion, a mustache, and a full head of black hair, graying slightly. One might easily mistake him for a college professor or a minister—and he has been both. After we spent some hours together, it was easy to see the artist emerge, for he regaled me with stories—his own, and those he tells for a living.

The son of European immigrants, Robert learned the art of storytelling from his mother, who told stories as she cooked dinner. From his father he developed his love of books. His earliest memory is of staring at the single candle on his brother's first birthday cake when he himself was three. His memories of the seasons are also strong:

As a child I remember being sensitive to the seasons. I was always uncomfortable in the summertime, with the heat and humidity, but I loved spring. I loved water, and the clear, snowy days that were rare in New Jersey.

His early winters on the East Coast were "delightful, very bright and clear and cold, very crisp." It was only much later—at age twenty-three, when he went with his wife, Mary Jo, to take up his first college teaching job in Minnesota—that the seasons began to be a problem for him. He became so depressed and physically ill the first Christmas there that he vowed he would move to California the next year, even though it was not a wise career decision to leave an academic position so soon after taking it.

He and his wife moved to northern California, choosing a place where there was a small amount of high fog. Robert enjoyed the mixture of sunlight and fog. He and Mary Jo had three children, all of whom suffered from a rare genetic illness. All died in infancy. Robert reacted to the loss of his children more with anger than with depression. He remembers raging at the unfairness of it, being angry at the universe and at God. Mary Jo was also grief-stricken and went into extensive therapy for several years to deal with the losses.

Robert completed his doctoral studies in theology and interviewed for a job in Niagara Falls. It was Christmastime when he flew up for the job interview, and he returned knowing that he had the job, yet weeping because he did not want to go back north. He remembers walking to the edge of Lake Ontario on a gray day and seeing the faint outlines of the Toronto skyline in the distance. "It was terrible," he recalls, "but that's where my job offer was." He loved teaching, however, so the couple lived in Niagara Falls for three winters—difficult times for himself and his wife. He went into Gestalt therapy and worked on his ambivalent feelings toward his father, whom he resembles. Although the therapy was helpful, he is doubtful whether he would have gone into it had it not been for the gloomy winter weather. Summers in Niagara Falls were a total delight. It was then that he came in contact with some outdoor storytellers, who were to shape his final career choice.

In January of his third winter, he returned to the San Francisco Bay area for a workshop. He walked through Golden Gate Park on a bright, sunny day, lay on the grass, and wept as he "felt the greenness," wondering, "What am I doing in upstate New York?" Robert and Mary Jo moved back to San Francisco and lived there for five years. By then he had dropped out of two tenure-track academic positions and was questioning his future. He later worked briefly as a Roman Catholic lay minister, but ruled that out as a realistic career option. Mary Jo, who had always had a love–hate relationship with San Francisco, was eager to leave the city where her children had died. Robert had not yet learned to take his winter difficulties seriously, for the couple then went to Seattle, one of the darkest cities in the United States. They moved in the summer, to a lovely house in the middle of a Douglas fir forest. All around the house were tall evergreens, and in the summer the sun streamed in through a high opening between the treetops. Robert did not realize that when winter came and the angle of the sun was low, the trees would block out all the light.

They spent two very difficult winters there. Robert recalls sitting by the window, watching the rain come down, and weeping. He thought of the opening of Dante's *Inferno* again and again, saying to himself, "Suddenly, in the middle of my life's journey, I find myself literally in a dark wood. I have failed in my work. My academic career is gone. I will never have a career in the ministry. But I have not failed as a person." That last observation was a core discovery for him. He came to feel that by comparison with the loss of his children, this midlife crisis was relatively insignificant. He also began to appreciate his parents, perhaps for the first time since adolescence; he came to see that they had loved him and felt good about him as a person. "In the midst of all the grayness," Mary Jo got a job offer to return to the Washington, D.C. area.

It was there that Robert finally decided to make storytelling his career. He would take people on tours to places that served as dramatic settings for his stories—for example, the British Isles and Canada. But his seasonal difficulties interfered with his ability to create. He would engage in "a surge of scheduling and planning that begins in the spring and goes wonderfully into early autumn. And then there is the real agony of going through the winter months." He would not have the energy to carry out his plans and would feel "incredible fatigue" as he dragged himself from one engagement to another. In addition, he would become physically sick with flu and colds, which would drag him down further.

Robert joined the NIMH Seasonal Studies Program at the urging of his wife. He had never really thought consciously that light might be important to his mood, "even though everything about my preoccupation with it should have led me to agree with her conclusion. It was so obvious, but I could not see it."

Robert did well on light therapy. Within a few hours of starting treatment, he felt dramatically better, and remained well through the winter. He was skeptical about the effect, and wondered whether it might not be a placebo. However, he became convinced that it was genuine after he went traveling without the lights a few times during the winter, and relapsed each time within days of stopping the treatment. He feels pleased that in the future he will not be at the mercy of intense periods of depression. On the other hand, he is worried that his creativity will be damped down if he is "too even" all year round. But this is not a serious concern for him, and he plans to use lights in future winters.

Robert has for some time been fascinated by stories of the far north—stories of winter journeys, tales told by Siberian shamans, and the legends of the Indians from Canada and the U. S. Northwest. Many of these stories embody the idea of light as a precious essence, connected with love and life, as darkness is connected with loss and despair. Robert has also studied Nordic and Celtic mythology, which is preoccupied with light. He told me the following stories in his deep, resonant voice, alternating among the drama of the story (in which he would become lost from time to time), its meaning to himself, and comments about how he achieves his effects. I relate the following stories as Robert related them to me.

The Selfish Seagull

This tale is told by the Nootka Indians of British Columbia.

When the world was created, gifts were given in the potlatch tradition of the Northwest Indians, in cedar boxes. In this imaginative story the animals all receive gifts of creation, the boxes are all opened, and they are shared. In this land of heavy cloud cover, one box that was not opened was that containing sunlight. It's an important aspect of this particular story that getting the sunlight out somehow requires pain. What happens is that Seagull, who has the light, is not willing to share it. Raven, who is the trickster of this culture, knows that Seagull has the sunlight, and tries to get it out of him by all possible means. He tries to flatter Seagull, to beg him, but no matter what he does, Seagull keeps saying, "It's mine, it's mine."

So Raven has a thought: Seagull is causing so much trouble that it would serve him right if something awful happened to him—if he got a thorn stuck in his foot. No sooner has Raven thought this than it happens, and Seagull cries out in pain. Raven then says, "Let me help you," and goes to pull the thorn out of Seagull's foot. The crucial part of the story is that he doesn't pull the thorn out; instead, he pushes it in farther, and then has the opportunity to say, "I'm sorry, but I can't see what I'm doing"—the hinge of the story—"I need more light if I'm to pull it out. Open the box." And then, in the form of storytelling, the box is opened only a little bit, and the scene has to be repeated. This happens a second and a third time, so the drama builds. But the key is that at each opening a lesser light comes out, followed by a greater light. At the first opening only the stars emerge; at the second, the moon; and only after the third opening does the sun come out. The world is filled with light. The story ends as other traditions would have it begin: In the beginning there was the light.

"And does Seagull get the thorn removed?" I asked, like a child after a bedtime story.

"There are different versions," he told me. "It depends how you choose to tell it. This story always troubled people in religious circles. They always felt it was cruel. But I knew somehow that it was valid, though I didn't know why. But now I realize that it was the connection between the lack of light and pain that caused me to resist changing it."

In an Estonian version of the story, Robert went on, there are four sets of light ranging in brightness from least to most adequate. The additional ones are the northern lights. As flickering lights, they are even less powerful than the stars. In this particular story a woman searches for her husband. The four sets of lights are a personification of her lovers, who range from least to most satisfactory, from the northern lights to the sun.

As I listened to Robert's stories—and he is a spellbinding story-teller—I thought of our research studies and how we have found that in order for light to have a powerful effect on mood, it has to be bright, approaching the intensity of sunlight streaming through a window. Lesser light, equivalent perhaps to starlight or moonlight, just doesn't work. So we reach the same conclusion by widely different approaches—an ancient folk tale or a modern scientific study.

Where the Spirits Go

The Ojibwa Indians say that the first day was seventy years long. The sun shone. There was joy until the first night. People were afraid, and some died.

Trickster was sad, and wanted to be with those friends who died. Then he saw a new light—a round, pale one—rise from the waters. Owl said the name of this light was "Moon."

Trickster paddled a canoe across the waters and saw that Moon was housed in the lodge of those who died. But they were not sad. They ate, danced, and laughed. Owl and Trickster disguised themselves and joined the feast. At dawn, Frog pulled Moon down from the lodge pole and hid it under a blanket, and all the spirits went to sleep.

But Trickster and Owl were awake. Trickster put each of the sleeping spirits into a moose-hide pouch and paddled the canoe across the lake. But Trickster could not wait to reach the Land of the Living, and opened the pouch to peek in. All the spirits flew high to the heavens, and floated back to the Lodge of the Dead.

Owl then perched on Trickster's canoe and spoke: "You will never trick them again into letting you into their Great Lodge. You will never see them again." Trickster was saddened, but then a little smile came into his heart. He said, "Owl speaks the truth, but I will now speak a deeper truth. Every night I—and all people—will fly across the Great Lake on the wings of Owl and Owl's brothers and sisters. We will not be welcomed into the Lodge of the Dead, but we will sleep outside. And we will hear the voices of the past. We will remember those we have lost. We will hear them laughing and dancing and telling stories. And the nights will be filled with memories and adventures for all people in the Land of the Living."

Trickster became quiet and still. Owl blinked, and said, "And what shall this be called?" A little smile came into Trickster's heart: "This shall be called . . . dreaming." And that is how dreaming came to be.

As I listened to this story, I thought about the association between darkness and loss, about the wish to recover loved ones who have departed. There is a universal need to find a way to come to terms with such losses. I thought of Robert's three children, lost in infancy. In the Ojibwa story, death is associated with the first sunset, or loss of the sun. It makes one wonder whether there is a relationship between the chemical changes that take place in the brain as a result of loss and sorrow, and those that result from darkness. Dylan Thomas, in a poem to his dying father, wrote:

> Do not go gentle into that good night.
> Rage, rage against the dying of the light.

There is a Scottish storyteller, so Robert told me, who in his tales of winter journeys uses the saying, "Where there is light there is life," at repeated points in the narrative to build up the drama, step by step.

Brother Wolf

There's a story that I tell, and it's one of my favorites, in which the feedback from the audience or workshop members is always the same. The heart of the story is a legend about St. Francis of Assisi speaking to a wolf who lives in the darkness and comes and devours people in a certain town. The townspeople live in dread of this wolf and consult St. Francis about their problem. St. Francis decides to go meet the wolf. Everyone is terrified, but he goes into the woods anyway.

When I describe that scene, I'm very clearly describing the darkness. And I'm describing how Francis goes into the woods without any light or weapons. He goes into the darkness—I always close my eyes when I get to this part of the story—and I say he goes to the part of the woods that *feels* the darkest. When he reaches the place that feels the darkest, he stops. He knows that if he reaches out in front of him he could touch the wolf. The two of them are silent until Francis speaks. He says just two words— "Brother Wolf."

The two of them understand each other. Francis comes back into town and tells the people that the way for them to deal with the wolf is to feed him. St. Francis then goes back to his own village. The people are confused about what he has said and they debate about it, but then night falls. The wolf comes into the village and prowls around the streets and alleys in the darkness. All the doors are shut, the windows are closed, and everything is barred and dark. Suddenly, as the wolf comes around a corner, a door opens and—I use this phrase because I see it so clearly—*light pours out*. Someone steps out and puts a platter of food in the roadway, and the wolf with burning eyes looks up at the person, then turns to the food and devours it.

The story goes on from there. But after it is done—and it is about twenty-five minutes long—three out of four people will always say that the image they recall most clearly is when the door opens and the light pours out. That image comes about twenty minutes into the story, and I really think that after being, essentially, in different levels of darkness throughout, I can really see the light. My eyes are open and I'm looking at my audience, but it is as if somewhere I've been in a dark night and I open a door, or I walk in and turn my light on. It just floods. It's overwhelming—there's an emotional response that is instantaneous with the appearance of light.

Robert regulates the amount of light that comes into his eyes as he tells this and other stories; it seems to influence his mood and how he conveys it to his audience. When he describes the darkness in his tales, he closes his eyes and feels it. When he talks about light, he opens his eyes and sees it. The most dramatic moment in this story, and in other stories of winter journeys, is coming upon bright light, suddenly and unexpectedly, in the midst of the dark landscape. I wonder whether the receptors in the eye, having been starved of light—and the chemical changes that light induces—might pour out these chemicals in response to the light that pours suddenly out of the darkness, flooding our senses.

Robert shared with me just a small sample of his life. When I think back over the forty-plus years that he covered in just a few hours, I am struck by his first memory—that of a three-year-old boy on a winter's day, staring at the flame on his brother's birthday cake. Only three, and already mesmerized by the light on a dark day!

As I think of Robert's tales, I think of all the people united within the pages of this book: Peggy driving through the dark New England countryside, tired and sad and craving cookies; Alan missing school on dark winter days; Neal, who used to be too tired to keep his appointments, now energetically selling light fixtures; Angela working on her book in front of her light box; Jessica picking wildflowers at high noon in the summer; and now Robert telling stories of winter journeys, of light pouring out of the darkness. These people, with their unusual sensitivity to darkness and light, tell us something about our world and our reactions to it that otherwise might have passed us by completely.

Epilogue

It is small wonder that we are affected by the physical world in which we live: the dome of the sky, alternately brilliantly blue or dark as sleep; the quality of the air, full of moisture or crisp and dry; heat and cold; the loveliness of the light or the oppressive shadows of a winter afternoon. We are affected by our physical environment because we have evolved under its influence over thousands of years. It orchestrates the internal rhythms of body and brain, the seasons of the mind.

In their infinite variety of nature, people, like other creatures, are all different. Some show little change with the revolving year, while others react to seasonal changes with exquisite sensitivity. There is no shortage of examples in the plant and animal world of creatures reacting to changes in light, heat, or moisture. People who experience marked seasonal changes have no reason to feel alone. Even among our fellow humans there are millions with such strong reactions. My colleagues and I have estimated that perhaps as many as 20 percent of the U.S. population—thirty-six million people—experience some diminished function or impaired quality of life in response to winter.

It is important for a seasonal person to realize that there are millions of others who suffer from the same changes and to have faith in the legitimacy of the messages that come from inside the body and mind. This was a major problem for people suffering from SAD before it was recognized by the medical establishment. A series of standard examinations and tests would be conducted in an attempt to diagnose the symptoms of SAD. When the results of these tests were negative, the sufferer would be left with the impression that the problem was not real or valid. Now we know that even without any positive chemical tests, it is possible to diagnose the condition of SAD and treat it. These discoveries are relatively new, so not all medical practitioners are aware of them. If you suffer from SAD and encounter such a practitioner, bring this information to his or her attention, and see whether you can resolve the problem together. If you encounter further skepticism, or a lack of open-mindedness about the powerful effects of the seasons and our capacity to reverse them, I suggest that you move on to another practitioner, rather than mistrust the messages that come reliably and powerfully from your mind and body.

In this book I have shown how you can evaluate the seasons of your own mind, how strongly they express themselves, and what form and pattern they take. If they are a problem for you, there is much that can be done about them. The physical environment can be changed—most obviously by adding extra light, but in many other ways as well. Likewise, the psychological environment can be modified to good effect. Stresses can be reduced. Friends and family members can help. Understanding the problem is valuable in its own right, and your view of the world and your relationship to it can be considered and modified, if you choose to do so. For all of us, it is vital to our mental health that we do not feel helpless—that we believe we can do something to influence our destinies and the way we feel. How fortunate it is, therefore, that seasonal people can do so much to improve their lives.

There is, however, a limit to the degree to which we can change ourselves, and there may be much—our seasonality included—that we do not wish to alter. Many may regard their seasonality as an important part of themselves, integral to their rhythms of joy and sorrow, to their creativity, and to the pulse that makes them feel alive. From such heightened sensitivity has come some of our most beautiful poetry and art. Had all such creative rhythms and fluctuations been flattened out by some omnipotent therapist, our lives would be the poorer for it.

I believe that we should use our seasonality to tune in to nature and to the creative forces within ourselves—that we should create with the seasons and share the products of our creation with others. This book is my seasonal creation, and if it brings you even a single shaft of light on a winter's day, my mission has been accomplished.

PART 4

Resources

Where to get further help for seasonal problems

Where to Purchase Light Fixtures

The technology of light fixtures is bound to change over time. Currently, most effective fixtures are metal light boxes (some with surrounding wooden frames), with fluorescent light bulbs in them. Although some of them emit ultraviolet wavelengths, there is no evidence at this time that ultraviolet light is of value in treating SAD. In fact, given its potentially harmful effects to the eyes and the skin, it is best to use light fixtures that screen out ultraviolet rays as thoroughly as possible.

The light fixtures vary in size and are correspondingly more or less portable. Some are positioned at an angle that causes them to give off more light than the traditional 2500-lux fixtures. Increasing the brightness enables people to obtain an antidepressant effect with shorter sessions. Standard fixtures, whether 2500-lux or 10,000-lux, appear to be quite safe. I recommend that you read Chapter 6 on light therapy for more information about how to use light therapy and precautions you might wish to take.

The suppliers with the widest distribution networks and best established track records for service and delivery to all parts of the United States are the following:

The SunBox Company
19217 Orbit Drive
Gaithersburg, MD 20879
Tel: 800-LITE-YOU (548-3968)
301-869-5980

Apollo Light Systems Inc.
352 West 1060 South
Orem, UT 84058
Tel: 800-545-9667
801-226-2370

Sphere One Inc.
432 Main St.
Silver Plume, CO 80476
201-746-9690

The dawn simulator and the Light Visor, both described in Chapter 6, can be obtained from The SunBox Company. The Light Visor can also be obtained from its manufacturer, Bio-Brite, and in the UK from OUTSIDE IN:

Bio-Brite, Inc.
7315 Wisconsin Ave., #1300 W
Bethesda, MD 20814-3202
Tel: 800-621-LITE (621-5483)
301-961-8557

OUTSIDE IN (Cambridge) Ltd.
Unit 21 Scotland Road Estate
Dry Drayton, Cambridge CB3 8AT
Tel: (0954)-211955
Fax: (0954)-211956

European sources for light fixtures are the following:

Finland

Auradent
Puutarhakatu 12
20100 Turku
Tel: (021)-233-1155
Fax: (021)-233-1148

France

Durolux
22 Rue Madiraa
92400 Courbevoie
Tel: (1) 47-68-90-80
Fax: (1)-43-33-41-21

Germany

SML Licht u. Bestrahlungssyteme
Schleidener Strasse 136
D-5100 Aachen
Tel: (02408)-80527
Fax: (02408)-80851

Ireland

LITECH
Westland House
1 Westland Square
Dublin 2
Tel: (01)-677-9199
Fax: (01)-677-9355

Italy

Natura-Lite s.r.l.
Via Luigi Kossuth 36
00149 Rome

Tel: (06)-526-2048
fax: (06)-526-2248

Norway

Miljo LYS A/S
Bromsvn, 9
3183 Horten
Tel: (0330)-44912
Fax: (0330)-47245

Sweden

Ratt Ljus AB
Osmundvagen 37
Box 11159
161 11 Bromma
Tel: (08)-250806
Fax: (08)-800665

Switzerland

Elec Handels
Eichenweg 33
CH-8121 Benglen
Tel: (01)-825-2414
Fax: (01)-825-2873

United Kingdom

FSL Ltd.
Unit 1
Riverside Business Centre
Victoria Street
High Wycombe
Bucks HP11 2LT

Tel: (0494)-526051/448727
Fax: (0494)-527005

OUTSIDE IN (Cambridge) Ltd.
Unit 21 Scotland Road Estate
Dry Drayton, Cambridge CB3 8AT
Tel: (0954)-211955
Fax: (0954)-211956

Sunbox Designs Ltd.
43 Woodberry Crescent
Muswell Hill
London N10 1PJ
Tel: (081)-444-9201/9218

Arthur McKay & Co. Ltd.
7/9 Arthur Street
Edinburgh EH6 5DA
Tel: (031)-554-0611

Practitioners and Research Programs for Supervision of Light Therapy

The following programs and individual practitioners have an active, ongoing interest in administering light therapy. All have demonstrated this interest, either by taking a course in light therapy or by doing research in the area. The list should certainly not be regarded as comprehensive, and as light therapy becomes better established as a recognized form of treatment, the list of practitioners competent to supervise it is bound to grow. Although I have tried to evaluate the knowledge, competence and interest of the practitioners and programs listed, I obviously cannot take responsibility for any unsuccessful outcome of consulting these individuals or programs.

United States

Alaska

Bruce Smith, Ph.D.
8550 Denali St., Suite 1306
Anchorage, AK 99503
Tel: 907-272-4741

Arkansas

Frederick Guggenheim, M.D.
Department of Psychiatry
University of Arkansas for Medical
  Sciences
4301 West Markham, Slot 589
Little Rock, AR 72205
Tel: 501-661-5483

California

La Jolla–San Diego

Daniel F. Kripke, M.D.
Department of Psychiatry
University of California at San Diego
Circadian Pacemaker Laboratory
Box 0667
9500 Gilman Dr.
La Jolla, CA 92093-0667
Tel: 619-534-7131

Barbara L. Parry, M.D.
Department of Psychiatry
University of California at San Diego
Box 0804
La Jolla, CA 92093
Tel: 619-543-5592

Los Angeles Area

David A. Sack, M.D.
3340 Los Coyotes Diagonal
Long Beach, CA 90908
Tel: 213-421-9311

Center for Mood Disorders
12301 Wilshire Blvd, Suite 210
Los Angeles, CA 90025
Tel: 213-207-8448

Robert H. Gerner, M.D.
1990 South Bendy Dr., #790
Los Angeles, CA 90025
Tel: 310-207-8448

Michael J. Gitlin, M.D.
300 UCLA Medical Plaza, #2200
Los Angeles, CA 90024
Tel: 310-206-5133

John P. Docherty, M.D.
National Medical Enterprises
2700 Colorado Ave.
Santa Monica, CA 90404
Tel: 310-998-6739

Colorado

R. Timothy Pollack, Ph.D.
Health Enhancement Center, Inc.
8370 West Coal Mine Avenue
Suite 107
Littleton, CO 80123
Tel: 303-972-0714

Connecticut

Francine C. Howland, M.D.
45 Trumbull St.
New Haven, CT 06510
Tel: 203-624-3516

Alan J. Sholomskas, M.D.
2 Church Street South
New Haven, CT 06519
Tel: 203-776-2077

Peritz Levinson, M.D.
Jada Lane
Greenwich, CT 06830
Tel: 203-869-0079

Neil Liebowitz, M.D.
Grove Hill Medical Center
300 Kensington Ave.
New Britain, CT 06051
Tel: 203-224-6289

Charles S. Mirabile
Box 683, Upper Main St.
Sharon, CT 06069
Tel: 203-364-0740

Daniel Romanoes, M.D.
Torrington Office Plaza, Suite 301
Torrington, CT 06790
Tel: 203-482-9321

D.C. Metropolitan Area

Seasonal Studies Program
National Institute of Mental Health
Building 10, Room 4S-239
9000 Rockville Pike
Bethesda, MD 20892
Tel: 301-496-2141
301-496-0500

Norman E. Rosenthal, M.D.
11110 Stephalee Lane
Rockville, MD 20852
Tel: 301-770-5647

Thomas A. Wehr, M.D.
National Institute of Mental Health
Building 10, Room 4S-239
9000 Rockville Pike
Bethesda, MD 20892
Tel: 301-530-7336

Dan A. Oren, M.D.
5612 Shields Drive
Bethesda, MD 20817
Tel: 301-231-4410

Frederick M. Jacobsen, M.D.
1301 20th St., N.W., #711
Washington, DC 20036
Tel: 202-234-1742

Florida

Donald L. Sherry, M.D.
3300 S.W. 34th Ave., #140
Ocala, FL 34474-7427
Tel: 904-854-7700

Robert G. Skwerer, M.D.
5600 Bee Ridge Rd.
Suite B
Sarasota, FL 34233
Tel: 813-377-2178

Georgia

Charles Melville, Ph.D.
25-B Lenox Pointe, N.E.
Atlanta, GA 30324
Tel: 404-266-8881

Charles B. Nemeroff, M.D., Ph.D.
Department of Psychiatry and
    Behavioral Sciences
Emory University School of
    Medicine
Box AF
Atlanta, GA 30322
Tel: 404-727-8382

George Johnson, M.D.
682 Lanier Dr.
Gainesville, GA 30505
Tel: 404-532-5640

Hawaii

Enrico G. Camara, M.D.
Department of Psychiatry
University of Hawaii
1356 Lusitana St., 4th Floor
Honolulu, HI 96813
Tel: 808-247-2191

Idaho

Winslow R. Hunt, M.D.
155 South Second Ave.
Pocatello, ID 83201
Tel: 208-232-3423

Illinois

Charmane I. Eastman, Ph.D.
Biological Rhythms Research
    Laboratory
Rush Presbyterian–St. Luke's
    Medical Center
1653 West Congress Parkway
Chicago, IL 60612
Tel: 312-942-8328

Michael Young, Ph.D.
Biological Rhythms Research
    Laboratory
Rush Presbyterian–St. Luke's
    Medical Center
1653 West Congress Parkway
Chicago, IL 60612
Tel: 312-942-8328

Richard H. Spector, M.D.
2850 W. 95th St., Suite 208
Evergreen Park, IL 60642
Tel: 708-424-2024

Indiana

Richard H. Spector, M.D.
833 W. Lincoln Highway, Suite 400
Schererville, IN 46375
Tel: 219-322-5662

Iowa

Bruce Pfohl, M.D.
Adult Outpatient Psychiatry Clinic
University of Iowa Health Center
200 Hawkins Dr.
#2887 JPP
Iowa City, IA 52242-1057
Tel: 319-356-1350

Kentucky

B. Kishore Gupta, M.D.
Department of Psychiatry
University of Louisville
133 Chenoweth Lane
Louisville, KY 40207
Tel: 502-895-6368

Louisiana

Department of Psychiatry
Louisiana State University
 Medical School
1501 Kings Highway
Shreveport, LA 71103
Tel: 318-674-6042

Maryland

Bethesda/Rockville. See listings
under "D.C. Metropolitan Area"

Baltimore Area

J. Raymond de Paulo, Jr., M.D.
Department of Psychiatry
Johns Hopkins University
 School of Medicine
Meyer 3-181
Baltimore, MD 21287-7381
Tel: 301-955-3246

The Affective Disorders Clinic
Johns Hopkins University School of
 Medicine

Meyer 3-181
Baltimore, MD 21287-7381
Tel: 301-955-3246

David Roth, Ph.D.
Shephard Pratt Hospital
6501 North Charles Street
Baltimore, MD 21285-6815
Tel: 410-938-3000 ext. 4219

Massachusetts

Amherst

Benjamin Levy, M.D.
University Health Services
University of Massachusetts
14 Amherst Rd., RFD #3
Amherst, MA 01003
Tel: 413-545-2337

Bruce Goderez, M.D.
18 Echo Hill Rd.
Amherst, MA 01002
Tel: 413-739-0882

Boston Area

Martin H. Teischer, M.D., Ph.D.
McLean Hospital
115 Mill St.
Belmont, MA 02178
Tel: 617-855-2970

Carol A. Glod, R.N., M.S.C.S.
McLean Hospital
115 Mill St.
Belmont, MA 02178
Tel: 617-855-2476

Janis L. Anderson, Ph.D.
Seasonal Affective Disorders Clinic
Brigham and Women's Hospital
221 Longwood Ave.
Boston, MA 02115
Tel: 617-732-4012

Dermott O'Rourke
C-R-C M-I-T
Massachusetts General Hospital
40 Ames St.
Cambridge, MA 02142
Tel: 617-253-3091

Michigan

Ann Arbor

Oliver G. Cameron, M.D., Ph.D.
University of Michigan
Riverview Building
900 Wall St.. J232
Ann Arbor, MI 48109-0722
Tel: 313-764-0267

Mark Demitrack, M.D.
University of Michigan Hospitals
UH 8D, Box 0116
Ann Arbor, MI 48109
Tel: 313-936-4860

Juan Lopez, M.D.
Mental Health Research Institute
Box 0720
Ann Arbor, MI 48109
Tel: 313-663-3141

Elizabeth Young, M.D.
Mood Disorders Program
Department of Psychiatry
University of Michigan Hospitals
1500 E. Medical Center Dr.
Ann Arbor, MI 48109
Tel: 313-936-2087

Kalamazoo

Pat Guilford, Ph.D.
Borgess Medical Center
Behavioral Medicine Services
1722 Shaffer St.
Kalamazoo, MI 49001-1643
Tel: 616-349-4460

Minnesota

Paul A. Arbisi, Ph.D.
Minneapolis Veterans Medical
  Center
One Veterans Drive
Minneapolis, MN 55417
Tel: 612-725-2074

Health Renewal Center
Psychology Consultants
Contact: Michael DeSanctis, Ph.D.
Gallery Professional Building
17 Exchange Street West
Suite 750
St. Paul, MN 55102-1036
Tel: 612-232-4120

Sandra C. Reese, Ph.D.
Family Counseling
2025 Stearns Way
St. Cloud, MN 56303
Tel: 612-255-2041

Missouri

Dale J. Anderson, M.D.
12520 Olive Blvd.
St. Louis, MO 63141
Tel: 314-576-6692

James K. Walsh, Ph.D.
Sleep Disorders Center
Deaconess Hospital
6150 Oakland Ave.
St. Louis, MO 63139
Tel: 314-768-3594

Montana

Michael J. Silverglat, M.D.
554 W. Broadway
Missoula, MT 59802
Tel: 406-721-6050

Nebraska

Robert G. Osborne, M.D.
2221 S. 17th St., Suite 110
Lincoln, NE 68502
Tel: 402-476-7557

Kay M. Shilling, M.D.
7602 Pacific St., Suite 302
Omaha, NE 68114
Tel: 402-393-4355

New Hampshire

James M. Claiborn, Ph.D.
80 Palomino Lane, Suite 203
Bedford, NH 03110
Tel: 603-624-2272

A. Frank, Ph.D.
North East Psychiatric Associates
14 Celina Ave.
P.O. Box 6010
Nashua, NH 03063-6010
Tel: 603-595-0601

Janet R. Wakefield, Ph.D.
White Mountain Mental Health
 Center
Box 559
Littleton, NH 03561
Tel: 603-444-5358

James R. Antisdel, M.D.
40 Bay St.
Manchester, NH 03104
Tel: 603-668-4079

Monadnock Family Services
454 Old Street Rd., Suite #303
Peterborough, NH 03458
Tel: 603-924-7236

Dr. Ravaris
Dartmouth Medical Center

One Medical Center Dr.
Lebanon, NH 03766
Tel: 603-650-5805

New Jersey

Benjamin Natelson, M.D.
Department of Neurosciences
New Jersey Medical School
185 South Orange Ave.
Newark, NJ 07103
Tel: 201-982-5208

Jeffrey T. Apter, M.D.
Princeton Psychiatric Centers
330 North Harrison St., Suite 6
Princeton, NJ 08540
Tel: 609-921-3555

Naomi Vilko, M.D.
Princeton Health Care Center
419 N. Harrison St.
Suite 206
Princeton, NJ 08540
Tel: 609-924-3225

Robert K. Davies, M.D.
47 Maple Street
Summit, NJ 07901
Tel: 609-252-0035

Robert Moreines, M.D.
Stuart Kushner, M.D.
Warren Commons
5 Mountain Blvd.
Suite 6
Warren, NJ 07060
Tel: 908-753-4444

Steven Resnick, M.D.
Suite 162
CN 5256
Princeton, NJ 08543
Tel: 609-683-1531

New York

New York City

Michael Terman, Ph.D.
Winter Depression Program
Columbia-Presbyterian Medical
    Center
722 West 168th St., Box 50
New York, NY 10032
Tel: 212-960-5714

Henry L. McCurtis, M.D.
146 Central Park West
New York, NY 10023
212-580-2222
and Department of Psychiatry
Harlem Hospital
506 Lenox Ave.
New York, NY 10037
Tel: 212-939-3060

Leslie L. Powers, M.D.
15 West 75th St., Suite 4B
New York, NY 10023
Tel: 212-724-5222

Lauren Gorman, M.D.
15 West 81st St.
New York, NY 10024
Tel: 212-548-0568

Norman Sussman, M.D.
Department of Psychiatry
New York University Medical Center
550 1st Ave.
New York, NY 10016
Tel: 212-737-7946

Rochester

Michael R. Privitera, M.D.
Mood Disorders Center
Department of Psychiatry
University of Rochester Medical
    Center

Brighton Campus Park
2024 West Henrietta Rd., Suite 6C
Rochester, NY 14623
Tel: 716-475-0440

Mildred D. Rust, M.D.
1360 Monroe Avenue
Rochester, NY 14618
Tel: 716-442-9601

Rockland County

James W. Flax, M.D.
11 Medical Park Dr., Suite 102
Pomona, NY 10970
Tel: 914-362-2557

Syracuse Area

Richard Kavey, M.D.
R.R. #2, 2922 Eager Rd.
Lafayette, NY 13084
Tel: 315-677-3486

Westchester County

Mohamed Yahia, M.D.
Inpatient Admission Units
FDR Veterans Administration
    Medical Center
Chappaqua, NY 10548
Tel: 914-238-3546

Joseph Deltito, M.D.
New York Hospital–Cornell
    University Medical Center
Anxiety and Mood Disorders
    Program
21 Bloomingdale Rd.
White Plains, NY 10605
Tel: 914-997-5967

North Carolina

William Simmons, M.D.
932 Hendersonville Rd.

Forest Center, # 101
Asheville, NC 28803
Tel: 704-274-1415

Dan G. Blazer, M.D., Ph.D.
Box 3005
Duke University School of Medicine
Durham, NC 27710
Tel: 919-684-4128

Jack D. Edinger, Ph.D.
Ambulatory Sleep Laboratory
Box 2908
Duke University Medical Center
Durham, NC 27710
Tel: 919-286-6934

Gail Marsh, Ph.D.
Box 2908
Duke University Medical Center
Durham, NC 27710-0000
Tel: 919-681-8777

Michael A. Hill, M.D.
Seasonal Disorders Clinic
Department of Psychiatry
University of North Carolina
Chapel Hill, NC 27599-7160
Tel: 919-966-3376

North Dakota

Robert Olson, M.D.
700 1st Ave. South
Fargo, ND 58103
Tel: 701-234-4093

Ohio

Ruth Ragucci, M.D.
11201 Shaker Blvd., #204
Cleveland, OH 44104
Tel: 216-721-6770

Gregory G. Young, M.D.
1735 Big Hill Rd.
Dayton, OH 45439
Tel: 513-293-2507

Oklahoma

David P. Crass, M.D.
1725 E. 19th St., Suite 604
Tulsa, OK 74104
Tel: 918-743-6694

Oregon

Sleep and Mood Disorders
   Laboratory
Department of Psychiatry
University of Oregon Health
   Sciences Center
3181 S.W. Sam Jackson Park Road
Portland, OR 97201
Tel: 503-494-5635
   Alfred J. Lewy, M.D., Ph.D.
   Robert L. Sack, M.D.
   Clifford M. Singer, M.D.

George C. D. Kjaer, M.D.
132 E. Broadway, Suite 303
Eugene, OR 97401
Tel: 503-686-2027

Pennsylvania

Philadelphia

George C. Brainard, Ph.D.
Department of Neurology
Jefferson Medical College
1025 Walnut St.
Philadelphia, PA 19107
Tel: 215-955-7644

Brenda Byrne, Ph.D.
Clorinda G. Margolis and Associates

1015 Chestnut St., #1500
Philadelphia, PA 19107
Tel: 215-592-8165

Pittsburgh

Michael Thase, M.D.
University of Pittsburgh
School of Medicine
3811 O'Hara St.
Pittsburgh, PA 15241
Tel: 412-383-1218

Edward Friedman, M.D.
University of Pittsburgh
School of Medicine
3811 O'Hara St.
Pittsburgh, PA 15241
Tel: 412-383-1210

Other

Frederick M. Brown, Ph.D.
Department of Psychology
The Pennsylvania State University
440 Moore Building
University Park, PA 16802
Tel: 814-865-1815

Leroy J. Pelicci, M.D.
748 Quincy Ave.
Scranton, PA 18510
Tel: 717-342-8633

Rhode Island

Mark S. Bauer, M.D.
Dept. of Psychiatry and Human
  Behavior
Brown University
Box G-VAH/116A2
Providence, RI 02912
401-457-3333

South Carolina

Timothy D. Brewerton, M.D.
Institute of Psychiatry

Medical University of South
  Carolina
171 Ashley Ave.
Charleston, SC 29425-0742
Tel: 803-792-4795

Tennessee

Kenneth O. Jobson, M.D.
Tennessee Psychiatry and
  Psychopharmacology Clinic
9401 Park West Boulevard
Knoxville, TN 37923
Tel: 615-690-8190

Department of Psychiatry
James H. Quillen College of
  Medicine
Box 70654
East Tennessee State University
Johnson City, TN 37614
Tel: 214-692-9660

Texas

College Station

Cynthia Desmond, Ph.D.,
  C.S.W.-A.C.P.
c/o Desart Hills
4201 Texas Ave. South
College Station, TX 77840
Tel: 409-846-4592

Dallas

John W. Cain, M.D.
A. John Rush, M.D.
Department of Psychiatry
University of Texas Southwestern
5323 Harry Hines Blvd.
Dallas, TX 75235-8898
Tel: 214-648-3111

Philip Becker, M.D.
Andrew Jamieson, M.D.
Sleep/Wake Disorders Center

8200 Walnut Hill Lane
Dallas, TX 75231
Tel: 214-696-8563

Howard Roffwarg, M.D.
8226 Douglas, #616
Dallas, TX 75240
Tel: 214-692-9660

El Paso

Jean R. Joseph-Vanderpool, M.D.
600 Sunland Park Drive
Building 6, # 100
El Paso, TX 79912
Tel: 915-833-5855

Houston

Stuart C. Yudofsky, M.D.
Professor and Chairman
Department of Psychiatry
Baylor College of Medicine
1 Baylor Plaza
Houston, TX 77030
Tel: 713-798-4945

Utah

Joanne L. Brown, Ph.D.
Cottonwood Counseling Center
525 East 4500 South, Suite F200
Salt Lake City, UT 84107
Tel: 801-266-6413

Vermont

Ray C. Abney, M.D.
Rt. 30 Brattleboro Professional
   Center
P.O. Box 1616
Brattleboro, VT 05302
Tel: 802-257-2442

John R. Edwards, M.D.
118 Pine Street

Burlington, VT 05401
Tel: 802-658-2762

Stephen M. Cohen, M.D.
118 Pine Street
Burlington, VT 05401
Tel: 802-864-5280

Edward A. Mueller, M.D.
Rutland Area Community Services
78 South Main St.
Rutland, VT 05701
Tel: 802-775-2381

Virginia

Bruce E. Baker, M.D.
150 Olde Greenwich Drive, Suite J
Fredericksburg, VA 22401
Tel: 703-898-5533

Tobin Jones, M.D.
1600 E. Little Creek Road, #346
Norfolk, VA 23518
Tel: 804-441-1717

See also listings under "D.C.
Metropolitan Area"

Washington

David H. Avery, M.D.
Harborview Medical Center, ZA-99
325 9th Avenue
Seattle, WA 98104
Tel: 206-223-3425

Michael Norden, M.D.
10740 Meridian Ave. N, Suite 101
Seattle, WA 98133
Tel: 206-361-7696

Keith L. Rogers, M.D.
2552 38th Ave.

Seattle, WA 98199
Tel: 206-286-1625

Wisconsin

Center for Affective Disorders
Department of Psychiatry
University of Wisconsin Hospital
and Clinics
600 Highland Drive
Madison, WI 53792
Tel: 608-263-6092
Nancy Barklage, M.D.
Stephen J. Weiler, M.D.
Ruth Benca, M.D.

Jan van Schaik, M.D.
1120 Dewey Avenue
Wauwatosa, WI 53213
Tel: 414-258-2600

Canada

Alberta

Chris P. Gorman, M.D., F.R.C.P.C.
704 3031 Hospital Drive, N.W.
Calgary, Alberta T2N 2T8
Tel: 403-270-8222

Carl A. Blashko, M.D., F.R.C.P.C.
Cedars Professional Park
2923 66th St.
Edmonton, Alberta T62 4C1
Tel: 403-461-4794

British Columbia

Raymond Lam, M.D., F.R.C.P.C.
Department of Psychiatry
University of British Columbia
2255 Wesbrook Mall, Room 2C-9
Vancouver, B.C. V6T 2A1
Tel: 604-228-7325

Manitoba

Mood Disorders Unit
PZ 202—PsycHealth Centre
771 Bannatyne Ave.
Winnipeg, Manitoba R3E 3N4
Tel: 204-787-7078

Nova Scotia

Gail Eskes, Ph.D.
Department of Psychology
Dalhousie University
Halifax, Nova Scotia B3H 4J1
Tel: 902-494-2211

C. Charles Mate-Kole, Ph.D.
Nova Scotia Rehab Centre
Dalhousie University
1341 Summer St.
Halifax, Nova Scotia B3H 4K4
Tel: 902-422-1787

Max Michalon, M.D.
Department of Psychiatry
Dalhousie University
Camp Hill Hospital
Abbie J. Lane Building
1763 Robie St.
Halifax, Nova Scotia B3H 3G2
Tel: 902-494-2211

Rachel L. Morehouse, M.D.,
F.R.C.P.C.
Sleep Disorders Laboratory
Dalhousie University
Room 4008, Abbie J. Lane Bldg.
1763 Robie St.
Halifax, Nova Scotia B3H 3G2
Tel: 902-496-4298

Ontario

Anthony J. Levitt, M.D.
Clarke Institute of Psychiatry

250 College St.
Toronto, Ontario M5T 1R8
Tel: 416-979-6868

Colin M. Shapiro, Ph.D., F.R.C.P.C.
Department of Psychiatry
The Toronto Hospital, Western
  Division
399 Bathurst St.
Toronto, Ontario M5T 2S8

Harvey Moldofsky, M.D.
Centre for Sleep and Chronobiology
University of Toronto
The Toronto Hospital, Western
  Division
399 Bathurst St.
EC 3D-022
Toronto, Ontario M5T 2S8
Tel: 416-369-5109

Meir Steiner, M.D., Ph.D.
Department of Psychiatry and
  Biomedical Sciences
McMaster University
Hamilton, Ontario
Tel: 416-522-4941

Edward R. Horn, M.D., F.R.C.P.C.
Royal Ottawa Hospital
1145 Carling Ave.
Ottawa, Ontario K1Z 7K4
Tel: 613-724-6500

Quebec

A-Missagh Ghadirian, M.D.
Seasonal Affective Disorders/Mood
  Disorders Clinic
McGill University
Royal Victoria Hospital
1025 Pine Ave. West
Montreal, Quebec H3A 1A1
Tel: 514-842-1231

Europe

Austria

Siegfried F. Kasper, M.D.
Department of Psychiatry
University of Vienna
Allgemeines Krankenhous der Stadt
  Wien
Währinger Gürtel 18-20
A-1090 Vienna
Tel: (43)-1-40-400-3568

Josef Schwitzer, M.D.
Christian Neudorfer, M.D.
Univ. Klinik fur Psychiatrie
Anichstrasse 35
A-6020 Innsbruck
Tel: (05222)-504-3631

Finland

Carl G. Hagfors, Ph.D.
Department of Psychology
University of Jyvaskyla
P.O. Box 35
40351 Jyvaskyla
Tel: (358)-41-602-851

France

Dan A. Waniek, M.D.
Laboratory of Biochemistry
Hospital Pitie–Salpêtrière
Ward, Inc. Eye Image Analysis
93400 Saint Ouen
Tel: (33)-42-514-570

Germany

Wilfried K. Kohler, Ph.D.
Heinrich-Hofman-Strasse 10
D-6000 Frankfort am Main
Tel: (069)-6301-5419

Iceland

Andrés Magnússon, M.D.
Department of Psychiatry
National University Hospitals
Box 10
121 Reykjavik
Tel: (354)-1-601-000

Ireland

Philip A. Carney, M.D.,
M.R.C.D.P.M.
Department of Psychiatry
University College Hospital
Galway
Tel: (353)-91-24222

Italy

Giuseppe Barbato, M.D.
Sezione di Psichiatria
Universita Degli Studi di Napoli
    Federico II
Via Sergio Pansini, 5
80131 Napoli (Naples)
Tel: (39)081-7462652/7463796

Alessandro Meluzzi, M.D.
Unita Sanitaria Locale Regione
    Piemonte
Responsabile Servizio di Psichiatria
Clinical Psychiatric University of
    Torino
10126 Torino (Turin)
Tel: (39)-11-655638

Giovanni Muscettola, M.D.
Department of Psychiatry
Medical School
University of Trieste
Via S. Cilino 16 Trieste

The Netherlands

Department of Biological Psychiatry
University of Groningen
Oostersingel 59
9713 EZ Groningen
Tel: (31)-50-612-034/039/056/067
Dominicus G. Beersma, Ph.D.
M. C. M. Gordijn
Ybe Meesters
Rutger H van den Hoofdakker
Cornelis A. van Houwelingen

Norway

Odd Lingjaerde, M.D.
Gaustad Sykehus
Boks 24, Gaustad
N-0320 Oslo 3
Tel: (47)-2-14-10-90

Trond Bratlid, M.D.
Asgard Hospital
N-9000 Tromsø
Tel: (47)-83-21000

Sweden

Roger I. Wibom
N.I.O.H.
Division of Neuromedicine IMN
S-17184 Solna
Tel: (46)-8-7309337

Torbjorn G. Akerstedt, Ph.D.
Karolinska Institute
Box 60205
S. 10401 Stockholm
Tel: (46)-8-340560

Johan Beck-Friis, M.D., Ph.D.
Department of Psychiatry
Karolinska Institute
Saint Gorans Hospital

S-11281 Stockholm
Tel: (46)-8-135000

Bengt F. Kjellman, M.D.
Department of Psychiatry
Karolinska Institute
Saint Gorans Hospital
S-11281 Stockholm
Tel: (46)-8-135000

Bjorn-Erik Thalen, M.D.
Karolinska Institute
Box 12500
S-11281 Stockholm
Tel: (46)-8-135000

Switzerland

Anna Wirz-Justice, Ph.D.
Psychiatrische Universitatsklinik
  Basel
Wilhelm Klein-Strasse 27
CH-4025 Basel
Tel: (061)-325-5111
Fax: (061)-325-5258

United Kingdom

Stuart Checkley, M.D.
Dean, Maudsley Hospital
De Crespigny Park
Denmark Hill
London SE5 8AF
Tel: (071)-703-5411
Fax: (071)-703-5796

Chris Thompson, M.D.
Department of Psychiatry
Royal South Hants Hospital
Graham Road
Southampton SO9 4PE
Tel: (0703)-634288 ext. 2533 or
  2535 (SAD clinic)

Stuart Montgomery, M.D.
Academic Department of Psychiatry
St. Mary's Hospital
Praed Street
London W2 1NY
Tel: (071)-725-6666
Fax: (071)-725-6609

G. Vincenti
Department of Mental Health
Friarage Hospital
Northallerton
N. Yorks DL6 1JG

John Eagles
Ross Clinic
Royal Cornhill Hospital
Cornhill Road
Aberdeen AB9 2ZF

Chris Lucas
Department of Child and Adolescent
  Psychiatry
University of Nottingham
Thorneywood Unit
Porchester Road
Nottingham NG3 6LF
(Children and adolescents only)

Japan

Tatsuro Ohta, M.D.
Department of Psychiatry
Nagoya University School of
  Medicine
65 Tsurumai-cho, Showa-ku
Nagoya 466
Tel: (81)052-741-2111 (Ext. 2256)

Kiyohisa Takahashi, M.D., Ph.D.
National Institute of Neuroscience
NCNP
4-1-1, Ogawahigashi, Kodaira
Tokyo 187
Tel: (81)-423-46-1714

Masako Okawa, M.D.
National Institute of Mental
  Health
1-7-3 Konodai, Ichikawa
Chiba 272
Tel: (81)-473-72-0141

Takuro Endo, M.D.
Departmant of Psychiatry
Jikei University School of Medicine
3-25-8 Nishishinbashi, Minato-ku
Tokyo 105
Tel: (81)-3-3433-1111

Support Groups for SAD and Mood Disorders

The National Organization for Seasonal Affective Disorder (NOSAD) was developed to support the interests of patients with SAD. Its membership is open to patients, friends, relatives, interested professionals, and any others who wish to further its goals. These goals include (1) disseminating information about SAD by means of a regular newsletter; (2) offering support groups to patients and their families in a manner that has been successful for many other medical and psychiatric illnesses; and (3) working toward goals that are important to people with SADfor example, insurance reimbursement for light fixtures.

The parent body was established in the Washington, D.C. metropolitan area, but members are eager to develop satellite groups across the country. If you are interested in finding more about NOSAD, or in starting your own local chapter of the group, further information can be obtained by writing to this address:

NOSAD
P.O. Box 40190
Washington, DC 20016

Other support groups that have a great deal to offer—including information about new research developments in the mood disorders, and about available support and facilities—include the following:

National Depressive and Manic
  Depressive Association (NMDA)
730 N. Franklin, #501
Chicago, IL 60610
Tel: 800-826-3632

Depression and Related Affective
  Disorders Association (DRADA)
Johns Hopkins University School
  of Medicine
Meyer 3-181
600 N. Wolfe St.
Baltimore, MD 21287-7381
Tel: 410-955-4647

In the United Kingdom:

SAD Association (SADA)
P.O. Box 989
London SW7 2PZ

The SAD Association is a voluntary organization and registered charity which informs the public and health professionals about SAD and supports and advises sufferers of the illness. SADA produces a newsletter three times a year and other publications, holds meetings, has a network of contacts and local groups, a lightbox hire scheme, and raises money for research into SAD.

For free basic information about SAD and its treatments, send a self-addressed envelope to SADA at the above address. For full details of SAD treatments, how to hire, buy, and use light fixtures, lists of contacts, telephone helpline, local groups, meetings, books, research updates, and general practitioner information, please send £5 (£3 concessions) to the above address.

Further Sources of Information

For further information about SAD and Light Therapy, you can write to one of these addresses.

Society for Light Therapy and
    Biological Rhythms
10200 West 44th Avenue
Suite 304
Wheat Ridge, CO 80033

DEPRESSION Awareness,
    Recognition, and Treatment
    (D/ART) Program
National Institute of Mental Health
5600 Fishers Lane, Room 10-85
Rockville, MD 20857
800-421-4211

Seasonal Studies Program
National Institute of Mental Health
Building 10, Room 4S-239
9000 Rockville Pike
Bethesda, MD 20892
Tel: 301-496-2141/496-0500

Sun Net
P.O. Box 10606
Rockville, MD 20850

For information on climatic conditions—daylength, amount of sunshine, and temperature—in different parts of the United States, contact this address:

The National Climatic Data Center
Federal Building
Asheville, NC 28801-2733
Tel: 704-CLIMATE (254-6283)

Dietary advice, menus, and recipes

As I've discussed in the section on diet and exercise in Chapter 7 of this book, there are currently at least three different approaches to treating the weight gain and fatigue associated with SAD. All three are represented below, and I encourage you to try whichever approach works best for you. These approaches include (1) calorie restriction with a high proportion of complex carbohydrates; (2) the Carbohydrate Addict's Diet®; and (3) a diet in which carbohydrate is balanced with protein, which I have referred to as the Paleolithic Diet.

Calorie Restriction with a High Proportion of Complex Carbohydrates

The following diets—1200, 1500, and 1800 calories—are designed for gradual weight loss in people whose ideal weights are 120, 150, and 180 pounds, respectively. Those whose ideal weights fall between these amounts may make calorie adjustments accordingly, allowing for 10 calories per pound of ideal weight per day. In practice, however, most people do fine on one of the three diets. The menus provided are just examples of the type of foods that will add up to the desired number of calories, while at the same time having appropriate proportions of the different major nutrients. If you wish to substitute your favorite foods for those mentioned below and would like to maintain the basic calorie and nutritional structure of the diets, you can easily accomplish this by contacting your local branch of the Diabetes Association and asking them to send you a copy of the Diabetic Exchange List. This lists those foods that are calorically and nutritionally interchangeable.

The diets below contain approximately 57 percent carbohydrate, 22 percent protein, and 21 percent fat. When you look them over, they may seem to contain too little protein. The reason for this is that there is a general tendency for us in the United States to eat more protein than necessary. Fat almost invariably accompanies the protein, especially protein derived from animal sources. For this reason, even if we stick to the less fatty animal proteins such as chicken or fish, we will still be getting too much fat if we consume large volumes of protein.

Remember, the total calorie counts include three snacks, and a list of suggested snacks is provided below. In addition, any items recommended as part of a meal can be held back and eaten between meals, if this is preferred. A list of "free beverages" that can be consumed at any time is also provided.

Menus for 1200 Calories

Day 1

Breakfast

1 cup cooked oatmeal
$1/4$ cup skim milk

Lunch

2 oz. roast beef with mustard on a large (2-oz.) roll
Large raw vegetable salad with 2 tblsp. reduced-calorie dressing

Dinner

1 cup Lentil Spaghetti Sauce (recipe, page 291)
1 cup cooked spaghetti
1 cup steamed zucchini

Day 2

Breakfast

2 slices toast
1 oz. cheese

Lunch

$1/2$ cup water-packed tuna with 1 tblsp. reduced-calorie mayonnaise
2 slices rye bread
2 cups raw vegetable sticks

Dinner

1 cup Sweet and Sour Apricot Chicken or Fish (recipe, page 291)
$^1/_2$ cup brown rice
1 cup steamed spinach and mushrooms

Day 3

Breakfast

$^3/_4$ cup cooked lentils with 1 oz. grated cheese

Lunch

1 oz. sliced turkey breast with mustard
2 slices rye bread
1 green pepper, raw, cut in strips

Dinner

2 oz. broiled fish with lemon and basil
1 large baked potato with $^1/_2$ cup fat-free, plain yogurt
1 cup steamed broccoli

Day 4

Breakfast

1 cup bite-sized shredded wheat
$^1/_2$ cup skim milk

Lunch

1 oz. lean ham
1 oz. cheese with mustard
1 6-inch pita bread pocket, filled with raw vegetables such as alfalfa
   sprouts, tomato, green pepper, cucumber

Dinner

2 cups Curried Barley and Lentil Soup (recipe, page 292)
1 slice pumpernickel bread
Large raw vegetable salad with 2 tblsp. reduced-calorie dressing

Day 5

Breakfast

1 cup cooked Wheatena cereal

Lunch

3 oz. boiled shrimp mixed with 1 cup diced raw vegetables (cucumber, green pepper, tomato), mixed with 1 tblsp. reduced-calorie mayonnaise, and stuffed into 1 6-inch pita bread pocket

Dinner

Medium chicken breast (1 piece), baked
1 cup lima beans
Large sliced tomato with vinegar

Day 6

Breakfast

1 bagel (2 oz.)
$^1/_3$ cup low-fat cottage cheese

Lunch

1 cup canned lentil soup
4 Ry-Krisp crackers
1 cup canned asparagus on lettuce with vinegar

Dinner

2 oz. broiled hamburger on hamburger bun with mustard
1 cup cole slaw made with 1 tblsp. reduced-calorie mayonnaise
$^1/_2$ cup fat-free, plain yogurt, flavored with vanilla and artificial sweetener

Day 7

Breakfast

2 slices toast
1 egg, fried in nonstick spray

Lunch

$^1/_3$ cup white beans with herbs and tomatos
$^2/_3$ cup brown rice
1 cup steamed broccoli

Dinner

3 oz. broiled lamb chop with garlic salt and rosemary

1 cup noodles with $^1/_2$ tsp. margarine, $^1/_3$ cup chopped tomato, and basil
1 cup steamed green beans

Menus for 1500 Calories

Day 1

Breakfast
1 cup cooked oatmeal

Lunch
3 oz. roast beef with mustard on a large (2-oz.) roll
Large raw vegetable salad with 2 tblsp. reduced-calorie dressing

Dinner
1 cup Lentil Spaghetti Sauce (recipe, page 291)
1 $^1/_2$ cups cooked spaghetti
1 cup steamed zucchini

Day 2

Breakfast
2 slices toast
2 oz. cheese

Lunch
$^1/_2$ cup water-packed tuna with 1 tblsp. reduced-calorie mayonnaise
2 slices rye bread
1 cup cream of tomato soup made with water
2 cups raw vegetable sticks

Dinner
1 cup Sweet and Sour Apricot Chicken or Fish (recipe, page, 291)
$^2/_3$ cup brown rice
1 cup steamed spinach and mushrooms

Day 3

Breakfast
1 cup cooked lentils

1 oz. grated cheese

Lunch

2 oz. sliced turkey breast with mustard and sliced tomato
2 slices rye bread
1 green pepper, raw, cut in strips

Dinner

3 oz. broiled fish with lemon and basil
1 large baked potato with $1/2$ cup fat-free, plain yogurt
1 cup steamed broccoli
1 slice bread

Day 4

Breakfast

1 $1/2$ cups bite-sized shredded wheat
1 cup skim milk

Lunch

2 oz. lean ham
1 oz. cheese with mustard and 1 tblsp. reduced-calorie mayonnaise
1 6-inch pita bread pocket, filled with raw vegetables such as
  cucumber, alfalfa sprouts, tomato, green pepper, etc.

Dinner

2 cups Curried Barley and Lentil Soup (recipe, page 292)
4 Wasa crackers
Large raw vegetable salad with 2 tblsp. reduced-calorie dressing

Day 5

Breakfast

1 cup cooked Wheatena cereal
1 cup skim milk

Lunch

6 oz. boiled shrimp mixed with $1/2$ cup diced raw vegetables (cucumber,
  green pepper, tomato, etc.), $1/2$ cup cooked macaroni, and 2 tblsp.
  reduced-calorie mayonnaise, and stuffed into 1 6-inch pita bread
  pocket

Dinner

Medium chicken breast (1 piece), baked
$^1/_2$ cup lima beans
1 large baked potato with $^1/_2$ tsp. margarine
1 medium sliced tomato with vinegar and basil

Day 6

Breakfast

1 bagel (2 oz.)
$^1/_3$ cup low-fat cottage cheese

Lunch

1 $^1/_2$ cups canned lentil soup
6 Ry-Krisp crackers
1 cup canned asparagus on lettuce with vinegar

Dinner

3 oz. broiled hamburger on hamburger bun with mustard
1 ear corn with $^1/_2$ tsp. margarine
1 cup cole slaw made with 1 tblsp. reduced-calorie mayonnaise
1 cup fat-free, plain yogurt, flavored with vanilla and artificial
  sweetener

Day 7

Breakfast

2 slices toast
1 egg, fried in nonstick spray
$^1/_2$ cup skim milk

Lunch

$^2/_3$ cup white beans with herbs and tomatoes
$^2/_3$ cup brown rice
1 cup steamed broccoli

Dinner

3 oz. broiled lamb chop with garlic salt and rosemary
1 $^1/_2$ cups cooked noodles with 1 tsp. margarine, $^1/_4$ cup chopped
  tomato, and basil
1 cup steamed green beans mixed with dill and $^1/_2$ cup fat-free, plain
  yogurt

Menus for 1800 Calories

Day 1

Breakfast

1 cup cooked oatmeal
1 cup skim milk
2 slices toast
2 tsp. margarine

Lunch

3 oz. roast beef with mustard on a large (2-oz.) roll
Large raw vegetable salad with 2 tblsp. reduced-calorie dressing

Dinner

1 $^1/_2$ cups Lentil Spaghetti Sauce (recipe, page 291)
2 cups cooked spaghetti
1 cup steamed zucchini

Day 2

Breakfast

2 slices toast
2 oz. cheese
$^1/_2$ cup bite-sized shredded wheat
$^1/_2$ cup skim milk

Lunch

$^1/_2$ cup water-packed tuna with reduced-calorie mayonnaise
2 slices rye bread
1 cup cream of tomato soup made with water
2 cups raw vegetable sticks

Dinner

1 $^1/_2$ cups Sweet and Sour Apricot Chicken or Fish (recipe, page 291)
1 cup brown rice
1 cup steamed spinach and mushrooms with 1 tsp. margarine

Day 3

Breakfast

1 cup cooked lentils
2 oz. grated cheese

Lunch

2 oz. sliced turkey breast with mustard
2 slices rye bread
1 green pepper, raw, cut in strips

Dinner

4 oz. broiled fish with lemon and basil
1 large baked potato with $1/2$ cup fat-free, plain yogurt
1 cup steamed broccoli
2 slices bread

Day 4

Breakfast

2 cups bite-sized shredded wheat
1 cup skim milk

Lunch

2 oz. lean ham
2 oz. cheese with mustard and 1 tblsp. reduced-calorie mayonnaise
1 6-inch pita bread pocket, filled with raw vegetables such as alfalfa
   sprouts, tomato, green pepper, cucumber, etc.

Dinner

2 cups Curried Barley and Lentil Soup (recipe, page 292)
6 Wasa crackers
Large raw vegetable salad with 2 tblsp. reduced-calorie dressing

Day 5

Breakfast

1 $1/2$ cups cooked Wheatena cereal
1 cup skim milk

Lunch

6 oz. boiled shrimp mixed with $1/2$ cup diced raw vegetables (cucumber,
   green pepper, tomato, etc.), $1/2$ cup cooked macaroni, and 2 tblsp.
   reduced-calorie mayonnaise, and stuffed into 1 6-inch pita bread
   pocket

Dinner

Large chicken breast (1 piece), baked
1 cup lima beans
1 large baked potato with 1 tsp. margarine
1 medium sliced tomato with basil, vinegar, and 1 tsp. olive oil

Day 6

Breakfast

2 bagels (2 oz. each)
$^2/_3$ cup low-fat cottage cheese

Lunch

1 $^1/_2$ cups canned lentil soup
6 Ry-Krisp crackers
1 cup canned asparagus on lettuce with 1 tblsp. reduced-calorie mayonnaise

Dinner

3 oz. broiled hamburger on hamburger bun with mustard
1 6-inch ear corn with $^1/_2$ tsp. margarine
1 cup cole slaw made with 1 tblsp. reduced-calorie mayonnaise
1 cup fat-free, plain yogurt, flavored with vanilla and artificial sweetener

Day 7

Breakfast

2 slices toast
1 tsp. margarine
1 egg, fried in nonstick spray
$^1/_2$ cup skim milk

Lunch

1 cup white beans with herbs and tomatoes
1 cup brown rice
1 cup steamed broccoli

Dinner

3 oz. broiled lamb chop with garlic salt and rosemary
1 $^1/_2$ cups cooked noodles mixed with 1 tsp. margarine, $^1/_4$ cup chopped tomato, and basil

1 cup steamed green beans mixed with dill and $^1/_2$ cup fat-free, plain yogurt

1 tsp. margarine over green beans

Allowed Beverages

Coffee, tea, club soda, seltzer water, water, diet soft drinks.

Snacks

In addition to your three meals, you may have three snacks per day. The following list provides only a few examples; many other snacks may have similar caloric and nutritional properties. Recipes are provided immediately below for the items with an asterisk, and under the recipes for the Paleolithic Diet further below for the items with a dagger.

$^1/_2$ cup Very Spicy Chick Peas*
2 rice cakes (may be flavored with apple or cinnamon)
$^1/_3$ cup kidney beans with chopped onion
4 Ry-Krisp crackers
1 Oat Bran Muffin*
3 cups Air-Popped Popcorn (no oil/salt)*
$^3/_4$ oz. matzoth
1 slice bread
$^1/_2$ cup Roseanne's Black Beans and Rice†
2 whole wheat crackers (may be topped with all-fruit jelly or applesauce)
1 Baked Fruit (apples, pears, peaches)*
$^1/_2$ cup Homemade Frozen Yogurt†
$^1/_2$ cup Malted†
Rice cakes with cottage cheese (low-fat, low-salt) and jelly
Small Twice-Baked Potato†
Stuffed Whole Wheat tortilla†
$^1/_2$ cup Yogurt Cream Cheese or Dip†
1 handful of 100% whole wheat pretzels with sesame seeds

Recipes

Air-Popped Popcorn

Use a hot air popper or put kernels in a brown paper bag and microwave. While hot, add onion powder, chili powder, oregano, or garlic powder (whatever spice you like), but try not to use salt.

Baked Fruit

Apples, pears, or peaches
All-fruit jelly
Cinnamon

Microwave fruit in 1 inch water. Add all-fruit jelly and cinnamon.

Oat Bran Muffins

2 $^1/_4$ cups Mother's Oat Bran cereal, uncooked
$^1/_4$ cup raisins (may omit if desired)
2 tsp. baking powder
$^1/_2$ tsp. salt (optional)
$^3/_4$ cup skim milk
$^1/_3$ cup honey
2 eggs, beaten
1 tblsp. vegetable oil

Heat oven to 425°F. Coat 12 medium muffin cups with nonstick spray or line with paper baking cups. In large bowl, combine cereal, raisins, baking powder, and salt. Add remaining ingredients; mix just until dry ingredients are moistened. Fill prepared muffin cups almost full. Bake 15 to 17 minutes or until golden brown. Makes 1 dozen muffins.

Very Spicy Chick Peas

2 tsp. olive oil
3 small garlic cloves, minced
1 tsp. minced fresh ginger
1 large onion, chopped
4 canned tomatoes packed in tomato juice*
3 tsp. coriander
$^1/_2$ tsp. cumin
$^1/_2$ tsp. cinnamon
$^1/_4$ tsp. salt
$^1/_4$ tsp. freshly ground black pepper
$^1/_4$ tsp. ground cloves
$^1/_8$ tsp. cayenne pepper
2 15-oz. cans chick peas, drained and rinsed

¹/₄ cup minced fresh parsley
*Reserve the tomato juice.

In a large, heavy skillet, warm the olive oil over moderately low heat. Add the garlic, ginger, and onion; cook, stirring occasionally, until softened (3 to 5 minutes). Add the tomatoes, breaking them into pieces with the spatula. Add ¹/₂ cup of the reserved tomato juice, along with the coriander, cumin, cinnamon, salt, black pepper, cloves, and cayenne pepper. Cook, stirring occasionally, for 5 minutes, then add the chick peas. Cook 10 minutes—if the mixture gets too thick, add more tomato juice. Add the parsley and toss.

Lentil Spaghetti Sauce

1 medium onion, chopped
1 clove garlic, minced
2 tblsp. oil
1 ¹/₂ cups dried lentils, washed
1 dried hot pepper, crumbled
1 tsp. salt (optional)
¹/₂ tsp. pepper
4 cups water and 2 beef bouillon cubes (or 4 cups fat-skimmed beef broth)
¹/₄ tsp. dried basil, crumbled
1 16-oz. can tomatoes
1 6-oz. can tomato paste
1 tblsp. vinegar

Saute onion and garlic in oil for 5 minutes. Add lentils, red pepper, salt, pepper, and water with bouillon cubes or beef broth. Cover and simmer 30 minutes. Add remaining ingredients and simmer uncovered for about 1 hour, stirring occasionally. Serve over regular or whole wheat spaghetti, or rice.

Sweet and Sour Apricot Chicken or Fish

Chicken breasts or fish filets
All-fruit apricot preserves
¹/₄ cup nonfat plain yogurt
Dijon or Grey Poupon mustard

Marinate chicken breasts or fish filets in all-fruit apricot preserves mixed with non-fat plain yogurt and mustard. Coat chicken breasts or fish filets and bake or grill.

Curried Barley and Lentil Soup

1 1/2 cup chopped onion
2 crushed garlic cloves
2 tsp. olive oil
1 1/2 tsp. curry powder
8 cups water
1/4 cup uncooked barley
1/2 cup uncooked lentils
1 tsp. salt
2 cups stewed tomatoes
1 cup chopped celery
1 tblsp. white vinegar

Place water, barley, and lentils in a 4-quart pot. Bring to a boil, cover, and reduce heat. Meanwhile, spray a nonstick skillet with vegetable cooking spray and heat until medium hot. Cook onions and garlic until lightly browned. Add oil and curry powder and continue cooking for 5 minutes. Add onions to barley–lentil mixture and simmer for 45 minutes. After 45 minutes, add tomatoes and celery and cook an additional 15 minutes. Remove from heat and let cool for 10 minutes. Blend in small batches in the food processor or blender. (Caution: Hot liquid tends to spurt, so be careful.) Return to pot, stir in vinegar, and reheat to serving temperature. Makes 8 cups.

The Carbohydrate Addict's Diet®

This 7-day Entry Meal Plan was kindly provided by Drs. Rachael and Richard Heller. According to them, it should immediately help cut carbohydrate cravings and start the weight loss process. If you find it helpful, you should then move on to one of four different eating plans, which have been individualized for your metabolic level along with the number of pounds you want to lose. Guidelines for how to tailor your follow-up diet for your own personal requirements are fully provided in the Hellers' book, *The Carbohydrate Addict's Diet* (Dutton, 1991).

There is no need to measure, count calories, or make food exchanges on the Carbohydrate Addict's Diet®. Unless otherwise noted below, all portions are average servings. Reward Meals® must be completed within a 60-minute period. All meals can be adapted to meet low-fat, very-low-fat, vegetarian, and/or low-salt guidelines.

Menus

Day 1

Breakfast

Cheese omelette (or egg substitute with low-fat cheese)
Sausage or bacon (regular or low-fat turkey)
Tea or coffee

Lunch

Tossed green salad with dressing (regular or low-fat)
Spicy shrimp with mushrooms
Iced or hot tea or coffee, seltzer, Perrier, or club soda

Reward Meal® Dinner

1/2 grapefruit
Caesar salad
Spaghetti with lots of meatballs
Garlic bread
Asparagus
Apple pie topped with scoop of ice cream or sherbet
Coffee, tea, wine, beer, or regular or diet soda

Day 2

Breakfast

Carbohydrate Addict's Light and Airy Muffins (recipe, page 296)
Tea or coffee

Lunch

Chef's salad (with strips of ham, chicken, turkey, and cheese)
Salad dressing (regular or low-fat)
Iced or hot tea or coffee, seltzer, Perrier, or club soda

Reward Meal® Dinner

Fresh fruit salad
Mixed salad with dressing (regular or low-fat)
Green beans almondine meatballs

Lean steak with broiled mushrooms
Whole grain roll with pat of butter (or low-fat substitute)
Slice of chocolate cake (regular or low-fat)
Coffee, tea, wine, beer, or regular or diet soda

Day 3

Breakfast

Scrambled eggs (or no-cholesterol egg substitute)
Sausage (regular or low-fat)
Cool cucumber slices
Tea or coffee

Lunch

Mixed greens with dressing (regular or low-fat)
Green and black olives
Chicken, turkey, or shrimp salad with sliced egg
Iced or hot tea or coffee, seltzer, Perrier, or club soda

Reward Meal® Dinner

Orange juice
Mixed salad with dressing (regular or low-fat)
Broccoli spears topped with cheese
Chicken Paprikash (recipe, page 297) on rice
Italian bread with butter (or low-fat substitute)
Chocolate pudding or low-fat fruited yogurt
Coffee, tea, wine, beer, or regular or diet soda

Day 4

Breakfast

Carbohydrate Addict's Bread (recipe, page 298)
Tea or coffee

Lunch

Finger salad (celery, green peppers, radishes, olives, mushrooms)
Salad dressing (regular or low-fat)
Cheeseburger (regular or low-fat turkey)
Sauteed green beans
Dill pickle
Iced or hot tea or coffee, seltzer, Perrier or, club soda

Reward Meal® Dinner

Tomato juice
Spinach salad with crumbled bacon, mushrooms
Salad dressing (regular or low-fat)
Green pepper steak with rice
French bread with butter (or low-fat substitute)
Fresh fruit salad
Brownies (regular or low-fat)
Coffee, tea, wine, beer, or regular or diet soda

Day 5

Breakfast

Carbohydrate Addict's Breakfast Crepes (recipe, page 299)
Tea or coffee

Lunch

Mixed salad with dressing (regular or low-fat)
Baked, broiled, or roasted chicken
Cheese-topped broccoli (regular or low-fat)
Iced or hot tea or coffee, seltzer, Perrier, or club soda

Reward Meal® Dinner

$^1/_2$ cantaloupe
Mixed salad with dressing (regular or low-fat)
Flounder (fried, baked, or broiled)
Baked potato with butter and sour cream (or low-cholesterol
    substitutes)
Whole grain roll with butter (or low-fat substitute)
Apple sauce
Strawberry shortcake with topping (low-fat or regular)
Coffee, tea, wine, beer, or regular or diet soda

Day 6

Breakfast

Ham and cheese omelette (or low-fat substitutes)
Sliced cucumber
Tea or coffee

Lunch

Mixed salad with dressing (regular or low-fat)
Hot dogs (regular or low-fat chicken)—remember, no buns until dinner
Sauerkraut, olives, and dill pickle
Iced or hot tea or coffee, seltzer, Perrier, or club soda

Reward Meal® Dinner

Wonton soup
Oriental salad with dressing (regular or low-fat)
Chicken with cashews or sweet and sour pork
Rice or noodles
Baked apple with topping (regular or low-fat)
Almond or fortune cookies
Coffee, tea, wine, beer, or regular or diet soda

Day 7

Breakfast

Breakfast Souffle (recipe, page 299)
Tea or coffee

Lunch

Tuna or salmon salad platter with olives, cucumber, tomato, and lettuce
Salad dressing (regular or low-fat)
Iced or hot tea or coffee, seltzer, Perrier, or club soda

Reward Meal® Dinner

Antipasto
$1/4$ honeydew melon
Sausage (regular or low-fat)
Lasagna (regular or vegetarian)
Garlic bread
Fresh strawberries with topping (regular or low-fat)
Coffee, tea, wine, beer, or regular or diet soda

Recipes

Carbohydrate Addict's Light and Airy Muffins

This recipe will give you a fluffy muffin that tastes a little like a popover. Serve warm or cold with butter, margarine, cream cheese, or low-carbohydrate preserves.

$^1/_2$ tblsp. polyunsaturated vegetable oil
4 eggs
$^1/_2$ tsp. cream of tartar
$^1/_4$ cup regular or low-fat cottage cheese
2 tblsp. soy flour*
1 package artificial sweetener
*May be purchased at most health food stores.

Preheat the oven to 300°F. Coat muffin cups with a little vegetable oil (or use butter, margarine, or pan spray). Separate the eggs very carefully, allowing no egg yolk to mix with the whites. Beat the egg whites with an electric mixer until frothy. Add the cream of tartar and continue beating just until stiff peaks form.

Combine egg yolks, cottage cheese, soy flour, and sweetener. Fold this mixture carefully into the egg whites. Fill each muffin cup two-thirds full of batter. Bake the muffins for about 30 minutes, until they are golden brown and spring back when touched with a finger. Makes 14 muffins.

Variation: To make Spice Muffins, stir $^1/_2$ tsp. cinnamon, $^1/_4$ tsp. ground ginger, and $^1/_8$ tsp. cloves into the soy flour before adding to the egg yolks.

Chicken Paprikash

2 tblsp. butter or margarine
2 tblsp. olive oil or polyunsaturated vegetable oil
1 to 2 tblsp. mild paprika
$^1/_2$ cup chopped onion
$^1/_2$ cup chopped green or red peppers
1 chicken (2 $^1/_2$ to 3 lbs.), cut into pieces
2 cups chicken stock, broth, or bouillon
1 tsp. flour
1 $^1/_2$ cup sour cream or low-cholesterol substitute

Melt the butter or margarine in a large, heavy frying pan over moderate heat. Add the oil and paprika; heat until hot but not smoking. Add the onion and peppers and saute for 2 minutes. Move the onion and peppers to the sides of the pan and add the chicken pieces, skin side down. Cook for about 3 minutes, until the skin begins to brown. Turn the pieces to brown the other side, cooking for about 3 minutes.

Stir in the chicken stock. Cover and simmer for 45 minutes to 1 hour, until the chicken is tender and the juices run clear when the meat is pierced with a fork. Transfer the chicken to a plate. Stir the flour into the sour cream and slowly stir the mixture into the pan. Cover the pan and simmer over low heat for 3 minutes. Stir, cover again, and simmer for an additional 2 minutes. Do not let the mixture boil. Pour the cream mixture over the chicken. Serves 3 to 4.

Carbohydrate Addict's Bread (with variations)

This is an unusual but delicious substitute for high-carbohydrate breads. Serve it with butter or margarine, or low-carbohydrate preserves.

Polyunsaturated vegetable oil, butter, or pan spray
3 eggs
$1/2$ tsp. cream of tartar
$1/4$ cup regular or low-fat cottage cheese
2 tblsp. soy flour
1 package artificial sweetener

Preheat the oven to 300 degrees. Oil a small loaf pan with vegetable oil, butter, or pan spray. Beat the egg whites with an electric mixer until frothy. Add the cream of tartar and beat until stiff peaks form, but the whites are still moist. Combine the egg yolks, cottage cheese, soy flour, and sweetener and fold into the egg whites. Do not overmix. Pour the mixture into the prepared pan and bake in the preheated oven for about 40 to 45 minutes, or until the loaf is lightly browned and springs back when touched with a finger. Makes 1 small loaf (about 4 x 7 inches).

Variations: To make Cinnamon Bread, stir $1/2$ tsp. cinnamon into the soy flour before adding the egg mixture. To make a Savory Onion Bread, saute $1/4$ finely diced onion in 1 tblsp. polyunsaturated vegetable oil, butter, or margarine. Cool and blot with paper toweling. Fold the onions into the egg mixture before it is turned out into the prepared bread pan.

Carbohydrate Addict's Breakfast Crepes

3 egg whites
$1/2$ tsp. cream of tartar
$1/4$ cup small-curd regular or low-fat cottage cheese
$1/4$ tsp. vanilla extract
$1/2$ package artificial sweetener
$1/2$ tblsp. vegetable oil, or pan spray

Beat the egg whites with the cream of tartar until stiff. Set aside. Combine the cottage cheese, vanilla extract, and sweetener, mixing well. Fold carefully into the egg whites, without mixing too thoroughly.

Oil a nonstick griddle or frying pan with a little vegetable oil or pan spray. Heat the pan over moderate heat. Form 4-inch crepes by spooning about 2 tblsp. of batter into the pan and spreading mixture into a thin round. Cook over moderate heat until the crepe sets and appears to be brown on the bottom. Turn and brown the other side. Repeat with the remaining batter. Makes 4 to 6 crepes.

Variation: To make blintzes, spread a tsp. of sour cream onto each crepe, and roll into a cylinder.

Breakfast Souffle

This breakfast dish is great served by itself or with bacon, ham, or sausage (or low-cholesterol breakfast meat substitute).

2 egg whites
$1/2$ tsp. cream of tartar
1 cup regular or low-fat cottage cheese
1 egg yolk
$1/2$ package artificial sweetener

Preheat the oven to 300 degrees. Oil a 9-inch round cake pan with a little butter, vegetable oil, or pan spray. Beat the egg whites until frothy with an electric mixer. Add the cream of tartar, and beat just until stiff peaks form. Combine the cottage cheese, egg yolk, and sweetener, mixing well. Fold gently into the egg whites, being careful not to mix too thoroughly.

Pour the souffle mixture into the buttered cake pan and bake in the preheated oven for 25 to 30 minutes. Turn the broiler up and brown the souffle under the broiler for 2 to 3 minutes, watching carefully to make sure it doesn't burn. Serves 2.

A Diet in Which Carbohydrate Is Balanced with Protein: The Paleolithic Diet

The object of the Paleolithic Diet is to provide more protein in relation to carbohydrate than is available from the two above diets. The specifications for this diet were put forward by Drs. S. Boyd Eaton and Melvin Konner in an article in the *New England Journal of Medicine*, and they followed up this concept with a popular book, *The Paleolithic Prescription* (see "Further Reading," below). The following menus and recipes were prepared along strict Paleolithic guidelines by a nutritionist, Bette Flax, who has adapted the proportions calculated by the scientists to modern ingredients and tastes. It is not necessary to calculate calories on this diet. Measurements are based on the needs of people of average weight and metabolism, and may need to be adjusted upward to downward according to your specific weight and metabolic rate.

A Note About Ingredients

In choosing ingredients to prepare the foods listed in the following menus, be sure to choose the following:

> Soups that are low in sodium (<100 mg per serving) and low in fat (<3 grams per serving)
> Cottage cheese that has 1 gram or less of fat per serving
> Jelly or syrup that is "all fruit"
> The following seasonings, which are good salt substitutes:
> > Mrs. Dash's saltless spices
> > McCormick's saltless spices
> > Parsley Patch saltless spices
> > Garlic powder/onion powder
> > Minced garlic/minced onion
> > Dill, basil, celery seed, oregano, black pepper, cayenne pepper, paprika
> The following sweetening agents:
> > Condensed frozen apple juice (use in frozen state)
> > Cinnamon
> > All-fruit jelly or syrup

Menus

Day 1

Breakfast
$^1/_2$ cup of plain yogurt, mixed with all-fruit jelly and $^1/_2$ cup shredded wheat
$^1/_4$ cup berries

Mid-Morning
Herbal tea

Lunch
$^1/_2$ whole wheat English muffin with 1 or 2 slices turkey, $^1/_2$ slice skim milk mozzarella, and tomato

Dinner
1 cup whole grain pasta, mixed with fish or seafood
2 to 3 oz. vegetables
Salad

Snack
Fruit
A Malted (recipe, page 305)

Day 2

Breakfast
1 individual container of low-fat yogurt with berries

Mid-Morning
Herbal tea

Lunch
Salad with grilled chicken and vegetables
Whole grain bread
Fruit

Dinner
Small piece of grilled chicken or fish
Baked sweet potato, mashed with cottage cheese, cinnamon, and nutmeg—rebaked

Broccoli
Salad

Snack

4 oz. of skim milk
Fruit

Day 3

Breakfast

2 or 3 mashed cooked egg whites with diced celery, carrot, and onion
(wet with 1 tsp. plain yogurt mixed with mustard), on a whole wheat
mini-pita with lettuce and cucumber

Mid-Morning

Herbal tea

Lunch

Salad with cooked egg whites, turkey, or shrimp and beans and
vegetables
Small Twice-Baked Potato (recipe, page 305)

Dinner

3 oz. Sweet and Sour Chicken or Fish (recipe given with restricted-
calorie diets, page 291)
$1/2$ cup couscous
1 cup vegetables

Snack

Fruit
Homemade Frozen Yogurt (recipe, page 305)

Day 4

Breakfast

$3/4$ cup low-fat/low-salt cottage cheese, with strawberries mixed with 2
tblsp. all-natural applesauce and cinnamon

Mid-Morning

Herbal tea

Lunch

Tuna wet with yogurt or vinegar
Lots of raw vegetables
Whole wheat bread

Dinner

Salad with filled poultry
$1/4$ cup beans
Lots of vegetables
All-natural applesauce

Snack

Fruit
4 oz. skim milk

Day 5

Breakfast

2 egg whites (beaten in microwave cup), with diced onions, peppers, etc., microwaved 1 $1/4$ minutes and served in whole wheat mini-pita with lettuce and tomato

Mid-Morning

Herbal tea

Lunch

2 oz. chicken or fish
Roseanne's Black Beans and Rice (recipe, page 305)
or Bette's Vegetarian Lasagna (recipe, page 306)
Salad
Fruit

Dinner

Chicken or turkey or fish chunks (stir-fried in white wine and no-salt chicken broth)
2 cups stir-fried vegetables with boiled new potatoes—use lots of seasonings

Snack

One piece of fat-free pound cake with berries, nonfat plain yogurt, and all-fruit syrup

Day 6

Breakfast

$1/2$ cup plain yogurt mixed with $1/2$ cup cottage cheese and all-fruit
    syrup
Whole wheat mini-pita
or Stuffed Whole Wheat Tortilla plus Yogurt Dip (recipes, page 307)

Mid-Morning
Herbal tea

Lunch
Grilled fish or chicken breast
Vegetables or salad
Fruit or one piece of whole wheat bread

Dinner
Steamed peppers, stuffed with ground cooked turkey, beans, $1/2$ cup
    wild rice, and marinara, and rebaked

Snack
Frozen nonfat plain yogurt, served over berries with all-fruit syrup

Day 7

Breakfast
1 piece whole wheat bread dipped in beaten egg whites (French toast)
    topped with All-Fruit Jelly and $1/4$ cup plain nonfat yogurt

Snack
Herbal tea

Lunch
Fruit salad mixed with $1/2$ cup low-salt or low-fat cottage cheese

Dinner
Egg White Omelette (recipe, page 307) stuffed with vegetables of
    choice

Snack
Fruit
4 oz. skim milk

Recipes

Homemade Frozen Yogurt

Nonfat plain yogurt
All-fruit syrup (to taste)
1 cup berries of your choice

Blend ingredients together. Put the mixture into the freezer in closed container.

Malted

4 oz. skim milk
$1/2$ cup strawberries (blueberries, raspberries)
1 capful vanilla extract
1 heaping tblsp. strawberry all-fruit syrup
Lots of ice cubes

Put into a blender and mix.

Small Twice-Baked Potato

Small potato
Onion (minced or fresh)
Mushrooms
1 heaping tblsp. nonfat plain yogurt
1 heaping tblsp. favorite mustard
1 heaping tblsp. low-fat, low-salt cottage cheese
$1/4$ cup (or less) skim milk

Heat oven to 450°F. Microwave potato for 4 minutes. Spoon out inside of potato and either mash by hand or put into a blender along with the remaining ingredients. Put mixture back into the potato skin. Bake for 10 minutes.

Roseanne's Black Beans and Rice

1 cup celery, chopped
1 large onion, chopped
1 large green pepper, chopped
2 cloves garlic, minced
2 tblsp. olive oil

2 1-lb. cans black beans
$^1/_2$ tsp. oregano leaves
1 tsp. salt (optional)
3 tblsp. lemon juice, or more (to taste)
4-oz. jar sliced pimentos
2 7-oz. or 3 5-oz. packages yellow rice dinner, prepared without fat

Saute celery, onion, green pepper and garlic in olive oil until tender. Add beans with their liquid, oregano and salt. Cover and simmer on low heat for about 15 minutes. Add entire jar of pimentos with their juice and heat for about 5 minutes. Add lemon juice to taste just prior to serving. Serve over yellow rice. Makes 6 to 8 servings.

Bette's Vegetarian Lasagna

Tomato and basil marinara sauce
Skim ricotta cheese
Mrs. Dash's seasonings
Garlic powder
Onion powder
Oregano
Pepper
Whole grain pasta noodles
Onions
Green, red, yellow Peppers
Fresh mushrooms
Zucchini/acorn squash
Eggplant
Frozen broccoli/cauliflower
Frozen carrots
Fat-free mozzarella cheese

Heat oven to 350°F. In a deep casserole dish, place the following layers: Layer of marinara sauce with heaping tblsp. of skim ricotta cheese. Layer of onions and mushrooms. Layer of lasagna noodles. Layer of same sauce. Layer of carrots (slightly steamed) and eggplant (slightly steamed in chunks). Layer of noodles. Layer of sauce. Layer of zucchini and acorn squash (slightly steamed). Layer of noodles. Layer of sauce. Layer of peppers (slightly steamed). Layer of noodles. Layer of sauce. Layer of broccoli and cauliflower (slightly steamed). Layer of noodles. Layer of sauce. Cover top with package of fat-free mozzarella cheese. Bake 30 to 45 minutes. Serve with salad.

Note: You can add ground turkey breast to sauce and cut down on some of the vegetable layers. Season marinara sauce with spices and herbs of choice. Season vegetables as well.

Stuffed Whole Wheat Tortilla

Heat oven to 425°F. To a whole wheat tortilla (which can be purchased at the dairy section of many stores), add marinara sauce with skim ricotta cheese, mushrooms, onions, peppers, etc., or 1 tblsp. low-fat/low-salt cottage cheese and all-fruit jelly or cinnamon. Bake for 10 to 15 minutes.

Yogurt Cream Cheese or Dip

Nonfat plain yogurt
Coffee filter

Place a coffee filter over the top of a deep glass, making sure that the sides of the filter are taped to the sides of the glass. Push filter down for room. Turn yogurt upside down on the top of the coffee filter and keep it in the refrigerator all night. In the morning, the yogurt left on top of the filter will now have the consistency of cream cheese. Add seasonings and use as cream cheese or as a dip with vegetables.

Egg White Omelette

Place spinach, mushrooms, onions, zucchini, or other vegetables of your choice in microwave for 1 minute, or until soft. Beat 3 egg whites and add vegetables. Melt 1 tsp. margarine on pan. Add omelette and cook.

A Note about Snacks

When you are snacking on the Paleolithic Diet, try not to have pure carbohydrate snacks. Instead, try to balance the carbohydrate with protein. The Stuffed Whole Wheat Tortilla described above is a good example of such a snack. Or try some of the Yogurt Cream Cheese or Dip on a whole wheat cracker. Low-fat tinned soups also work well on this diet. If you're craving bread, perhaps half a toasted English muffin with a piece of part-skim mozzarella cheese will satisfy the craving. In other words, on this diet you are trying to avoid having too much carbohydrate without the balancing effects of the other major dietary nutrients, protein and fat.

Further reading

This is not intended to be a comprehensive bibliography, but rather a list of some texts that you might find useful and interesting. For an extensive list of articles on SAD and light therapy, I refer you to the first two scholarly works, each of which lists hundreds of references.

Part 1: Seasonal Syndromes

Blehar, M.C., and Lewy, A.J. "Seasonal Mood Disorders: Consensus and Controversy," *Psychopharmacology Bulletin*, 26(4): 465–494, 1990.
Oren, D.A., and Rosenthal N.E. "Seasonal Affective Disorders." In: *Handbook of Affective Disorders*, 2nd edition, E.S. Paykel, ed., pp. 551–567, Edinburgh: Churchill Livingstone, 1992.
Rosenthal, N.E., and Blehar, M.C., eds. *Seasonal Affective Disorders and Phototherapy*. New York: Guilford Press, 1989.
Thompson, C., and Silverstone, T., eds. *Seasonal Affective Disorders*. London: CNS Neuroscience Press, 1989.

Part 2: Treatments

Light Therapy

Lewy, A.J., Sack, R.L., Miller, S., and Hoban, T.M. "Antidepressant and Circadian Phase-Shifting Effects of Light," *Science*, 235: 352–354, 1987.
Lewy, A.J., Sack, R.L., and Singer, C.M. "Treating Phase Typed Chronobiologic Sleep and Mood Disorders Using Appropriately Timed Bright Artificial Light," *Psychopharmacology Bulletin*, 21: 368–372, 1985.
Rosenthal, N.E., Sack, D.A., Gillin, J.C., Lewy, A.J., Goodwin, F.K., Davenport, Y., Mueller, P.S., Newsome, D.A., and Wehr, T.A. "Seasonal

Affective Disorder: A Description of the Syndrome and Preliminary Findings with Light Therapy," *Archives of General Psychiatry, 41*: 72–80, 1984.

Rosenthal, N.E., and Wehr, T.A. "Towards Understanding the Mechanism of Action of Light in Seasonal Affective Disorder," *Pharmacopsychiatry, 25*(1): 56–60, 1992.

Sack, R.L., Lewy, A.J., White, D.M., Singer, C.M., Fireman, M.J., and Vandiver, R. "Morning vs. Evening Light Treatment for Winter Depression," *Archives of General Psychiatry, 47*: 343–351, 1990.

Terman, M., Remé, C.E., Rafferty, B., Gallin, P.F., and Terman, J.S. "Bright Light Therapy for Winter Depression: Potential Ocular Effects and Theoretical Implications," *Photochemistry and Photobiology, 51*(6): 781–791, 1990.

Terman, M., and Terman, J.S. *Light Therapy for Winter Depression: Report to the Depression Guidelines Panel, P.H.S. Agency for Health Care Policy and Research.* Bethesda, MD: U.S. Public Health Service.

Wirz-Justice, A., Graw, P., Kräuchi, K., Gisin, B., Jochum, A., Arendt, J., Fisch, H.-U., Buddeberg, C., and Pöldinger, W. "Light Therapy in Seasonal Affective Disorder is Independent of Time of Day or Circadian Phase, " *Archives of General Psychiatry*, in press.

Diet and Exercise

Carper, Jean. *The All-in-One Calorie Counter.* New York: Bantam Books, 1974.

Eaton, S.B., and Konner, M.J. "Paleolithic Nutrition: A Consideration of its Nature and Current Implications," *New England Journal of Medicine, 312*: 283–289, 1985.

Eaton, S.B., Shostak, M., and Konner, M.J. *The Paleolithic Prescription.* New York: Harper & Row, 1988.

Goor, Ron, Goor, Nancy, and Boyd, Katherine. *The Choose to Lose Diet.* Boston: Houghton Mifflin, 1990.

Heller, Rachael F., and Heller, Richard F. *The Carbohydrate Addict's Diet: The Lifelong Solution to Yo-Yo Dieting.* New York: Dutton, 1991.

Wurtman, Judith J. *The Carbohydrate Craver's Diet.* Boston: Houghton Mifflin, 1983.

Wurtman, Judith J. *Managing your Mind and Mood through Food.* New York: Rawson Associates, 1986.

Psychotherapy and Advice to Friends and Family

Burns, David D. *Feeling Good: The New Mood Therapy.* New York: Signet, 1981.

Papolos, Demitri F., and Papolos, Janice. *Overcoming Depression.* New York: Harper & Row, 1987.

Storr, Anthony. *The Art of Psychotherapy.* New York: Methuen, 1979.

Jet Lag, Shift Work, and General Information about Light

Hyman, Jane. *The Light Book*. Los Angeles: Jeremy P. Tarcher, 1990.
Moore-Ede, Martin. *The Twenty-Four Hour Society*. Reading, MA: Addison-Wesley, 1993
Oren, D.A,, Reich, W., Rosenthal, N. E., and Wehr, T.A. *How to Beat Jet Lag: A Practical Guide for Air Travelers*. New York: Holt, 1993.

Part 3: Celebrating the Seasons

Boorstin, D. J. *The Discoverers*. New York: Vintage Books, 1983.
Cameron, 1. *Antarctica: The Last Continent*. London: Cassell, 1974.
Cook, F.A. "Medical Observations among the Esquimaux," *New York Journal of Gynaecology and Obstetrics*, 4: 282–296, 1894.
Dewhurst, K. "A Seventeenth-Century Symposium on Manic–Depressive Psychosis," *British Journal of Medical Psychology*, 35: 111–125, 1962.
Eliade, Mircea. "Experiences of the Mystic Light." In: *Mephistopheles and Androgyne*. New York: Sheed and Ward, 1965.
Eliade, Mircea. *The Myth of the Eternal Return, or Cosmos and History*. Translated by W. R. Trask. Bollingen Series XLVI. Princeton, NJ: Princeton University Press, 1954.
Esquirol, J.E.D. *Mental Maladies: Treatise on Insanity*. New York: Hafner, 1965.
Frumkes, G. "A Depression Which Recurred Annually," *Psychoanalytic Quarterly*, 65 :351–364, 1946.
James, William. *The Varieties of Religious Experience*. New York: University Press, 1963. (Originally published, 1902)
Jamison, Kay Redfield. "Mood Disorders and Seasonal Patterns in Top British Writers and Artists," *Psychiatry*, 52(2): 125–134, 1989.
Jamison, Kay Redfield. *Touched with Fire: Manic–Depressive Illness and the Artistic Temperament*. New York: Free Press, 1993.
Johnson, T.H., ed. *The Complete Poems of Emily Dickinson*. Boston: Little, Brown, 1960.
Jones, Jack Raymond. *The Man Who Loved the Sun: The Life of Vincent van Gogh*. London: Evans Brothers, 1966.
Marsh, Michael. *Philosophy of the Inner Light* (Pendle Hill Pamphlet 209). Pendle Hill, PA: Pendle Hill Publications, 1976.
Manner, Knud, ed. *Selected Letters of Gustav Mahler*. London: Faber & Faber, 1979.
Stone, 1., ed. *Dear Theo: The Autobiography of Vincent van Gogh*. New York: Signet, 1969.
Wechsberg, J. "Mørketiden," *The New Yorker*, March 18, 1972.

Self-assessment mood scale for SAD (SAM SAD)*

*The Self-Assessment Mood Scale for SAD (SAM-SAD) is adapted from the Structured Interview Guide for the Hamilton Depression Rating Scale—Seasonal Affective Disorder version, by J. B. W. Williams, M. J. Link, N. E. Rosenthal, and M. Terman, 1988. ©Norman E. Rosenthal, 1993.

Compared to how you feel **when you are in an even or normal mood state,** how would you rate yourself on the following items **during the past week?**

0 = Not at all
1 = Just a little
2 = More than just a little
3 = Quite a bit, moderately
4 = Markedly or severely

I have been feeling. . .	Before starting treatment	After 1 week of treatment	After 2 weeks of treatment	After 3 weeks of treatment	After 4 weeks of treatment
down and depressed					
less interested in doing things					
less interested in sex					
less interested in eating					
that I've lost some weight					
that I can't fall sleep at night					
that my sleep is restless					
that I wake up too early					
heavy in my limbs or aches in back, muscles, or head, more tired than usual					
guilty or like a failure					
wishing for death or suicidal					
tense, irritable, or worried					
sure I'm ill or have a disease					
that my speech and thought are slow					
fidgety, restless, or antsy					
that morning is worse than evening					
that evening is worse than morning					
unreal or in a dream state					
suspicious of people/paranoid					
preoccupied/obsessed that I must check things a lot					
physical symptoms when worried					
Standard depression score	——	——	——	——	——

Compared to how you feel **when you are in an even or normal mood state**, how would you rate yourself on the following items **during the past week?**

0 = Not at all
1 = Just a little
2 = More than just a little
3 = Quite a bit, moderately
4 = Markedly or severely

Supplemental Symptoms Chart

I have been feeling. . .	Before starting treatment	After 1 week of treatment	After 2 weeks of treatment	After 3 weeks of treatment	After 4 weeks of treatment
like socializing less					
that I have gained weight					
that I *want* to eat more than usual					
that I *have* eaten more than usual					
that I crave sweets and starches					
that I sleep more than usual					
that my mood slumps in the afternoons or evenings					

Supplemental depression score _____   _____   _____   _____   _____

Total depression scores   _____   _____   _____   _____   _____
(Add standard to supplementary scores)

The Columbia eye check-up for users of light therapy*

You may wish to have your opthamalogist or optometrist use the chart on page 316 to record the results of your eye check-up before, and at intervals during, light therapy.

The Amsler grids on page 317 should be used to record the results after you look at the larger grid on page 318.

---

*This set of ocular tests was specified for patients in the Winter Depression Program at the New York State Psychiatric Institute, Columbia-Presbyterian Medical Center. The development team included: Pamela F. Gallin, M.D., Brian Rafferty, A.B., and Michael Terman, Ph.D., of Columbia University, Ronald M. Burde, of the Albert Einstein College of Medicine; and Charlotte E. Remé, M.D., of the University of Zürich, Switzerland. Note that the examining doctor should include a summary note indicating any problematic ocular condition. For further information, see: M. Terman et al. *Photochemistry and Photobiology* (1990) 51:781–791. © 1993, New York State Psychiatric Institute.

PATIENT	_____	EXAMINED BY	_____
ADDRESS	_____	ADDRESS	_____
PHONE	_____	PHONE	_____
REFERRED BY	_____	DATE OF EXAM	_____

CHECKLIST

RETINA

Detachment	+	−
Diabetic retinopathy	+	−
Retinal vasculitis/Chorioretinal inflammation	+	−
Vascular retinopathies	+	−
Central serous retinopathy	+	−
Degenerative disease of the macula	+	−
Tapeto-retinal degenerations	+	−
Solar/radiation retinopathy	+	−
Drug-induced retinopathy	+	−
Post-traumatic retinopathy	+	−

EYE COMPLAINTS

Photophobia	+	−
Glare	+	−
Dry eyes	+	−
Blurred vision	+	−
Metamorphopsia	+	−
Color vision (poor, good)	+	−
Night vision (poor, good)	+	−
Other complaints:		

OTHER

Inflammatory diseases of anterior segment/uveal tract	+	−
Glaucoma	+	−
Cataracts	+	−
Optic nerve affections	+	−
Keratoconjunctivitis sicca	+	−
Hypothyroidism	+	−
hormone supplement (yes, no)	+	−
stable (yes, no)	+	−

CURRENT MEDICATIONS

Antidepressants (tricyclic)	+	−
Neuroleptics (phenothiazine)	+	−
Lithium	+	−
Tryptophan or melatonin	+	−
Psoralens	+	−
Antimalarial/antirheumatics	+	−
Diuretics (hydrochlorothiazide)	+	−
Porphyrins	+	−
Tetracycline	+	−
Sulfonamides	+	−
Other photosensitizers:		

EXAMINATION

Best corrected visual acuity

	R	L
V_{SC}	_____	_____
V_{CC}	_____	_____	Wearing _____

_____

Ocular motility (9 cardinal directions of gaze)

         R   L

Intraocular pressure (applanation), noting time of day: _____

        R_____   L_____

Amsler grid (Use to record results when you look at larger grid on next page)

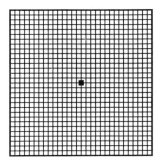

R normal/abnormal (specify)   L normal/abnormal (specify)

Pupillary reactions

R			L		
direct	+	–	direct	+	–
direct	+	–	direct	+	–

Slit lamp examination

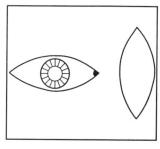   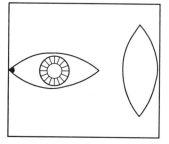

            R   L

Ocular fundus (check which): direct _____ indirect_____ mydriasis_____

          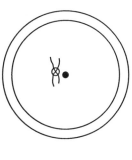

R c/d = _____   R c/d = _____

Patient's observation grid

How to use the Amsler Grid. If you wear glasses for near vision, be sure to use them for this test. In a well-lit room, hold the chart in front of you at arm's length. Place the palm of your free hand over one eye, so it is completely blocked. Look only at the center black dot on the display, while you examine the chart carefully for any perception of wavy lines or blank areas. (If there are no problems, you should see the entire chart as a perfectly aligned piece of graph paper.) Then switch hands, and test the other eye. The results of this test should be recorded on a photocopy of the two smaller grids on the previous page, for right and left eyes separately. For wavy lines, the image should be drawn as you see it; for blank patches of space, a smooth line should be drawn around the appropriate areas.

Index

About the Author

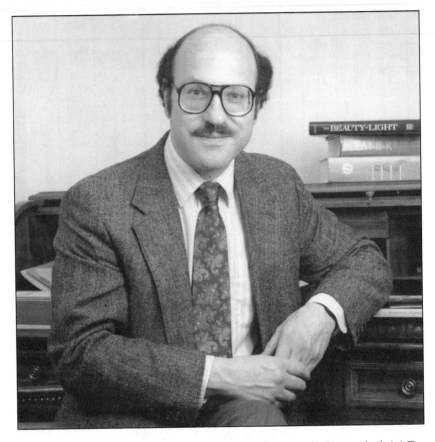

A pioneer in the field of seasonal studies, Norman E. Rosenthal, M.D., is director of light therapy studies at the National Institute of Mental Health. Internationally recognized for his outstanding contribution to the understanding and treatment of depression, he is in popular demand by the media because of his capacity to make his work accessible to the general public. Widely published, he is co-author of *How to Beat Jet Lag: A Practical Guide for Air Travelers*.